Colorectal Surgery

Handbooks in General Surgery

Kirby I. Bland • Michael G. Sarr
Markus W. Büchler • Attila Csendes
O. James Garden • John Wong
Editors

Colorectal Surgery

Handbooks in General Surgery

Springer

Editors
Kirby I. Bland, MD
Fay Fletcher Kerner Professor
and Chairman
Department of Surgery
Deputy Director
Comprehensive Cancer Center
University of Alabama School
of Medicine
Birmingham, AL, USA

Markus W. Büchler, MD
Professor of Surgery
and Chairman
Department of General
and Visceral Surgery
University of Heidelberg
Heidelberg, Germany

Attila Csendes, MD, FACS (Hon)
Professor of Surgery
and Chairman
Department of Surgery
University Hospital
Santiago, Chile

Michael G. Sarr, MD
James C. Mason Professor
of Surgery
Department of Surgery
Mayo Clinic College
of Medicine
Rochester, MN, USA

O. James Garden, MBChB, MD,
FRCS (Ed), FRCP (Ed),
FRACS (Hon)
Regius Professor of Clinical
Surgery
Department of Clinical and
Surgical Sciences
The University of Edinburgh
Royal Infirmary of Edinburgh
Edinburgh, UK

John Wong, BSc (Med (Syd)),
MBBS(Syd),
PhD (Syd), MD (Hon (Syd)),
FRACS, FRCS (Edin), FRCS
(Glasg), FACS (Hon)
Chair Professor
Department of Surgery
The University of Hong Kong
Queen Mary Hospital
Hong Kong, China

ISBN 978-1-84996-443-2 e-ISBN 978-1-84996-444-9
DOI 10.1007/978-1-84996-444-9
Springer London Dordrecht Heidelberg New York

British Library Cataloguing in Publication Data

A catalogue record for this book is available from the British Library

Library of Congress Control Number: 2010933598

First published in 2009 as part of General Surgery: Principles and International Practice, edited by Kirby I. Bland, Markus W. Büchler, Attila Csendes, O. James Garden, Michael G. Sarr & John Wong, ISBN: 978-1-84628-832-6

Printed on acid-free paper

Springer is part of Springer Science+Business Media (www.springer.com)

Preface

The editors designed the original textbook, *General Surgery: Principles and International Practice,* from which this shorter paperback monograph on colorectal surgery was taken to be an accessible, concise, and state-of-the-art volume that explores and documents evolutionary principles in the practice of surgery. This work is aimed at the general surgeon and the resident in training. The scientific community continues to witness extraordinary advances in the therapy of both benign and malignant surgical diseases of various organ sites. Much of this progress has been evident over the past decade with new concepts and techniques of management that allow the surgeon to integrate this discipline with medicine, pharmacology, immunology, biostatistics, pathology, genetics, medical and radiation oncology, and diagnostic radiology and imaging. Further, each of these major disciplines contributes a small component for the diagnostic and therapeutic approaches to clinical care; hence the comprehensive planning, integration, and provision of patient care throughout the preoperative, intraoperative, and postoperative phases of care remains essential in the successful practice of our specialty.

The editors acknowledge that the aim of this work is to provide an illustrative, instructive, and comprehensive review that depicts the rationale of basic operative principles essential to surgical therapy. In organizing this monograph, the editors chose authors renowned in the disciplines for illustrating, forming, and depicting in a comprehensive fashion the surgical therapy expectant for metabolic, infectious, endocrine, and neoplastic abnormalities in adult and pediatric patients **from a truly international and multi-continental perspective.** The editors and authors were chosen carefully from across geographies and also from multi-cultural and diverse locations. While the authors consider this text to be inclusive regarding the technical and operative conditions for perioperative care in this field, its purpose should not be intended to replace standard textbooks of surgery nor should it be considered complete in its coverage of pathophysiologic disorders. In contrast, this monograph is organized to familiarize practicing surgeons, residents, and fellows with state-of-the-art surgical principles and techniques essential to contemporary practice. Therefore, the tenor of this monograph on colorectal surgery has been developed to coexist with other major surgical reference texts that are dedicated—some in more comprehensive fashion—to the therapy of individual organs of systemic diseases. This monograph is much more a "working text" for the practicing surgeon with emphasis on diagnosis and treatment of colorectal disorders. Along with this monograph, nine other paperback monographs are available and focus on the general principles of surgery, trauma, critical care, esophagus and stomach, small bowel, liver and biliary, pancreas and spleen, oncology, and endocrine organs, all adapted from the primary textbook—*General Surgery: Principles and International Practice.*

The chapters in this monograph on colorectal surgery include a condensed bibliography of highly selective journal articles, reviews, and text. In this manner of attempting to be concise, we hope to provide a precise focus for the education of the reader relative to accepted surgical principles involved in patient care. Moreover, the editors have sought to provide a counterpoint view for the selection of therapy by presenting at the opening of each chapter a list of "Pearls and Pitfalls" that highlight particular concerns or controversies. The chapters provide pertinent, though not exhaustive, summaries of anatomy and physiology, a history of surgical illness, and stages of operative approaches with relevant technical considerations outlined in an easily understandable manner. Complications are reviewed when appropriate for the organ system, diseases, and problem. The text is supported amply by line drawings and photographs that depict anatomic or technical principles. The editors have made every attempt to minimize duplicative or repetitive discussions except when controversial or state-of-the-art issues are presented. Moreover, the editors have attempted to ensure that accurate presentations and illustrations depict properly the most complex problems confronted by the general surgeon.

Finally, in an attempt to address advances in contemporary concepts, the text has been organized to address in detail expeditious, safe, and anatomically accurate operations and incorporate standard as well as evolving surgical principles and techniques. These principles have been tested in the clinics of valid scientific knowledge and are well supported by the time-tested approaches that have been provided by practicing surgeons. The editors are excited to be able to respond to the challenge of developing a truly international text and are indeed hopeful that our readers will find this focused monograph on colorectal surgery to be a repository of insight, useful, and timely information.

Kirby I. Bland
Michael G. Sarr
Markus W. Büchler
Attila Csendes
O. James Garden
John Wong

Contents

Contributors

Mario A. Abedrapo Moreira, MD
Department of Surgery, Clinical Hospital, University of Chile, Santiago, Chile

Simon P. Bach, MD, FRCS
Clinical Lecturer and Honorary Registrar, Division of Colorectal Surgery, Department of General Surgery and Trauma, John Radcliffe Hospital, Oxford, UK

Anne Marie Boller, MD
Fellow, Division of Colon and Rectal Surgery, Department of Surgery, Mayo Clinic Foundation, Rochester, MN, USA

Raul Martin Bosio, MD
General Surgery Resident, Department of Surgery, University of Toledo, Toledo, OH, USA

Graham Branagan, MS, FRCS
Specialist Registrar and Consultant, Department of Surgery, Salisbury District Hospital, Salisbury, UK

Fábio Guilherme Campos, MD, PhD
Department of Gastroenterology, University of São Paulo Medical School, São Paulo, Brazil

Sue Clark, MD, FRCS
The Polyposis Registry, St. Mark's Hospital Harrow, UK

Richard Cohen, MBBChir, BSc, MD, FRCS
Consultant, Colorectal Surgeon, Department of Colorectal Surgery, University College Hospital, London, UK

Lisa M. Colletti, MD
Professor of Surgery, Department of Surgery, University of Michigan Medical School, Ann Arbor, MI, USA

Mark D. Duncan, MD, FACS
Associate Professor of Surgery, Department of Surgery, Johns Hopkins Bayview Medical Center, Baltimore, MD, USA

Daniel L. Feingold, MD, FACS
Assistant Professor of Surgery, Section of Colon and Rectal Surgery, Columbia University, New York, NY, USA

Ian G. Finlay, MB ChB, BSc FRCS
Consultant, Colorectal Surgeon, Department of Coloproctology, Glasgow Royal Infirmary, Glasgow, UK

Robert D. Fry, MD
Chairman, Department of Surgery, Hospital of the University of Pennsylvania, Philadelphia, PA, USA

Susan Galandiuk, MD
Director, Section of Colon and Rectal Surgery and Price Institute of Surgical Research, University of Louisville School of Medicine, Louisville, KY, USA

Robert Gryfe, MD, PhD, FRCSC
Colorectal Surgical Oncologist, Department of Surgery, Mount Sinai Hospital University of Toronto, Toronto, Canada

Angelita Habr-Gama, MD, PhD
Professor of Surgery, Department of Gastroenterology, University of São Paulo, São Paulo, Brazil

Richard J. Heald, M.Chir, FRCS
Director of Surgery, Pelican Cancer Foundation, North Hampshire Hospital, Basingstoke, UK

Yik-Hong Ho, MBBS Hons (Qld), MD (Qld), FRCS Ed, FRCS (Glasg), FRACS, FAMS, FI CS
Professor and Head of Surgery, Department of Surgery, School of Medicine, James Cook University, Townsville, Queensland, Australia

David W. Larson, MD
Assistant Professor of Surgery, Department of Surgery, Division of Colon and Rectal Surgery, Mayo Clinic Foundation, Rochester, MN, USA

Andrew Latchford, BSc, MRCP
Research Fellow, The Polyposis Registry, St. Mark's Hospital, Harrow, UK

Anne Y. Lin, MD
Assistant Professor of Surgery, Section of Colorectal Surgery, Washington University School of Medicine, St. Louis, MO, USA

Thomas H. Magnuson, MD
Professor, Department of Surgery, Johns Hopkins Bayview Medical Center, Baltimore, MD, USA

David J. Maron, MD
Assistant Professor of Clinical Surgery, Department of Surgery, Hospital of the University of Pennsylvania, Philadelphia, PA, USA

Robin S. McLeod, BSc, MD, FRCSC, FACS
Professor of Surgery, Department of Surgery & HPME, University of Toronto, Toronto, Canada

Genevieve B. Melton-Meaux, MD
Assistant Professor, Department of General Surgery, Johns Hopkins Bayview Medical Center, Baltimore, MD, USA

Brendan John Moran, MCh, FRCSI, FRCS
Consultant, Colorectal and General Surgeon, Department of General Surgery, North Hampshire NHS Trust, Basingstoke, UK

Melinda M. Mortenson, MD
Surgical Oncology Fellow, Department of Surgical Oncology, University of Texas M D Anderson Cancer Center, Houston, TX, USA

Chrispen D. Mushaya, MBChB(UZ), FCS(ECSA)
Department of Surgery, The Townsville Hospital, Townsville, Australia

Heidi Nelson, MD
Professor of Surgery, Division of Colon and Rectal Surgery, Mayo Clinic College of Medicine, Rochester, MN, USA

Santhat Nivatvongs, MD
Professor of Surgery, Division of Colon and Rectal Surgery, Mayo Clinic College of Medicine, Rochester, MN, USA

Robin K. S. Phillips, MS, FRCS
Professor and Director, The Polyposis Registry, St. Mark's Hospital, Harrow, UK

Theresa W. Ruddy, MD
Department of General Surgery, Rush University, Medical Center, Chicago, IL, USA

Theodore J. Saclarides, MD
Professor of Surgery, Department of General Surgery, Rush University Medical Center, Chicago, IL, USA

Deborah Schrag, MD, MPH
Elizabeth and Felix Rohatyn Chair for Junior Faculty, Department of Medicine, Memorial Sloan-Kettering Cancer Center, New York, NY, USA

Deborah Schrag, MD, MPH
Elizabeth and Felix Rohatyn Chair for Junior Faculty, Department of Medicine, Memorial Sloan-Kettering Cancer Center, New York, NY, USA

Anthony J. Senagore, MD MS MBA
Professor, Department of Surgery, College of Human Medicine, Michigan State University, Lansing, MI, USA

Francis Seow-Choen, MBBS, FRCSEd, FAMS, FRCS
Senior Consultant, Colorectal Surgeon, Seow-Choen Colorectal Center, Mt. Elizabeth Medical Centre, Singapore

Gonzalo Soto Debeuf, MD
Department of Surgery, Clinical Hospital, University of Chile, Santiago, Chile

Jenny Speranza, MD
Assistant Professor, Division of Colorectal Surgery, Department of Surgery, Cleveland Clinic Florida, Weston, FL, USA

Paul H. Sugarbaker, MD, FACS, FRCS
Director of Surgical Oncology, Peritoneal Surface Oncology Program, Washington Cancer Institute, Washington Hospital Center, Washington, DC, USA

Kok-Yang Tan, MBBS (Melb), MMed (Surgery), FRCS (Edin), FAMS
Associate Consultant, Colorectal Service Department of Surgery, Alexandra Hospital, Singapore

Kumaran Thiruppathy, MBBS (Lon), MRCS, BSc (Hon)
Department of General Surgery, University College, London Hospital, London, UK

Joe J. Tjandra, MD, FRACS, FRCS, FRCPS, FASCRS
Late Associate Professor of Surgery, Department of Colorectal Surgery, Royal Melbourne Hospital, Victoria, Australia

Steven D. Wexner, MD, FACS, FRCS, FRCS(Ed)
Chairman, Department of Colorectal Surgery, Cleveland Clinic Florida, Weston, FL, USA

Richard L. Whelan, MD
Associate Director, Section of Colorectal Surgery, Columbia University, New York, NY, USA

Alastair Windsor, MBBS, MD, FRCS, FRCS (Ed)
Colorectal Surgery, Consultant, Department of Surgery, University College Hospital, London, UK

Bruce G. Wolff, MD
Professor of Surgery Chair, Division of Colon and Rectal Surgery, Mayo Clinic College of Medicine, Rochester, MN, USA

W. Douglas Wong, MD, FRCS(C), FACS
Chief, Colorectal Service, Department of Surgery, Memorial Sloan-Kettering Cancer Center, New York, NY, USA

Henry Yeh, MD
Department of Colorectal Surgery, Epworth and Royal Melbourne Hospitals, Melbourne, Australia

Part I
Benign

1
Large Bowel Obstruction

Angelita Habr-Gama and Fábio Guilherme Campos

Pearls and Pitfalls

- Differentiation of mechanical large bowel obstruction (LBO) from colonic pseudo-obstruction is crucial.
- Colonoscopic examination is a beneficial diagnostic and potentially therapeutic modality.
- The most frequent cause of LBO is colorectal cancer, and the most frequent site is the sigmoid colon followed by splenic flexure.
- Volvulus of the sigmoid colon is the second most frequent cause of LBO and occurs most commonly in elderly, chronically constipated patients.
- Timing, grading, site of obstruction, competency of the ileocecal valve, presence of ischemia or perforation, presence of locally advanced or metastatic disease, and operating skill influence the prognosis of patients and choice of the procedure.
- Obstructing right colon cancer can be treated usually with primary resection and anastomosis; however, a protective ileostomy should be considered in selected patients.
- Obstructing left colon cancer is more likely to necessitate resection with end colostomy; in selected patients, a primary resection and anastomosis may be considered.

K.I. Bland et al. (eds.), *Colorectal Surgery*,
DOI 10.1007/978-1-84996-444-9_1,

- Subtotal colectomy with ileorectostomy may be an acceptable operation in selected elderly patients with an obstructing left colon cancer.
- On-the-table colonic lavage can be used to facilitate resection and primary anastomosis for an obstructing left colon when the proximal colon looks reasonable; the presence of feces in the colon does not appear to increase the rate of complications.
- Sigmoid volvulus may be treated successfully by endoscopic decompression unless there is associated ischemia; however, elective resection should be considered in the future.
- LBO secondary to diverticular disease is rare and may be managed by a one-stage procedure when conservative management fails.

Large Bowel Obstruction

Large bowel obstruction (LBO) is a common condition that may be caused by mechanical conditions such as colorectal cancer, volvulus, diverticular disease, fecal impaction, inflammatory or vascular diseases, hernias, adhesions, carcinomatosis, or by functional disturbances (pseudo-obstruction). This chapter focuses on the clinical features, diagnosis, and management of LBO.

Clinical Features

The classic symptoms of LBO include obstipation, abdominal pain, and marked abdominal distension. Vomiting occurs generally late in the evolution of the condition. These symptoms and clinical findings depend on several factors, such as rapidity of the onset of the obstruction, cause and degree of obstruction, presence of co-morbid conditions, and the competency of the ileocecal valve. When a closed loop LBO is present, either by a colonic volvulus or a competent ileocecal valve, colonic distension is greater and is associated with a markedly increased risk of ischemia and perforation. Perforation may occur in the region of the neoplasm or proximally in areas of distended ischemic colon, most frequently in the thin-walled cecum. Many surgeons consider a closed loop LBO to be a surgical emergency. If the ileocecal valve is incompetent, patients are more likely to present with findings similar to small bowel obstruction and are less likely to present with ischemic colonic complications.

On physical examination, usually there is marked abdominal distention, often without much discomfort or tenderness to palpation. Auscultation may demonstrate obstructive bowel sounds, but with chronic obstruction, the bowel sounds may be diminished. On palpation, usually no mass is evident with a colonic volvulus or with an obstructing colon cancer (the colon cancer may be relatively small, <10 cm), but with diverticulitis, the suggestion of a mass and local tenderness may be present. On digital rectal or proctoscopic examination, a rectal or a low sigmoid tumor, presence of impacted feces, or evidence of extrinsic compression may be identified.

In addition to the clinical examination and routine laboratory evaluations, plain abdominal radiographs are helpful in determining the next diagnostic and therapeutic approach. The presence and location of gaseous distension of the colon, the diameter of cecum, fluid levels, association with small bowel dilation, and the presence or absence of gas in the rectum are essential for evaluation of LBO (Fig. 1.1). If this study is inconclusive or if more information is sought, a multislice CT with intravenous and rectal contrast is a useful method for diagnosing the cause and site of obstruction. If CT is not available, water-soluble contrast enema can be used. Oral gastrointestinal contrast examination provides no useful information and should not be used.

General Principles of Management

The majority of patients with mechanical LBO require an urgent or emergent operation; indeed complete LBO should be considered a surgical emergency. The timing of operative

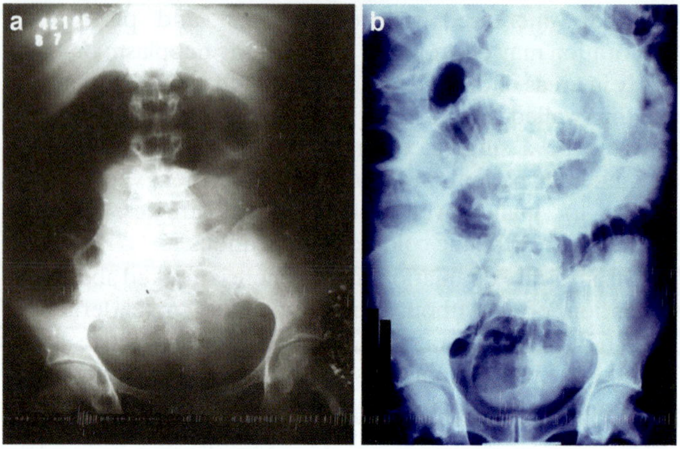

FIGURE I.I. **a.** Complete closed loop obstruction with gross distension of the cecum and right colon. **b.** An incomplete LBO with distension of small bowel.

intervention is dependent on the diagnosis, the general condition of the patient, the presence of a competent ileocecal valve, and signs of ischemia and perforation.

The first step in the treatment is fluid and electrolyte resuscitation. A nasogastric tube is advised to prevent further entry of orally ingested gas into the colon. When operative intervention is required, it is important to assume that adequate resuscitation efforts have been initiated and that appropriate prophylactic measures are taken. Perioperative broad-spectrum antibiotics, prophylaxis for deep vein thrombosis, and an indwelling urinary catheter are important. The patient is placed preferably in a lithotomy position, and a midline incision performed. After opening the peritoneum, the abdominal cavity should be inspected carefully and the cause of obstruction and as well the viability of the involved bowel segments must be confirmed. In patients with massive luminal distension, decompression with a suction tube helps the manipulation of the bowel. If the small bowel is also distended, its contents should be decompressed back into the stomach and aspirated through the nasogastric tube.

Specific Causes of LBO and Treatment

Colorectal Cancer

Colorectal cancer (CRC) is the most common cause of LBO. In about 10% of patients with CRC, acute intestinal obstruction may be the presenting diagnosis. Obstruction is more common in the left colon due to its more solid contents, smaller luminal diameter, and less distensible bowel wall. The splenic flexure and sigmoid colon are the most common sites for obstruction. Patients presenting with an obstructing CRC have an increased risk of perioperative morbidity and mortality. Perforation occurs in 15% of patients and is associated with decreased long-term disease-free and overall survival, often because of both the perforation and locally advanced disease.

Treatment: For many years, a three-stage procedure was considered to be the best approach for an obstructing CRC. In the first stage, the colon was decompressed proximally by an external stoma. Colonic resection is then performed at a second stage, and the bowel continuity re-established in the third stage of this approach. With this approach, however, about 30% of patients were never able to undergo the third stage due to patient refusal, prohibitive medical comorbidities, or development of an advanced malignancy. Currently, the majority of surgeons agree that primary resection, with or without immediate restoration of colonic continuity, can be performed safely under favorable conditions.

There is now consensus that primary right colectomy and immediate anastomosis is a safe alternative in the majority of patients with an obstructing or near-obstructing right colon cancer. Contraindications of primary resection with anastomosis are an unstable patient, presence of intraperitoneal sepsis, or concern about the viability of the bowel. Under these circumstances, the tumor should be resected, an end ileostomy performed, and the proximal end of the transverse colon closed or brought out as a mucous fistula near or at the same site as the ileostomy to facilitate restoration of intestinal continuity.

Intestinal bypass of the obstructing segment or loop ileostomy should be reserved for patients with fixed, large neoplasms with extensive local invasion or for patients with a prohibitively high risk for a prolonged anesthetic. Despite the acceptance that radical operations for obstructing right colon cancer are safe, mortality and morbidity in emergent operations is greater than that observed for elective operations.

The optimal operative strategy for an obstructing left colon cancer remains controversial. Opinions are divided between initial decompression by a colostomy followed by resection or an immediate resection with or without a primary anastomosis. Factors that may affect the operative approach may include the surgeon's experience, the clinical condition of the patient, and availability in the hospital resources.

The *three-stage procedure* (Fig. 1.2) is associated with higher overall cost, longer hospital stay, considerable cumulative morbidity, and a mortality rate of 31%. Currently, the tendency is to reserve this approach for high-risk patients or for situations where surgical expertise in emergent colorectal procedures is lacking. In contrast, resection without primary anastomosis (the classic *two-stage procedure*) as described by Hartmann or Mickulicz (Fig. 1.3) has the advantages of early resection of the cancer, relief of obstruction without the risk of anastomotic complications, a shorter overall hospital stay, and faster recovery. Disadvantages of the two-stage approach include the cost and morbidity of the second operation, and the necessity of another hospitalization and recovery period. Nevertheless, this two-stage approach is probably the most commonly performed approach for left-sided obstructing CRCs and appears especially suited for patients with a perforated left colon cancer and those patients with a compromised nutritional or medical state. This Hartmann's operation is generally reserved for neoplasms located in the high rectum or low sigmoid colon when the remaining rectal stump can be closed. For neoplasms in the upper sigmoid or descending colon, resection with exteriorization of both ends brought out through separate wounds is generally advocated to facilitate later restoration of intestinal continuity.

A *one-stage procedure* of segmental resection with primary anastomosis has been advocated increasingly over the

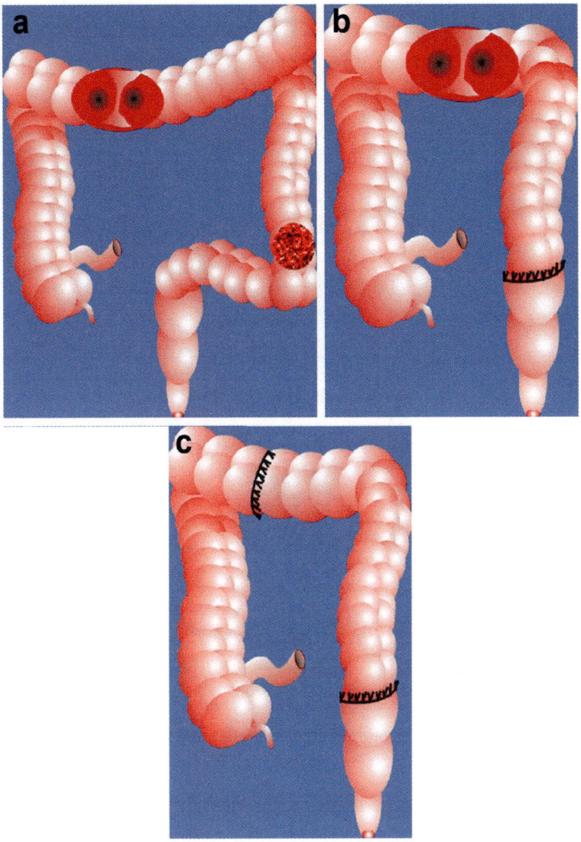

FIGURE 1.2. Three-stage procedure for obstructed left colon cancer. **a.** colostomy; **b.** resection; **c.** colostomy closure.

past few years despite alleged concerns of anastomotic complications in an unprepped bowel or the presence of bacterial contamination (Fig. 1.4).

The use of *intraoperative colonic lavage* has engendered acceptance of resection with primary anastomosis. This procedure is time-consuming, requires take down of one or both colonic flexures, and can be messy; however, operative mortality with this approach is low (4%), which compares favorably with the overall morbidity of the two-stage colostomy

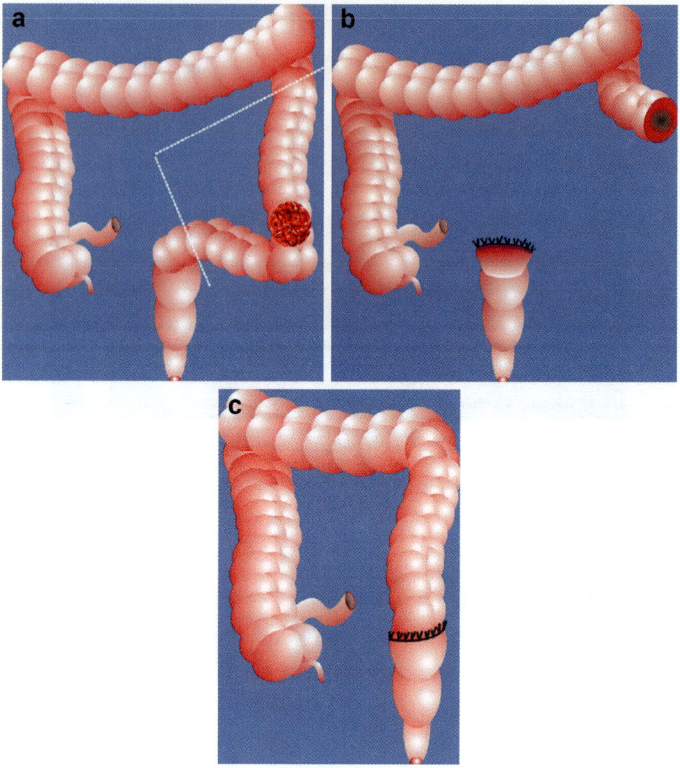

FIGURE 1.3. Two-stage procedure for obstructed left colon cancer. Hartmann's operation. **a** and **b.** Resection and colostomy; **c.** Colostomy closure.

decompression procedures. Comparisons of this approach to the two-stage approaches are limited by selection bias, because patients undergoing two-stage are generally sicker with more medical comorbidity. Although several controlled trials have demonstrated that mechanical bowel preparation may not be necessary prior to an elective primary colonic anastomosis, the need for fecal evacuation in an obstructed colon is believed necessary but not proven.

Subtotal colectomy with ileosigmoidostomy or ileorectostomy is another form of one-stage procedure (Fig. 1.5). This

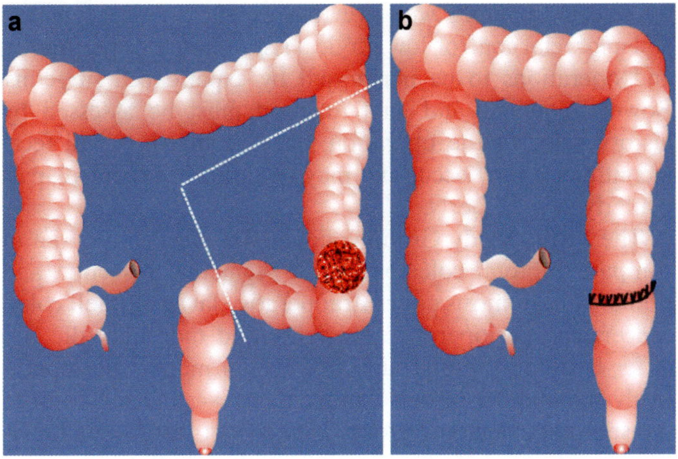

FIGURE 1.4. Segmental resection and primary anastomosis.

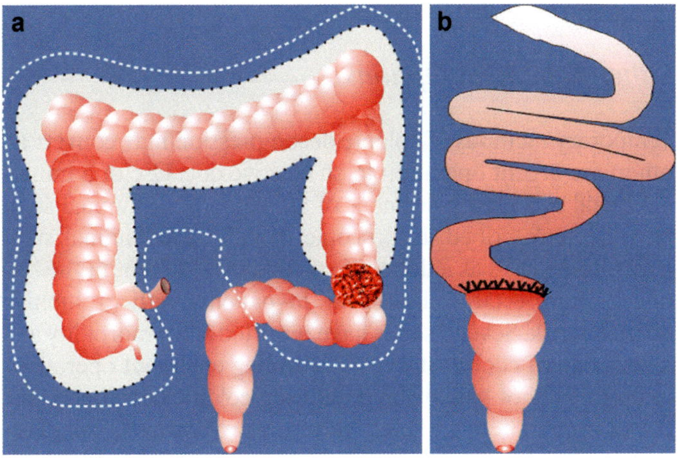

FIGURE 1.5. Subtotal colectomy with primary ileosigmoid anastomosis.

approach is the most appropriate operation for patients with synchronous right and left colon cancers, or when the cecum has serosal tears or ischemia related to the LBO. This approach is more difficult technically and should be reserved for selected patients with previous excellent bowel function and anorectal control, low surgical risk, absence of peritonitis, and operations to be performed by experienced surgeons. Bowel frequency and anal function must be assessed by history prior to the operation, because diarrhea and fecal incontinence may occur and may be difficult to control, particularly in the elderly.

The Scotia Study Group conducted a prospective trial to compare subtotal colectomy with segmental resection and primary anastomosis after intraoperative lavage for left colon cancer. The perioperative mortality and morbidity did not differ between these groups; however, 4 months postoperatively, the number of bowel movements was much greater in the subtotal colectomy group. Thus, at our institution, favorable short-and long-term results with subtotal colectomy have encouraged our use of this approach but only in selected patients with obstructing colon cancer.

Other Treatment Options

Temporary methods of colonic decompression may convert an otherwise urgent operation to an elective one. Use of a transanal rectal tube and placement of an expandable luminal stent have been described. Endoscopic metallic endoluminal stent may also be used as a definitive palliative treatment in the setting of unresectable disease or in patients with prohibitive operative risk. Several series have reported a low morbidity and a high rate of clinical success in avoiding emergent operations in up to 94% of patients and allowing colonic decompression, bowel preparation, and elective resection; however, complications such as stent migration, pain, bleeding, intestinal perforation, and recurrence of obstruction have been reported.

Volvulus

Volvulus is defined as the abnormal rotation of a segment of bowel around its mesentery resulting in a complete or partial obstruction. The incidence of colonic volvulus varies depending on the region of the world, the socioeconomic status, age, and the presence of mental handicaps. In Western Europe and North America, volvulus accounts for only 2–5% of all LBOs with 80% of those occurring in the sigmoid colon. Among certain populations in Africa, Iran, and Eastern Europe, however, volvulus is the most common cause of intestinal obstruction.

Sigmoid Volvulus

Predisposing factors for sigmoid volvulus include both congenital and acquired conditions. In all cases, redundancy of the bowel, an elongated mesocolon, and approximated points of fixation are present. In developed countries, sigmoid volvulus is seen most frequently in elderly, institutionalized, or chronically constipated patients treated with excessive use of laxative, psychotropic, or sedative drugs. Dietary factors such as ingestion of an excessively large bulk diet may also explain the differences in geographic distribution of the disease. In countries as in South America where Chagas' disease is frequent, sigmoid volvulus represents the most frequent complication of megacolon.

Complete volvulus requires torsion of the intestine of more than 180°. When the rotation is less than 90°, there is a simple twisting of the sigmoid colon over the rectum. A rotation of more than 180° around its mesenteric axis is followed by axial torsion of the bowel above the posterior fixation point. The magnitude of this axial torsion is twice that observed in the mesentery, as demonstrated by Groth, who suggested this to be the most important factor in producing intestinal obstruction.

Once obstruction occurs, the proximal colon distends with air and fluid, the extent of which depends on the competency of the ileocecal valve. As distension of the proximal colon and/or the volvulated colon increases, occlusion of intramural vessels can result in ischemia. As transmural ischemia develops, peritonitis with perforation may follow, either in the proximal colon (if the ileocecal valve is competent) or in the volvulated segment. Plain roentgenograms generally demonstrate a large, air and fluid-filled loop of bowel projecting into

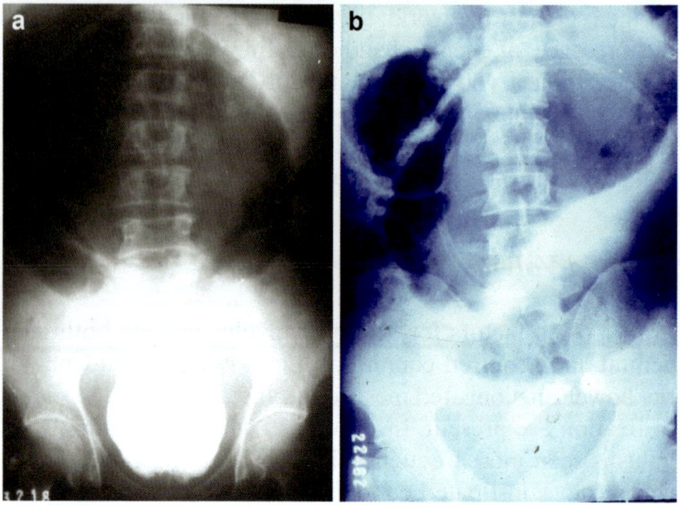

FIGURE 1.6. **a.** Sigmoid volvulus; **b.** sigmoid volvulus with radiologic signs of peritonitis.

the right upper quadrant with loss of haustrations and the presence of other air-fluid levels in the abdomen (Fig. 1.6). Depending on the competence of the ileocecal valve, there may be multiple distended loops of small bowel. Contrast enema studies demonstrate the typical bird-beak deformity.

Treatment: When there is no clinical or radiologic signs of peritonitis, conservative management is usually indicated initially. Endoscopic reduction of the sigmoid volvulus is based on the knowledge that the obstruction due to axial torsion causing distention can be decompressed effectively and de-torsed via an intraluminal approach. This technique requires passage of a nasogastric or rectal tube into the volvulated loop using the sigmoidoscope. The decompression tube should be left in place for several days to prevent recurrence of the volvulus; frequent irrigation ensures tube patency. Endoscopic decompression allows the opportunity for bowel preparation and elective operation. The overall success of endoscopic tube decompression initially is around 75–90%.

Emergent laparotomy is indicated in patients with evidence of ischemia, perforation, or failed endoscopic reduction. The choice of surgical procedure depends on the viability of the colon. When the sigmoid colon is viable and the colon proximal to the volvulus is viable and not too dilated, good results with resection and primary end-to-end anastomosis as an emergency procedure have been obtained in good risk, selected patients. In the presence of ischemia of the sigmoid colon, a Hartmann's procedure is the procedure of choice without primary anastomosis. Exteriorization of the colon distal to the volvulated segment is usually not possible, and therefore closure of the rectal stump is preferable.

Cecal Volvulus

Cecal and right colon volvulus represent only 1–10% of all acute causes of LBO and is less common than sigmoid volvulus. A cecal volvulus arises from an axial twist of the cecum on its mesentery, resulting in obstruction with the potential for vascular compromise and gangrene. Typically, cecal volvulus involves the terminal ileum, cecum, and the ascending colon, and on abdominal radiography, the dilated obstructed loop projects into the left upper quadrant. This type of cecal volvulus must be differentiated from a cecal bascule in which the cecum folds anteriorly and superiorly onto the ascending colon. Excessive mobility of right colon, typically due to congenital anomalies of fixation (the so-called floppy cecum), is prerequisite for the development of cecal volvulus.

Treatment: Spontaneous resolution of a cecal volvulus occurs in less than 2% of patients, and thus some form of intervention is necessary. When there is no sign of peritonitis, treatment options include colonoscopic decompression, cecopexy, cecostomy, and ileocolonic resection.

Although colonoscopic decompression has been reported with success, favorable results have not been obtained uniformly. While this conservative approach may be appropriate for selected patients with contraindications for operative intervention, laparotomy is required for the majority of patients. If the dilated segment of bowel is non-viable after reduction, resection is the appropriate treatment. Primary anastomosis or end ileostomy with distal mucous fistula may be performed according to the clinical condition of the patient and operative findings (peritonitis, contamination, and the quality of proximal bowel).

When the colon is viable after reduction, the optimal treatment remains controversial. Simple reduction without other intervention is associated with an inordinately high rate of recurrence. Cecopexy is advocated by some surgeons, although recurrence rates of up to 30% have been reported unless a very wide, long, peritoneal flap-based fixation is performed. Tube cecostomy has the advantage of fixation of the bowel to the abdominal wall while also allowing maintenance of cecal decompression. Whereas recurrence rates are low, morbidity is increased compared with other procedures. Overall, we favor colectomy with primary anastomosis in young or relatively healthy patients, and reserve cecopexy and cecostomy for elderly, poor risk patients.

Acute Colonic Pseudo Obstruction

Acute colonic pseudo obstruction or Ogilvie's syndrome is a condition characterized by symptoms and signs of LBO but without any mechanical obstruction. It is characterized by acute, massive dilation usually limited to the cecum and right colon. Without prompt colonic decompression, the dilated colon may result in perforation, peritonitis, and death. The syndrome may be a primary condition caused by an underlying motility disorder such as familial visceral myopathy or a disorder affecting the innervation of smooth muscle. Secondary pseudo-obstruction is much more frequent and may be the result of metabolic disturbances, cardiovascular disease (especially complicating myocardial infarctions), the postoperative state after orthopedic, urologic, or renal transplantation surgery, or conditions that are inflammatory, neurologic, or endocrine-related. Additional contributing factors include opiates, psychotropics, anticholinergics, and chemotherapic agents.

Patients with acute colonic pseudo-obstruction present with abdominal distension and progressive discomfort which may develop acutely or gradually. Clinical features may be similar to those observed in mechanical obstruction.

Plain abdominal radiographs demonstrate diffuse gaseous distension of the colon. Often there are few or absent fluid levels. The diameter of the cecum correlates with the risk of perforation and determines timing and aggressiveness of intervention. When the diameter is less than 10 cm, management may be conservative, with placement of a nasogastric tube, fluid and electrolyte resuscitation, identification of contributing factors, and serial abdominal x-rays. Rectal tube decompression and pharmacologic stimulation of the motility of the bowel with neostigmine have demonstrated effectiveness.

Colonoscopy is useful as an aid to diagnosis, allows decompression, and facilitates luminal tube placement for continued decompression. Colonoscopic decompression or aggressive neostigmine therapy is indicated for patients with a cecal diameter of ≥10 cm. Colonoscopy is our preferred initial approach and may be performed without mechanical bowel preparation and with minimal insufflation of air. Colonic decompression with placement of a colonic tube provides initial success in up to 80% of patients; however, repeated colonoscopy may be necessary for recurrences.

Laparotomy is required for patients who do not response to conservative methods and for those with signs of perforation or ischemia. If at laparotomy a small cecal perforation with little spillage is encountered, a tube cecostomy may be used. The success rate of tube cecostomy has been reported as 100% and has the lowest mortality rate among the operative procedures. These cecostomy tubes need to be of a large diameter and require frequent irrigation to clear the lumen of stool to allow ongoing decompression. For patients with free perforation or ischemic colon, resection of the segment and exteriorization are usually necessary. These procedures have high rates of complications and mortality due to both the presence of the complication itself and to the presence of other medical conditions, and thus a primary ileocolostomy should be undertaken only in selected patients. Percutaneous cecostomy has been proposed, although it is associated with as yet undefined risk of complications.

Diverticular Disease of the Colon

Intestinal LBO is quite rare in diverticular disease of the colon, occurring in less than 10% of all cases. It may occur in patients with acute diverticulitis with a peridiverticular abscess, pericolic annular fibrosis in chronic disease, or by angulation and consequent adhesive fixation of the inflamed bowel to the lateral wall of the pelvis. Small bowel obstruction may also occur if a segment of bowel adheres to the inflamed sigmoid colon.

Patients with obstruction caused by an acute episode of diverticulitis and an associated abscess may be treated with intravenous antibiotics, bowel rest, and image-guided percutaneous drainage. For those patients with a complete LBO, emergent laparotomy is usually required. The most frequently used operative intervention is resection of the diseased segment with immediate anastomosis with or without a diverting loop ostomy depending on operative findings, patient condition, and preference of the surgeon.

Other Causes of Large Bowel Obstruction

Fecal Impaction

Fecal impaction is more common in elderly patients, those who have been bedridden for an extended time, or institutionalized patients. This type of fecal impaction is a common complication of Chagasic megacolon and in younger

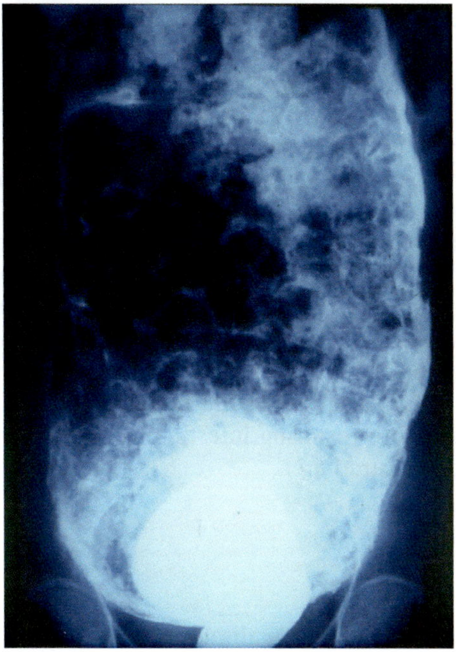

FIGURE 1.7. Megacolon with fecaloma.

patients with megarectum (Fig. 1.7). Symptoms include chronic constipation with frequent small liquid feces and occasional incontinence. Abdominal palpation may detect an abdominal mass, usually in the left iliac fossa. A hard bolus of feces usually can be also felt by digital examination of the rectum.

Treatment usually consists of digital manipulation, enema with oil or paraffin, magnesium sulfate, or phosphate enema. These methods generally are successful, although in some patients, disimpaction under general anesthesia may be necessary. Rarely, laparotomy is required to prevent or treat the complications of fecal impaction, such as complete intestinal obstruction or stercoral perforation.

Ischemic Stricture

Ischemia of the colon may be caused by occlusion of the inferior mesenteric artery by thrombosis, embolus, low output states, iatrogenic causes such as aortic surgery or therapeutic embolization, or after an episode of ischemic colitis. Despite these causes, vascular occlusion rarely is a cause of complete LBO. Treatment consists of wide resection of the ischemic segment back to healthy vascularized bowl; primary restoration of continuity depends on local conditions and overall patient health. After aortic surgery in which the inferior mesenteric artery has been occluded, cognizance of an adequate vascular supply of the remaining colon should be confirmed before restoring intestinal continuity after resection of the strictured area.

Crohn's Disease

LBO caused by Crohn's disease is also extremely rare, although strictures of the large colon are common. When LBO occurs, differentiation from CRC may be difficult or impossible even after colonoscopic examination. Sometimes the diagnosis of Crohn's disease is made only at laparotomy or after resection. Treatment consists of segmental resection if the stricture is localized or total colectomy in the presence of extensive disease. A primary anastomosis is for LBO complicating Crohn's disease is not recommended often due to the high incidence of anastomotic dehiscence.

Radiation Damage

In contrast to small bowel obstruction, LBO is extremely rare after radiation therapy. The distal colon may, however, become obstructed by a fibrous stricture, usually in the proximal rectum after pelvic irradiation. Operation must be carried out with caution because of adhesions, fibrosis, and difficult manipulation of the rectum in the pelvis. Inadvertent enterotomy is not a rare event. Resection may be technically impossible and a diverting stoma may be the procedure of choice.

Selected Readings

Bokey EL, Chapius PH, Fung C, et al. (1995) Postoperative morbidity and mortality following resection of the colon and rectum for cancer. Dis Colon Rectum 38:480–487

Habr-Gama A, Haddad J, Simonsen O, et al. (1976) Volvulus of the sigmoid colon in Brazil: a report of 230 cases. Dis Colon Rectum 19:314–320

Lopez-Kostner F, Hool GR, Lavery I (1997) Management and causes of acute large-bowel obstruction. Surg Clin N Amer 77:1265–1286

Martinez-Santos C, Lobato RF, Fradejas JM, et al. (2002) Self-expandable stent before elective surgery vs. emergency surgery for the treatment of malignant colorectal obstructions: comparison of primary anastomosis and morbidity rates. Dis Colon Rectum 45:401–406

Rabinovici R, Simansky DA, Kaplan O, et al. (1990) Cecal volvulus. Dis Colon Rectum 33:765–769

The SCOTIA Study Group (1995) Single-stage treatment for malignant left-sided colonic obstruction: a prospective randomized clinical trial comparing subtotal colectomy with segmental resection following intraoperative irrigation. Br J Surg 82:1622–1627

Smothers L, Hynan L, Fleming J, et al. (2003) Emergency surgery for colon carcinoma. Dis Colon Rectum 46:24–30

Tuech JJ, Becouarn G, Cattan F, Arnaud JP (1996) Volvulus du côlon droit. Plaidoyer pour l'hé micolectomie droite. J Chir 133:267–269 carried out with caution because of adhesions, fibrosis and difficult manipulation of the rectum in the pelvis. Inadvertent enterotomy is not a rare event. Resection may be technically impossible and a diverting stoma may be the procedure of choice.

Selected Readings

[illegible] Gorgun E[illegible] Fung [illegible] et al [illegible] Preoperative [illegible] morbidity and mortality following resection of [illegible] and factors [illegible] Dis Colon Rectum [illegible]
[illegible]

2
Chronic Ulcerative Colitis

Simon P. Bach and Neil J. Mortensen

Pearls and Pitfalls

- Ulcerative colitis (UC) patients admitted in relapse should be managed jointly by an "aggressive" physician and a "conservative" surgeon.
- If emergency surgery is required, a subtotal colectomy and end ileostomy should be performed. Leave a long closed sigmoid stump within the subcutaneous tissues at the lower pole of the wound. Decompress the rectum with a Foley catheter.
- Thromboprophylaxis should be strongly considered in all patients admitted with UC due to the increased risk of deep venous thromboses and thromboembolic events.
- Surveillance colonoscopy is performed optimally with the patient in remission to avoid sampling regenerative areas with histological features that might be misconstrued as dysplasia. Also, report recent cyclosporin treatment to the pathologist in order to facilitate the diagnosis of "pseudodysplasia".
- Incomplete endoscopic excision of any dysplastic colonic lesion within an area of colitis or the discovery of flat dysplasia in association with or remote from a dysplastic mass (regardless of resectability) is an indication for proctocolectomy. High grade flat dysplasia is a relatively rare indication for colectomy and patients with low grade flat dysplasia should be observed.

K.I. Bland et al. (eds.), *Colorectal Surgery*,
DOI 10.1007/978-1-84996-444-9_2,

- The ileal pouch-anal anastomosis should ideally be positioned 2–3 cm above the anal margin. In practice this distance is roughly equivalent to the length of the distal two phalanges of the index finger.

Basic Science

Ulcerative colitis (UC) is characterized by chronic mucosal and submucosal inflammation of the colon and rectum. While the etiology of UC is yet to be elucidated, several associations are observed. There is a family history of either UC or Crohn's in 15% of patients. It is hypothesized that a hierarchy of inflammatory bowel disease (IBD) genes exist. One level may confer susceptibility to IBD in general, separate genes specify for UC or Crohn's while others modulate clinical features, such as disease distribution and the presence of extra-intestinal manifestations. Genetic influences are likely to interact with environmental factors. For instance UC occurs more commonly in non-or ex-smokers. Presentation is more frequent in the winter months, possibly as a result of an infectious agent. Appendicectomy is associated with a reduced risk of developing UC. Whether surgery is protective or patients destined to develop UC experience appendicectomy less frequently remains unclear. A unifying hypothesis is that UC follows an inappropriate, genetically determined response by the mucosal immune system to unspecified luminal antigens.

Clinical Presentation

UC is a relapsing and remitting disease confined to the colon and rectum. Disease activity is highly variable, ranging from chronically active colitis to a "burnt out" disease with protracted remission. Sex distribution is equal. Most patients present between 15 and 30 years of age although in a small proportion it occurs for the first time in their 60s and 70s, usually with localized proctitis. Onset of loose bloody stools with mucus and pus is usually gradual and reflects underlying inflammation of the colorectal mucsa. Abdominal cramping, bloating and increased stool frequency indicate more widespread enteric involvement. Patients may experience urgency or urge incontinence. Stool frequency is a particularly good indicator of disease severity. Systemic symptoms of anorexia, malaise and weight loss are similarly useful when assessing severity as are signs of tachycardia, fever, abdominal distension and tenderness. It should be remembered that steroid treatment may mask many of these findings.

Diagnosis of Ulcerative Colitis

***Blood Tests*:** Anemia, leukocytosis and thrombocytosis indicate severe disease. Hypokalemia and dehydration may complicate prolonged diarrhea. Poor nutritional intake results in hypoalbuminemia. C reactive protein (CRP) > 45 mg/l or erythrocyte sedimentation rate (ESR) > 30 mm/h are additional markers of disease severity.

***Stool Microscopy and Culture*:** Stools should be examined for *E. coli*, *Campylobacter*, *Salmonella* or *Entamoeba histolytica* in addition to *Clostridium difficile* toxin. Cytomegalovirus (CMV) is detected following intestinal biopsy and immunohistochemical staining (seronegativity negates the need for this test).

***Radiological Diagnosis*:** Plain films are largely used to evaluate colonic calibre and to rule out perforation. A diameter of > 6 cm is considered abnormal.

***Endoscopic Diagnosis*:** Although there is a risk of perforation in acute disease, initial endoscopic assessment provides an accurate tissue diagnosis and helps determine the extent and severity of inflammation. In the acute setting, flexible sigmoidoscopy is usually the investigation of choice, being relatively easy and safe to perform. Ultimately the colon should be surveyed until macroscopically normal tissue is reached. In UC, circumferential inflammation extends proximally from the anal verge. This is in contrast to Crohn's colitis where 40% of patients demonstrate rectal sparing. The pattern of involvement in UC is rectum alone in approximately 40%, left colon in 40% and total colitis in 20%. The distribution of disease is not static and may increase or decrease after initial assessment. Biopsies taken from normal and abnormal areas avoid underestimating the extent of colonic involvement, although the significance of microscopic inflammation proximal to macroscopic disease remains uncertain. Mucosa affected by UC initially exhibits a granular appearance with loss of vascular markings secondary to intramural edema. Bleeding often occurs spontaneously or following contact with the endoscope. Numerous shallow erosions or microulcers may be apparent, and their size and extent mirror disease severity. Repeated cycles of relapse and remission lead to clumps of hyperplastic, regenerating mucosa interspersed between areas of ulceration that give rise to "pseudopolyps" otherwise termed "inflammatory polyps". Clinicians should be aware that *bone fide* UC may present initially with features suggestive of Crohn's disease. Prominent inflammation of the transverse colon in severe UC gives an impression of rectal sparing, and partial treatment with steroid enemas may compound this effect. Fissuring or transmural ulceration is another feature of fulminant UC. Lastly, one quarter of patients with active subtotal UC exhibit discontinuous inflammation at the appendiceal orifice. This appendiceal "skip lesion" is considered to be a normal variant of UC.

***Histological Diagnosis*:** UC is characterized by isolated mucosal inflammation; the muscularis propria and serosa remain unaffected except in fulminant disease. Inflammatory cells congregate within crypts and alongside dilated vessels of the lamina propria. Secondary infection of inflammatory debris within the crypt lumen is thought to drive the formation of crypt abscesses. While these lesions are characteristic of UC they are a non-specific feature of large intestinal inflammation. Crypt abscesses can point directly into the intestinal lumen or alternatively rupture in a submucosal plane causing ulceration. Crypt architecture is distorted and goblet cells are lost giving rise to mucin depletion. These histological features may become unevenly distributed as the patient improves giving a false impression of segmental disease. A degree of crypt distortion will usually persist once remission is achieved. This is a histopathological hallmark of UC.

***Differential Diagnoses*:** Infectious colitides usually arises as a result of an isolated infection that is self limiting within a period of 14 days and of insufficient duration to cause crypt distortion.Immunocompromised hosts, such as AIDS and UC patients, treated with immunosuppressive agents are prone to develop longer lasting infection, often of viral origin. Protozoal infections also have a tendency to persist if untreated. It is estimated that in 10–20% of patients with relapsing UC, pathogens are seen on stool testing. It remains unclear whether these pathogens trigger or mimic relapse but some will respond to appropriate antibiotic therapy. Fulminant colitis complicated by CMV infection may respond to antiviral treatment using gancyclovir. Major differential diagnoses are outlined in Table 2.1.

***Assessing the Severity of Ulcerative Colitis*:** Complete assessment of disease activity involves evaluation of symptoms, physical examination, measurement of laboratory indices and endoscopy. Scoring systems draw together key elements of this assessment to stratify patients according to their disease severity. They provide a basis for the consistent delivery of treatment protocols, especially within randomized controlled trials. Truelove and Witts first classified relapses of UC according to criteria listed in Table 2.2.This system is easy to remember and may aid identification of the sick patient.

Special Features of Ulcerative Colitis

***Extra-intestinal Manifestations*:** 20% of patients with UC manifest associated conditions of the joints, liver, eyes or skin. IBD-associated peripheral arthritis is the commonest extra-intestinal manifestation of UC. It produces a transient and asymmetrical inflammation of the large joints (knees, ankles,

TABLE 2.1. Differential diagnoses of ulcerative colitis.

Infectious	Bacterial	*Campylobacter, Escherichia coli, Clostridium difficile, Salmonella, Shigella, Yersinia, Chlamydia*or *Gonococcus*
	Viral	Rotavirus, CMV, Herpes simplex
	Protozoal	*Entamoeba histolytica, Cryptosporidium* or *Giardia*
Non-infectious	Drug induced	NSAIDs eosinophilic infiltrate – eosinophilic infiltrate
	Diverticular	Characteristic distribution, rectal biopsies are normal
	Ischemic	Rectal biopsies should be normal
	Radiation	History of radiation and telangiectasia
	Microscopic colitis	Triad of watery diarrhea, endoscopically normal mucosa and collagenous or lymphocytic infiltrate (most pronounced in the proximal colon). Minority of cases associated with drug ingestion or coeliac disease

TABLE 2.2. Classification of disease severity in ulcerative colitis (Modified from Truelove and Witts, 1955).

	Mild	Moderate	Severe	Fulminant
Stools per day	<4	4–6	>6	>10
Rectal bleeding	Infrequent	Intermediate	Frequent	Continuous
Temperature	<37.5°C	Intermediate	>37.5°C	>37.5°C
Heart rate	<90 bpm	Intermediate	>90 bpm	>90 bpm
Hemoglobin	>10 g/dl	Intermediate	<10 g/dl	Transfusion
ESR	<30 mm/h	Intermediate	>30 mm/h	>30 mm/h

elbows, wrists). Synovitis mirrors the course of colitis and is cured by colectomy. The axial skeleton may be affected by ankylosing spondylitis (AS) or isolated sacroiliitis. AS is a seronegative arthropathy of the sacroiliac and vertebral facet joints. Its prevalence in UC is 1–5% and two thirds of affected individuals are HLA-B27 positive. Axial arthritis does not resolve following successful treatment of colitis.

Primary sclerosing cholangitis (PSC) is a serious condition that causes fibrous stricturing of the entire biliary tree in 5% of patients with UC. Asymptomatic elevation of alkaline phosphatase may be the first indication of liver disease. Abdominal pain, intermittent episodes of jaundice and pruritus develop later. The diagnosis is confirmed by a characteristic magnetic resonance cholangiopancreatography (MRCP) or endoscopic retrograde cholangiopancreatography (ERCP) and compatible liver biopsy. Hepatic failure gradually ensues over a 5–10 year period and it is independent of the course of colitis. Biliary stenting and rarely, surgery may be required to relieve obstruction, and orthotopic liver transplantation can be performed in end-stage disease. Unfortunately, a significant proportion of patients develop cholangiocarcinoma which has a very poor prognosis. The risk of colorectal cancer is also increased 10-fold compared to those with UC alone.

Iritis, episcleritis and anterior uveitis complicate UC relatively rarely. Prompt access to specialist services and appropriate treatment with topical and/or oral corticosteroids leads to resolution of symptoms in the majority of cases without any permanent damage.

Pyoderma gangrenosum is a skin condition occasionally associated with UC. Painful violaceous plaques merge to form solitary ulcers with an undermined purple border. Any area can be affected but the lower limbs are especially vulnerable as are any previously injured areas of the skin. Systemic steroid therapy or intralesional steroid injection have been used to treat this for many years although the condition will slowly improve following colectomy. More recently, tacrolimus ointment (an immune modulator that inhibits calcineurin) has been used with some success. Cyclosporin and infliximab also show activity in this disorder. Erythema nodosum produces tender red nodules on the shin that are also prone to ulceration. Treatment includes bed-rest and anti-inflammatory medication.

***UC and Neoplasia*:** Large bowel malignancy ultimately complicates UC in 5% of patients. Risk becomes clinically significant once the disease has been present for 8–10 years. Subsequent risk accumulates at a rate of 0.5–1.0% per year. It is estimated that 2% will develop cancer at 10 years, 8% at 20years and 18% after 30 years. The magnitude of risk may be decreasing due to the effects of screening, prophylactic surgery and anti-inflammatory maintenance therapy. Nonetheless, a family history of colorectal cancer combined with pancolitis mark subjects at high risk. Frequency and severity of relapse are also considered significant factors. Those with PSC are at highest risk of colorectal cancer.

The best surrogate for development of colorectal cancer in UC is the discovery of dysplasia in large intestinal mucosal biopsies. This provides the rationale for colonoscopic surveillance. Dysplasia associated with UC is classified microscopically as either low, (LGD) or high, (HGD) grade depending upon the degree of cytological and architectural disturbance. Endoscopic classification depends upon whether the lesion is raised or flat with further subdivision of raised lesions according to their macroscopic appearance. Raised areas resembling conventional adenomas are designated as adenoma-like lesions or masses (ALMs). These pedunculated or sessile polyps are usually amenable to endoscopic resection. Areas that demonstrate pronounced irregularity are termed dysplasia-associated lesions or masses (DALMs). These include plaques, velvety patches, areas of nodular thickening and broad based masses. Such lesions are typically not endoscopically resectable in their entirety. Sporadic adenomas may be encountered within non-inflamed portions of the colon. These are managed in a conventional way.

The majority of UC related lesions (~80%) are ALMs and in such cases COMPLETE local excision and surveillance yields a good prognosis, irrespective of the degree of dysplasia.

Continued surveillance will identify further ALMs in 50–60% of patients and flat dysplasia may occur in a small proportion (< 5%). DALMs are usually more challenging to remove endoscopically due to their irregular morphology. Ultimately, completeness of endoscopic resection will govern prognosis, and categorizing lesions as ALMs or DALMs is perhaps of secondary importance. This management strategy must be under pinned by careful endoscopic assessment of the whole colon by an experienced practitioner with facility to use dye-spray techniques. Adherence to these principles uncovers otherwise "occult" colonic lesions. Indications for procto-colectomy following the discovery of a dysplastic mass are (1) incomplete excision of that mass or (2) discovery of multifocal flat dysplasia of any grade at sites either near to or remote from the index lesion. Biopsy samples must be taken beyond the perimeter of a sessile mass to uncover patients who possess a wider field change. The incidence of underlying malignancy in those who undergo proctocolectomy for DALM is in the order of 30–40%.

The finding of HGD in otherwise flat mucosa is an indication for proctocolectomy as the risk of underlying malignancy is in the order of 40%. This is a relatively unusual finding as isolated HGD is more often associated with some form of discernable lesion. Management of LGD in the absence of a macroscopic lesion is more controversial as its natural history is still hotly debated. It should be appreciated that there is significant inter-observer variability in the reporting of LGD even amongst experienced gastroenterological histopathologists. One problem is that biopsies taken from regenerative mucosa following an exacerbation of UC may be mistaken for LGD. Some institutions favor immediate proctocolectomy for LGD based upon studies demonstrating a 20% risk of occult malignancyatpresentationwith50% disease progression in 5 years. A more conservative approach consists of intensified surveillance with colonoscopy at 6-monthly intervals even in cases of multifocal flat LGD.

Thorough endoscopic examination by an experienced clinician obviates the need for routine colectomy for LGD.

Dye-spray techniques help to identify malignant lesions that are otherwise invisible. This strategy has been safely adopted in specialist centers with rates of disease progression between 3 to 10% at 10 years. The patient's attitude towards surgery, risk of occult cancer and increased endoscopic surveillance should also be taken into account and used to guide treatment in these circumstances.

***Screening for Malignancy*:** Colonoscopy is advocated for patients with long-standing colitis. Surveillance programs have been derived empirically and much heterogeneity exists in the application and delivery of this service. Evidence based guidelines produced in the UK recommend that patients with pancolitis start surveillance 8–10 years following the onset of symptoms. Examinations are recommended every 3 years during the second decade of UC, 2-yearly in the third and annually in the fourth. Smaller intervals reflect the notion of an exponential rise in cancer incidence over time although this view has recently been challenged. Patients with isolated left sided disease may begin surveillance later at 15–20 years. Due to the higher risk of malignancy in patients with PSC, annual surveillance is recommended from the outset. Guidelines in the UK state that random biopsy samples (2–4 in number) should be taken at 10 cm intervals throughout the colon and rectum. Another favorable strategy is to perform careful inspection of the whole colon with dye-spray, targeting macroscopically abnormal areas for biopsy. Colonoscopy should optimally be performed with the patient in remission as regenerating mucosa may display atypical features that mimic dysplasia, although in practice this is often difficult to achieve. Cyclosporin treatment may also cause pseudodysplasia and the pathologist should be informed where this drug has been used.

***Thromboembolism*:** Patients with UC have a threefold increased risk of developing pulmonary embolism compared to normal controls. This risk is manifest at a young age. Thrombocytosis, dehydration, nutritional deficiencies, presence of inflammatory cytokines, immobility and surgery have all been implicated. Antithrombotic stockings and prophylactic heparin should be prescribed routinely for inpatients with UC, especially those undergoing surgery. Pneumatic calf compression devices are used intra-operatively.

Treatment for Ulcerative Colitis

Treatment of patients with UC is dependent upon disease location (proctitis vs. left sided disease vs. pancolitis), severity(mild, moderate, or severe) and the presence of complications. Medical treatment is aimed at inducing and then maintaining remission. Surgery is usually considered appropriate for those with refractory disease or where neoplastic lesions are found within the colon. In children, growth retardation can prompt colectomy in order to correct malnutrition.

Medical Treatment

Aminosalicylates constitute first line therapy for both the induction and maintenance of remission in mild to moderate UC. They are thought to exert topical anti-inflammatory and immunomodulatory effects. Mesalazine inducesremissionin 70%of patients with mild to moderate UC at a dose of 4g/day, although at 6 weeks this figure drops to 30%. In predominantly left sided disease, steroid (prednisolone 5 mg) or mesalazine (1 g daily) are also administered topically per rectum. Suppositories reach the upper rectum and foams to the distal sigmoid (these preparations may be combined) while enemas extend up to the splenic flexure. Patients who fail to respond after2weeks are given oral prednisolone 20 mg daily which is then reduced over the course of a month as symptoms improve. Mesalazine is continued to maintain remission. Two-year therapy may be appropriate for those with left sided disease whereas indefinite therapy is considered for patients with pancolitis. 5-ASA compounds reduce relapse rates from 80% to 30–50% and in addition the incidence of neoplastic transformation may also be reduced.

Moderate flares of UC are treated using oral prednisolone (40 mg daily). A reducing dose is continued for 4–6 weeks. Hospitalization with administration of parenteral hydrocortisone (200–400 mg/day) or prednisolone (60 mg daily) should be considered in those who do not improve or have severe disease from the outset. Aminosalicylates are generally poorly tolerated in this type of patient. Antidiarrheal agents may precipitate megacolon and should also be avoided. With steroid therapy clinical improvement typically occurs over 7–14 days. Those who promptly relapse are treated with azathioprine or 6-mercaptopurine. There is evidence to suggest that these drugs are effective in reducing corticosteroid dose and may also help maintain remission in patients with UC. They may take 3 months to reach full activity. Non-responders have their diagnosis reconfirmed by stool culture and sigmoidoscopy with biopsy. Intravenous cyclosporin may help avoid surgery in those with refractory UC. More than 50% of patients respond over 2–5 days. Oral cyclosporin must then be used to maintain remission and allow tapering of steroids and establishment of azathioprine. Infliximab may similarly be used to treat severe steroid resistant flares. Three infusions at 0, 2 and 6 weeks are recommended for induction. Responders receive maintenance therapy with infliximab infusions every 8 weeks.

Surgical Treatment

About 25% of patients with UC ultimately require colectomy. Patients usually submit to surgery during a particularly severe exacerbation of the disease or following a protracted period of ill-health and steroid dependence. In the acute setting, colectomy most often follows failure of medical treatment for severe and extensive colitis. Toxic dilatation (colon > 6 cm), perforation and hemorrhage are less common indications for colectomy. The decision to operate is taken jointly and involves daily communication between the gastroenterology and surgical teams. Patients receiving high-dose intravenous steroids, and who have a stool frequency of > 8 per day on the third treatment day are likely to require colectomy. Similarly, those with a stool frequency of 3–8 stools per day who have a CRP > 45 mg/l are unlikely to settle. Failure to respond after 5–7 days or any significant deterioration during this period is an indication for colectomy. Patients who initially respond but promptly relapse with the reintroduction of diet are also likely to require colectomy.

In the acute setting, ile-pouch anal anastomosis (IPAA) surgery should be avoided. It is customary to instead perform subtotal colectomy with an end ileostomy. The diseased rectum is left in situ, for resection at a later date once the patient has regained health and steroids have been withdrawn. Emergency colectomy may be performed using an open or laparoscopic approach. The colon is mobilised and vessels taken relatively close to the bowel wall. The sigmoid stump is stapled and left long allowing it to be secured with sutures in the subcutaneous space at the lower pole of the wound. Any stump dehiscence will then result in an easily manageable fistula rather than a pelvic abscess.

Occasionally the stump must be left short in cases of sigmoid hemorrhage. In all cases, a Foley catheter is used to decompress the rectum for a period of 3 or 4 days.

Three operative strategies are in common use for the definitive surgical treatment of UC patients. (1) Proctocolectomy plus end ileostomy removes all diseased tissue at the expense of a permanent stoma. This option is undertaken in patients with poor sphincter function. It is also used in those patients who are happy with their ileostomy following subtotal colectomy and do not wish to consider a pouch. (2) Subtotal colectomy plus ileorectal anastomosis (IRA) is a compromise procedure in which a minimally diseased rectum is retained. The rectum must be distensible and retain its capacity to act as a reservoir. This can be confirmed using flexible sigmoidoscopy or a contrast enema. There should be no evidence of colonic dysplasia or malignancy. These criteria are seldom met and this option is rarely used. Function is difficult to predict following IRA and one quarter of patients suffer from unacceptable stool frequency as a consequence of persistent rectal inflammation. Long-term endoscopic follow up of the retained rectum is essential due to the risk of malignant change. (3) Finally, IPAA has become the standard of care for patients with ulcerative colitis who ultimately require colectomy. This approach is popular with patients as it avoids the necessity for a long-term stoma. Pouch surgery aims to deliver 5 or 6 semi-formed bowel motions per day, with no night time evacuation and no incontinence. Successful outcomes are built upon sensible patient selection, clear pre-operative counseling, an operative strategy appropriate to the patient and expedient management of any complications.

Patient Selection for Ileal Pouch Surgery

***Age*:** Large case series have shown that surgical complications and pouch preservation rates appear to be independent of age at operation, whilst continence and quality of life are generally a little worse with advancing years. IPAA surgery is performed routinely in well motivated elderly individuals without symptomatic disturbance of the anal sphincters.

***Indeterminate Colitis*:** A definitive histopathological diagnosis of UC or Crohn's is not always possible following colectomy for colitis. In 10–15% of all surgical specimens a diagnosis of indeterminate colitis (IndC) is made. A diagnosis of Crohn's disease will be made subsequently in 4–15% of patients initially labeled as IndC. Clinicians make every effort to define this population prior to embarking upon ileal pouch surgery. While the majority of patients with IndC obtain good results from IPAA surgery, pelvic sepsis and pouch failure may occur more frequently. This is largely due to the emergence of patients with Crohn's disease. At 10 years, 85% of those with IndC retain their pouch. The consensus amongst most surgeons is that patients with *bona fide*IndC are suitable candidates for pouch surgery if fully informed of the risks involved. Special attention should be paid to any suspicious history of pelvic sepsis or perineal fistula as these patients are more likely to manifest Crohn's and in our opinion should not be considered for IPAA surgery.

***Crohn's Colitis*:** Crohn's disease remains an absolute contraindication to IPAA as the overall failure rates approach 50%. There may be a role for pouch surgery in a highly selective group of patients with Crohn's colitis who possess a normal anus, have no small bowel disease and are prepared to accept the increased risks of failure and reoperation.

***Dysplasia or Cancer in the Proctocolectomy Specimen*:** The presence of dysplasia or potentially curable cancer either within the colon or high in the rectum does not preclude IPAA. Mucosectomy and a hand-sewn pouch-anal anastomosis rather than stapling are considered for patients with multiple tumors or multifocal dysplasia especially when these lesions encroach upon the rectum. Following mucosectomy dysplastic cells may survive deep within the muscular rectal cuff and these may re-present as "pouch tumors". For this reason, reconstructive pouch surgery is probably inadvisable when dealing with low rectal tumors.

Technique of Ileal Pouch Surgery

***Pouch Design*:** Parks and Nicholls originally devised a triple limb "S"-shaped pouch. This was relatively complicated to construct and suffered from kinking of the efferent limb if left too long. Alternative designs have included the high capacity "W" pouch, the "H" pouch and the "J" pouch. The majority of surgeons now favor the J pouch due to ease of construction, economical use of terminal ileum and reliable emptying. Functional results are equal to those of other reservoir designs. The pouch is formed from the terminal 40 cm of ileum using several applications of a linear, cutting stapler to join the antimesenteric borders of two 20 cm ileal limbs.

***Mucosectomy vs. Double Stapling*:** Stripping of the columnar mucosa above the dentate line has been advocated in order to prevent recurrence of UC. Mucosectomy, combined with a per-anal hand-sewn anastomosis allows precise placement of the pouch-anal anastomosis at the dentate line. This technique is more complex to perform and may be associated with higher rates of sphincter damage and incontinence. Mucosectomy also entails excision of the anal transition zone (ATZ), an area of cuboidal epithelium richly innervated by sensory nerve endings that mediate anal sampling reflexes. The "double stapled" IPAA technique preserves this theoretically important area with no requirement for prolonged anal dilation. A transverse stapler fired from above, separates the rectum from the top of the anal canal. The stapling instrument should be positioned 2–3 cm above the anal margin, a distance roughly equivalent to the length of the distal two phalanges of the index finger. This helps to avoid an error of judgement that places the anastomosis too high resulting in a pouch-rectal anastomosis. A circular EEA stapler inserted via the anus joins the ileal reservoir to the upper anal canal. Many surgeons favor the double staple technique as this is a simpler operation and may have a lower risk of failure.

One, Two or Three Stage IPAA: To date, most surgeons have favored the creation of a temporary defunctioning loop ileostomy following IPAA surgery as this avoids catastrophic pelvic contamination in the event of anastomotic dehiscence. Pouch failure rates from St Marks were higher in patients without a covering stoma; 15% versus 8%, although Toronto have published contrasting figures with less than 1% of one-stage pouches failing. To omit a defunctioning ileostomy is an exercise in risk management. Large series indicate that anastomotic separation occurs in approximately 5–15% of patients while complication rates for ileostomy closure range from 10% to 30%. Small bowel obstruction, wound infection and anastomotic leakage are most prevalent. In practice, stomas are omitted in approximately 15% of cases based upon the perceived risks (steroids, nutrition, age, anemia etc.), uneventful surgery and discharge arrangements.

Laparoscopic IPAA: Conventional open surgery utilizes a long midline incision for access to the splenic flexure and pelvis. The laparoscopic approach is more elegant as trauma to the abdominal wall is minimized. In the short term, wound related complications, such as pain and infection, may be reduced. Over a more protracted period the risk of symptomatic adhesions and incisional herniation may be diminished. There is little doubt that cosmetic appearance is enhanced. To date, rigorous assessment of these endpoints using large clinical trials has been hindered by the relative complexity of these techniques. Accelerated recovery programs have delivered reduced hospital stays for elective IPAA patients somewhat negating the benefits of laparoscopic over open surgery in this regard.

Acute Complications of IPAA

***Acute Sepsis*:** Fever in a patient recovering from IPAA surgery should arouse suspicion of pelvic sepsis. This remains a relatively common acute complication and failure to react in a timely fashion is likely to compromise pouch function and may lead to its eventual failure. Septic complications usually result from anastomotic dehiscence or the presence of an infected pelvic hematoma. Digital examination may reveal the anastomotic defect or localized tenderness overlying an indurated or fluctuant mass. CT or MRI can be used to gauge the extent of sepsis. A trial of broad spectrum antibiotics is appropriate for relatively small abscesses. More sizeable collections are considered for radiological drainage. Failure to settle would prompt examination under anesthesia. The anus is inspected using an Eisenhammer anal speculum (Seward, London, UK). Anastomotic breakdown is usually detected without difficulty. The underlying area is then probed to determine the extent of any associated abscess cavity and suction applied to clear its contents. Larger defects may be amenable to digital examination followed by placement of a catheter for irrigation and drainage. Regular re-examination under anesthesia may be required to be confident that the cavity remains clean. The vagina must also be inspected for evidence of fistulation, especially if the IPAA was stapled.

Re-laparotomy is reserved for cases where CT-guided drainage and minor surgery have failed to control sepsis and also for those who deteriorate quickly with signs of generalized peritonitis. Major leaks require a proximal diverting loop ileostomy to be formed if one is not already in place. Consideration should be given to exteriorizing of the pouch if complete anastomotic disruption has occurred. If gross ischemia occurs, it is best to resect and exteriorize the ileum.

Rates of pelvic sepsis are much higher for patients with UC undergoing IPAA than for those with familial adenomatous polyposis (FAP) who are subject to the same operation. High dose corticosteroids (systemic equivalent of > 40 mg prednisolone per day) have been implicated in the causation of anastomotic failure. Steroids may impair healing at the anastomosis, promote infection or merely label patients in poor clinical condition. It is customary to avoid IPAA formation and instead perform subtotal colectomy in those patients who are acutely unwell and receiving high dose corticosteroids.

Hemorrhage**:** Primary intraluminal hemorrhage may follow formation of a sutured or stapled pouch and it is therefore important to carefully inspect the mucosal surface before the pouch-anal anastomosis is constructed. Reactionary intraluminal hemorrhage, within 24 h of surgery is likely to originate from the suture or staple lines. Irrigation of the pouch with a 1:200,000 adrenaline solution controls the majority of clinically significant hemorrhages. Continued bleeding necessitates a return to the operating room. The pouch is inspected using an Eisenhammer speculum, proctoscope or sigmoidoscope. Suction and irrigation are used to accurately locate the bleeding point which is then sutured or injected with 1:100,00 adrenaline solution. Secondary hemorrhage is less common and usually heralds pelvic sepsis. The pouch should be inspected in theater with special attention to the ileoanal anastomosis for evidence of localized anastomotic breakdown. Bleeding points are under-run and collections drained, preferably via the original defect. A small mushroom or Foley catheter may then be placed trans-anally into the cavity.

Intra-abdominal hemorrhage may arise from mesenteric vessels or the pelvic side wall. The rectal stump may bleed following hand-sewn pouch-anal anastomosis. In exceptional circumstances inspection of the lower pelvis is facilitated by detachment of the pouch. The stump is approached endo-anally using a Lone Star retractor (Lone Star Medical Products Inc, Houston, TX). The pouch may then be exteriorized as a left iliac fossa mucous fistula if re-anastomosis is considered unsafe. Uncontrollable pelvic hemorrhage requires packing of the cavity with a follow-up 48 h later.

Chronic Complications and Outcome Following IPAA

***Mucosal Adaptation and Pouchitis*:** Pouchitis is a relapsing, acute-on-chronic inflammatory condition presenting with diarrhea (maybe bloody), urgency, abdominal bloating, pain or fever. The etiology is unknown although recurrent UC in areas of colonic metaplasia and bacterial overgrowth are possible mechanisms. Interestingly, this condition does not seem to affect pouches in patients with FAP. Patients with new symptoms suggestive of pouchitis should be investigated by endoscopy and biopsy. Endoscopic appearances are similar to those of UC. Histologically signs of acute inflammation (polymorphonuclear leucocyte infiltration) with superficial ulceration, superimposed onto a background of chronic inflammatory changes are typical. Once the diagnosis is established then it would be reasonable to instigate empirical therapy for relapses.

The cumulative probability of pouchitis, determined on the basis of symptomatology, endoscopy and histopathology is in the order of 20% at 1 year, 30% at 5 years and 40% at 10 years. Differential diagnoses include undiagnosed Crohn's disease, especially in the presence of prominent ulceration, with pre-pouch ileitis or fistula formation. Alternatively, bacterial/ viral infections, cuffitis, pelvic sepsis, a low volume reservoir, pouch outlet obstruction and incomplete emptying, can produce similar symptoms. Stool examination, MRI and isotope or contrast pouchogram may help to elucidate the nature of malfunction.

Most cases respond to oral metronidazole or ciprofloxacin. Two thirds of patients develop further attacks and 5% become chronic sufferers. Maintenance therapy may be effective for those who promptly relapse although prolonged treatment with metronidazole is inadvisable due to the risk of peripheral neuropathy. The probiotic VSL-3 may be taken orally with some evidence that relapse rates are decreased. Those who fail to respond may be offered oral or rectal corticosteroids. Oral or topical mesalazine may also be used. Consideration should be given to removing the pouch where function is very poor as a consequence of chronic pouchitis. Chronic pouchitis accounts for 10% of all pouch failures.

***Cuffitis*:** The ATZ forms a relatively small proportion of the anal canal. Conventional double-stapled restorative proctocolectomy therefore leaves 1.5–2.0 cm of columnar epithelium above the ATZ (Fig. 2.1). Recurrent UC within the columnar cuff is termed "cuffitis" and it arises in 9–22% of patients. Cuffitis may lead to increased stool frequency, bloody

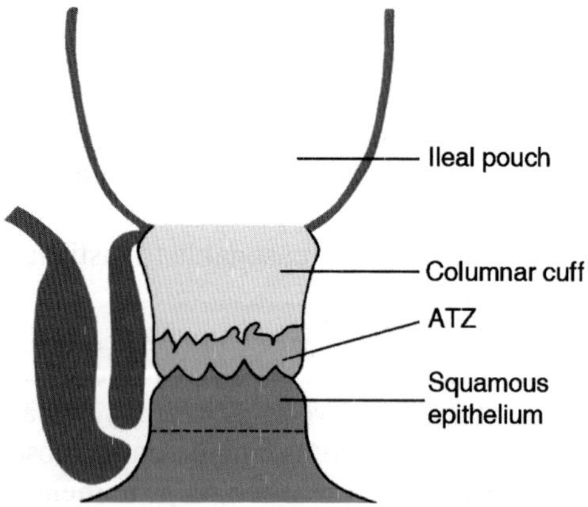

FIGURE 2.1. Distribution of epithelial subtypes in a typical double-stapled pouch-anal anastomosis (Reprinted from Thompson-Fawcett et al., 1998. Copyright 1998. With permission from Wiley).

discharge, urgency and discomfort. Mesalazine suppositories may be helpful in improving these symptoms. Dysplasia or carcinoma may theoretically arise within unresected columnar mucosa. Reports do exist of adenocarcinomas situated below the level of the IPAA but these lesions are generally associated with the presence of severe dysplasia or malignancy within the original proctocolectomy specimen. Routine surveillance of the anal canal is not advocated for the first 10 years following IPAA unless the patient has a previous history of dysplasia or malignancy.

***Small Bowel Obstruction*:** In a large series from Toronto, the risk of small bowel obstruction (SBO) outside of the perioperative period was reported as 6% at 1 year, 14% at 5 years and 19% at 10 years. Laparotomy was required in one third of patients, and in the majority of cases small bowel was adherent to the pelvis or a previous stoma site. About 20% of patients who underwent laparotomy and adhesiolysis developed further episodes of SBO. One quarter of these had a further laparotomy. A water soluble contrast enema may help to determine the site, nature and degree of obstruction. This investigation may also be of therapeutic benefit. Alternatively, CT scan with oral contrast provides similar information.

***Chronic Pelvic Sepsis*:** Pelvic sepsis is estimated to complicate 10–20% of IPAA procedures. Long term manifestations of pouch sepsis include a variety of fistulae (pouch-anal anastomotic, pouch vaginal, pouch perineal or proximal pouch) and anastomotic stenosis. Functional outcome is likely to be worse and long term ileostomy may be required.

Fistulae arising between the IPAA and vagina occur relatively rarely. Operative trauma, postoperative pelvic sepsis and undiagnosed Crohn's disease are all implicated. Unsuspected Crohn's should be actively sought as rates of healing are worse (25% vs. 48%) and pouch failure more common (33% vs. 14%) amongst this subgroup. Principals of management include local drainage of the tract using a seton with fecal diversion in selected cases based upon the degree of uncontrolled sepsis. Several options are available to the surgeon for definitive treatment. Transanal ileal advancement flap is appropriate for a pouch that remains mobile with success rates reported in the order of 50%. Transabdominal advancement of the ileoanal anastomosis with closure of the defect is necessary when the pouch cannot be mobilized from below. Per-anal access to fistulae arising within the anal canal may be difficult, especially where an anastomosis has been placed at the anorectal junction. For this reason the transvaginal route is favored by some as access is easier and damage to the anal sphincters may be avoided. Fistulae that arise as a consequence of previously unrecognized Crohn's disease may be treated with infliximab, although recurrence remains a problem.

Anastomotic stricture may complicate leakage, tension or ischemia at the IPAA. It is important to perform an adequate examination under anesthesia prior to ileostomy closure in addition to the pouchogram. For those using the pouch, symptoms of straining, diarrhea and anal or abdominal pain suggest stricturing of the anastomosis. It may be possible to attempt dilatation at the time of pouchoscopy. Alternatively, application of Hegar's dilators under anesthesia treats most cases successfully. Particularly long or tight strictures may not respond to these measures and further biopsies should be taken to exclude Crohn's disease. Per-anal pouch advancement is considered once all sepsis has been eradicated if the pouch is not tethered. This technique is also used to close fistula tracks situated at the level of the stricture. Otherwise re-laparotomy and mobilization of the pouch with re-anastomosis is the sole option.

***Sexual Dysfunction*:** Erectile function is a parasympathetic response mediated by the erigent nerves, while ejaculation is a sympathetic event mediated by the hypogastric nerves. These structures may be damaged during pelvic dissection as they lie behind the parietal facial envelope, close to the mesorectal plane. One may avoid contact with the pelvic nerves using a close rectal dissection. This approach is highly vascularized and for this reason many surgeons prefer to dissect in the more anatomical mesorectal plane. Sexual dysfunction affects 3% of men following pouch surgery and for this reason sperm banking should be recommended. Sildenafil (Viagra) has been shown to help erectile dysfunction but will not impact upon retrograde ejaculation.

***Fecundity and Pregnancy*:** UC commonly affects young females of reproductive age. Neither the disease itself nor the medical treatments currently available (apart from salazopyrin in men) are thought to compromise fertility. Fertility rates are lower in women who have had pouch surgery when compared those who undergo medical management. About 40% of women will have difficulty becoming pregnant following IPAA. It may be possible to delay proctectomy until a family has been established or alternatively anti-adhesion products may combat tubal obstruction.

Vaginal delivery has been associated with occult sphincter injury in 30% of patients. Females with an ileal pouch might risk incontinence following vaginal delivery. The Cleveland Clinic have reported that sphincter injury occurs more frequently in those who choose vaginal delivery rather than cesarean section with rates of 50% and 13% respectively but no difference in pouch function was apparent at 5 years. For the duration of the pregnancy, stool frequency, incontinence and pad usage gradually increase with pouch function returning quickly to normal in most cases. It seems reasonable to conclude that while vaginal delivery confers no functional disadvantage in the medium term there is concern that sphincter integrity is indeed compromised. Long-term implications remain unmeasured and therefore uncertain.

***Pouch Failure*:** Complication rates for IPAA of about 30–40% are relatively high. Fortunately, most of these problems can usually be resolved. Pouch excision or indefinite retention of a defunctioning stoma defines failure. Institutional pouch failure rates have notably fallen over the past 20 years presumably following improvements in patient selection and surgical technique. Long term failure occurs with a frequency of 5–10%. A consistent theme that emerges from the large institutional series is that early pouch failure is associated closely with the occurrence of perioperative pelvic sepsis while that occurring later is often secondary to poor function or following an unexpected diagnosis of Crohn's disease. The success of redo pouch surgery for UC has improved with approximately half to three quarters of patients now retaining a functional pouch in the long term. When considering revision, it is necessary to evaluate the sphincters, assess pelvic soft tissue compliance, make a judgement regarding the likely diagnosis (Crohn's or UC) and determine the patient's general health and wishes. It is clear that redo-IPAA surgery may benefit patients with an excessively long efferent ileal spout or those with a tortuous stricture. It is perhaps less clear whether revision is as beneficial to those with ongoing septic complications. Even in the best hands, redo-IPAA surgery carries an appreciable morbidity rate. Not surprisingly outcomes are worse both in terms of overall failure and function when compared to first time surgery; nonetheless this procedure remains a valid alternative to a defunctioning stoma or pouch excision.

When faced with the proposition of removing an ileoanal pouch should be considered that 62% of 68 cases treated at St. Marks suffered significant morbidity and one patient died. The single most common complication following pouch excision was non-healing of the perineal wound. Readmission within 5 years was the norm with 20% of patients requiring reoperation for small bowl obstruction, stoma complications or hemorrhage.

Selected Readings

Bernstein CN (2006) Natural history and management of flat and polypoid dysplasia in inflammatory bowel disease. Gastroenterol Clin North Am 35:573–579

Lim CH, Dixon MF, Vail A, et al. (2003) Ten year followup of ulcerative colitis patients with and without low grade dysplasia. Gut 52:1127–1132

Parks AG, Nicholls RJ (1978) Proctocolectomy without ileostomy for ulcerative colitis. Br Med J 2:85–88

Rubio CA, Befrits R (2004) Low-grade dysplasia in flat mucosa in ulcerative colitis. Gastroenterology126:1494; author reply 1494–1495

Rutter MD, Saunders BP, Schofield G, et al. (2004) Pancolonic indigo carmine dye spraying for the detection of dysplasia in ulcerative colitis. Gut 53:256–260

Rutter MD, Saunders BP, Wilkinson KH, et al. (2006) Thirty-year analysis of a colonoscopic surveillance program for neoplasia in ulcerative colitis. Gastroenterology 130:1030–1038

Thompson-Fawcett MW, Warren BF, Mortensen NJ (1998) A new look at the anal transitional zone with reference to restorative proctocolectomy and the columnar cuff. Br J Surg 85:1517–1521

Travis SP, Farrant JM, Ricketts C, et al. (1996) Predicting outcome in severe ulcerative colitis. Gut 38:905–910

Truelove SC, Witts LJ (1955) Cortisone in ulcerative colitis: final report on a therapeutic trial. Br Med J 2:1041–1048

Yu CS, Pemberton JH, Larson D (2000) Ileal pouch-anal anastomosis in patients with indeterminate colitis: long-term results. Dis Colon Rectum 43:1487–1496

3
Crohn's Disease of the Small Bowel and Colon

Jenny Speranza and Steven D. Wexner

Pearls and Pitfalls

- Crohn's disease is a transmural inflammatory condition of the GI tract.
- The disease can affect the entire GI tract from the mouth to the anus and present a myriad of extraintestinal manifestations.
- Medical therapy is the principal treatment for exacerbations and active disease.
- Surgery is indicated when the patient is refractory to medical therapy, has intractable adverse sequelae of medical management, or desires to discontinue medical therapy.
- Bowel conservation is a fundamental tenet of surgery.
- Presenting features include: abdominal pain, fever, diarrhea, weight loss, anorexia, vomiting, chronic malnutrition, and fatigue.
- Affects the young in 2nd and 3rd decades of life but also has a bimodal distribution and equal gender predominance.
- Distal ileal involvement is most common at 41%, small bowel disease in 27%, colonic involvement in 27%, and isolated perianal involvement in 3.4% of patients.
- Diagnosis is most often made with a combination of physical exam, contrast radiographic studies, endoscopy, and histopathology.
- Histopathology of the small bowel will exhibit "fat wrapping"; mesenteric thickening and granulomas are pathognomonic.

K.I. Bland et al. (eds.), *Colorectal Surgery*,
DOI 10.1007/978-1-84996-444-9_3,

- Colonoscopic exam may grossly reveal skip areas, linear deep ulcerations, and stricture formation. Histologically granulomas will be definitive of Crohn's disease.
- Surgical intervention is used to treat the complications of the disease such as perforation, abscess, and fistula.
- Intraoperative ureteric catheters are advised in surgical patients with severe inflammation presenting with a large phlegmon.
- Bowel margins should be resected to grossly normal tissue.
- The mesentery should be carefully thinned and suture ligated to avoid hematoma formation.
- The quality and length of both resected and retained bowel should be accurately documented during surgery.
- Whenever possible intra-abdominal abscesses should be percutaneously drained prior to surgery to assist in control of inflammation.
- Strictureplasty should always be considered in patients with recurrent or extensive disease and in patients who have or are in imminent danger of having short bowel syndrome.
- Isolated colonic disease with rectal sparing may be best treated by subtotal colectomy with ileorectal anastomosis.
- Segmental colectomy should only be done in selected cases since recurrence has shown to be increased as compared to proctocolectomy.
- Severe perianal disease will ultimately necessitate proctectomy in 25% of patients with perianal involvement.

Introduction

Crohn's disease was originally described in 1932. Crohn's disease is a transmural inflammatory condition that can affect the entire gastrointestinal tract from the mouth to the anus with a myriad of extraintestinal manifestations. Although there have been suggestions of immunologic, genetic, and environment effects, the etiology is still unknown. Medical therapy is the mainstay of treatment at the current time.

Although efficacy is variable, side effects of such therapy may be extreme. Surgery is reserved to treat complications of the disease, complications of medical therapy or the intractability of disease despite medical therapy. Since there are many components of care required in treating Crohn's patients, it is best that such patients be treated in a tertiary center with a multi-specialty approach to the disease.

Presentation

Crohn's disease typically presents with abdominal pain, distension, nausea, vomiting, chronic diarrhea, weight loss, fever, and general malaise. On physical examination, a tender mass in the right lower quadrant often signifies the presence of terminal ileal/small bowel disease. Although quite rare (1–3%), duodenal involvement will present with duodenal or gastric outlet obstruction. When Crohn's disease is isolated to the colon, patients can have pain, diarrhea, bloody bowel movements, and anemia, along with extraintestinal manifestations. Enterocolonic fistula is usually a result of small bowel disease and the colon is otherwise normal. If there is perianal involvement, there can be multiple fistulous tracts, linear ulcerations and abscesses, enlarged skin tags, and stricture of the anal canal. Perianal disease often precedes the onset of small bowel disease by several years. Perianal involvement is more common in patients with colonic manifestations than with small bowel disease.

Epidemiology

Crohn's disease usually presents in the 2nd and 3rddecades of life, although a bimodal distribution has been described with the second onset in the 5th and 6th decade of life. The incidence is 1–6 per 100,000 population. The prevalence is higher among Ashkenazi Jews (10 cases per 100,000 persons per year) and in cooler climates areas, such as Scandinavia, the United Kingdom, Germany, and the northern United States. Genetics have also been implicated since the disease has been shown to affect first-degree relatives. Women and men seem to be equally affected. The distribution of Crohn's disease is varied 41% of patients will have distal ileal involvement, 27% have small intestine involvement only, 27% have colonic involvement, and 3.4% have anorectal involvement.

Diagnosis

A patient often presents to the colorectal surgeon with an established diagnosis. At that time it is important to determine the extent and activity of the disease. This analysis can often be accomplished by radiographic and endoscopic studies. A small bowel series can determine extent of small bowel disease, giving location and assessing stricture and fistulous disease. CT scan with oral and intravenous contrast can help define enterocutaneous fistulas, as well reveal and possibly drain localized abscesses. A contrast enema can identify colonic strictures, fistulae, cobblestoning, and ulceration. Colonoscopic examination is vital when assessing the colon, as well as to intubate the terminal ileum and obtain biopsies throughout the colon. Findings on colonoscopy often reveal rectal sparing, stricture formation, skip areas, deep linear ulceration, and fissures. Although granulomas identified by endoscopic biopsies will confirm the diagnosis, they are rarely found. Upper endoscopy is also important in evaluating the esophagus, stomach, and duodenum. Endoanal ultrasound can evaluate fistulous disease using hydrogen peroxide to further delineate complex fistulae. MRI is useful in further identifying complex perianal disease.

Histopathology

On macroscopic exam the bowel appears thick-walled, granular, and friable. "Fat wrapping" is often seen encroaching from the mesentery toward the antimesenteric border of the bowel. The mesentery may be thickened and foreshortened with adenopathy adjacent to diseased small bowel. Strictures frequently reveal deep linear ulcerations on the mucosal surface. Microscopic granulomas are pathognomonic for Crohn's disease, although they are present in only two-thirds of all patients. Transmural inflammation is also pathognomonic of the entity.

Medical Management

The goals of medical treatment of Crohn's disease are to treat manifestations of the disease, while minimizing the morbidity of the therapeutic agents. Therapy is aimed at minimizing inflammation with medication and providing nutritional support. Sulfasalazine and 5-ASA compounds can help induce and maintain remission of disease. Antibiotics, such as metronidazole and ciprofloxacin, are beneficial in treating perianal disease. Corticosteroids are used for acute exacerbation of disease, but have detrimental side effects and are not intended for long-term use for suppression. Immunosuppressant agents, 6-MP, azathioprine, methotrexate, and cyclosporine are used when first-line agents are not effective. These agents have been shown to induce remission, but also have multiple side effects. Infliximab has been shown to promote healing of Crohn's fistulas, but administration of this medication requires careful surveillance due to serious adverse effects. Total parenteral nutrition can be beneficial in strengthening the malnourished patient.

Surgical Indications

Indications for surgery include patients, abscesses, obstruction, perforation fistulization, resistance to or intolerable complications of medical treatment, and growth retardation. Approximately 80% of patients with Crohn's disease require surgery within 20 years of onset. The cumulative rate of intestinal resection was shown to be 44%, 61%, and 71% at 1, 5, and 10 years after diagnosis, respectively. Because short gut syndrome can become a potential danger with repeated bowel resections, bowel-preserving surgery and avoiding surgery until it is an absolute necessity are major tenets for treating Crohn's disease.

Pre-Operative Planning

CT scan of the abdomen can allow for preoperative percutaneous drainage of abscess collection. This step can help decrease inflammation and sepsis, in addition to providing total parenteral nutrition, to improve the patient's nutritional status and wound healing ability prior to surgical intervention. Patients should undergo stoma marking by a stoma therapist prior to the procedure. Mechanical bowel prep is given if the patient is not obstructed. In the presence of severe inflammation and phlegmon, we employ the use of ureteric catheters to help identify and avoid the ureters.

Surgical Management

Small Bowel

Surgery for small bowel disease is the primary modality for treatment of complications of Crohn's disease, such as strictures, fistulae, abscess, and phlegmon. Bowel preservation is the principle goal of management. The bowel should be evaluated from the ligament of Treitz to the ileocecal valve; measurement should be documented for disease extent and normal bowel. Bowel resection limits are evaluated by gross examination. Histologic margins have not been proven to affect recurrence. Fazio et al. prospectively examined two groups of patients having margins of small bowel that were not diseased grossly with either a 2 cm or 12 cm margin.

No significant difference in recurrence rates between the two group was noted. When dividing thickened Crohn's mesentery, it is important to score the peritoneum and carefully palpate vessels. Suture ligating can help ensure hemostasis, as the vessels in this thickened tissue have a tendency to retract, with subsequent hematoma formation and further loss of small bowel.

When treating strictured small bowel, Heineke-Mikulicz type strictureplasty is preferred in short segment disease (Figs. 3.1–3.3). If there are multiple short strictures in a small segment of bowel, it may be advantageous to resect a continuous piece of bowel rather than having numerous stricture plasties in one area. For long-segment strictures, resection or long stricture plasty are two options. Long stricture plasty is as safe and effective as short strictureplasty. Shartari et al. followed 62 patients undergoing strictureplasty for jejunoileal disease over a 20-year period. Twenty-one patients underwent long strictureplasty, while 41 patients received strictureplasty. No significant differences were found in the 3, 5 and 10 year

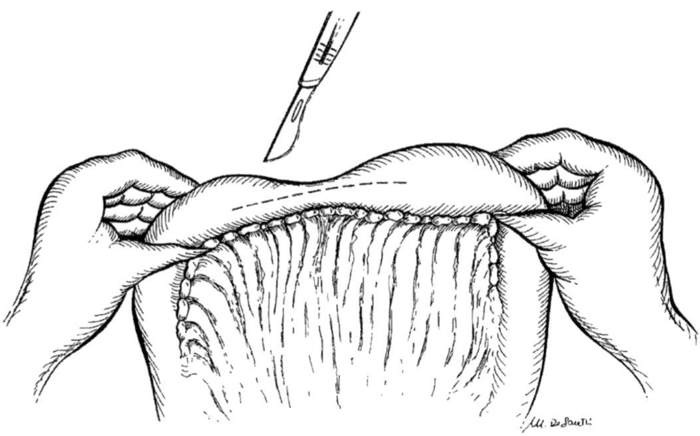

FIGURE 3.1. A longitudinal incision over the stricture, on the antimesenteric border of the small bowel, extends 3–5 cm beyond the edges of the stricture on each side (Reprinted from Wexner et al., 2001. With permission).

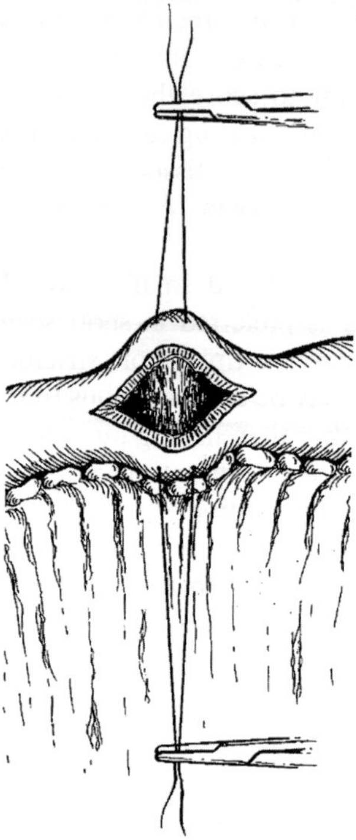

FIGURE 3.2. The lumen is spread apart and inspected (Reprinted from Wexner et al., 2001. With permission).

disease free rates for the long and short strictureplasty. For disease involving fistulous communications to adjacent organs, skin, or bowel, the basic premise is to resect the diseased bowel and to repair the involved organ, if possible. The "bystanding" organ need not be resected if there is no gross disease; in such circumstances, a wedge resection or suture closure may suffice.

When gastroduodenal disease is present, the complication is usually a stricture of the duodenum causing an outlet obstruction. Although this is a rare event, a gastrojejunostomy can be created with or without vagotomy.

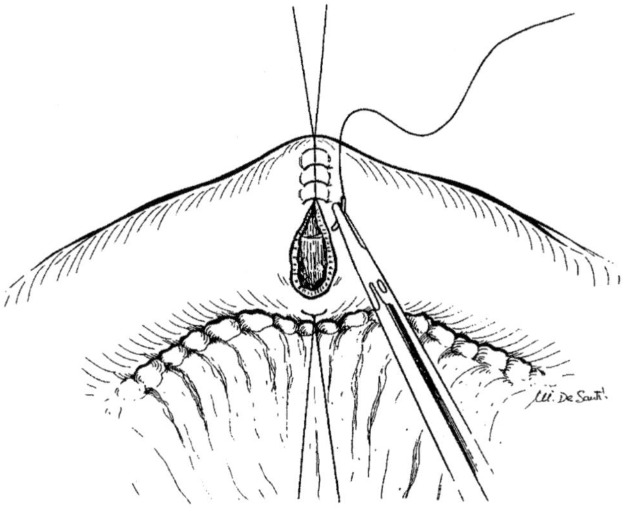

FIGURE 3.3. A Heineke-Mikulicz-type stricturoplasty. The longitudinal incision is closed transversely using a single layer of interrupted polydioxan 3–0 sutures (Reprinted from Wexner et al., 2001. With permission).

Surgical Management

Colonic Crohn's

With colonic involvement, surgical intervention is dependent on the severity and location of the disease. In the emergent setting of toxic colitis, total abdominal colectomy with end ileostomy is warranted. Colectomy with ileorectal anastomosis may be warranted if there is rectal sparing and otherwise normal small bowel. Segmental colectomy can be performed in select cases, such as terminal ileal disease, with limited involvement of the right colon. Segmental colectomy can also be used in cases of ileosigmoid fistulas, when the ileum is diseased and the colon is normal. Although the above options of segmental colectomy are occasionally feasible, segmental colectomy has been shown to have a significantly shorter time to recurrence and increased risk of recurrence, compared with proctocolectomy. Fichera et al followed 55 patients who underwent segmental colectomy, 49 total abdominal colectomy, and 75 proctocolectomy. Total proctocolectomy patients had significantly lower morbidity, lower risk of recurrence, and longer time to recurrence.

Surgical Management

Perianal Crohn's

Perianal Crohn's should be treated based on the presenting signs and symptoms. Patients with chronic fistulae and perianal disease may need temporary diversion of the fecal stream. Treatment of mild disease such as an abscess will require incision and drainage, which can be accomplished with a small incision and use of a drain or Mallenkot catheter. Fistula tracts should be identified either by examination under anesthesia, endoanal ultrasound, or MRI. Once the tract is known, a seton of 0 Ethibond can be placed within the tract while the sepsis and inflammation abate. These setons can be left in place for long periods of time to provide effective drainage and limit possible incontinence from fistulotomy. Fistulotomy should only be used for patients with a documented minor amount of sphincter involvement. For definitive treatment of transsphincteric fistulas in patients with Crohn's disease, the endorectal advancement flap has been applied with good results (Shatari et al.,2004). Joo et al. evaluated outcomes of 31 endorectal advancement flaps between January 1991 and December 1995.Theresults were found to be more favorable if there was no small bowel Crohn's disease (25% versus 87% of patients with no small bowel involvement). Asymptomatic skin tags and hemorrhoids should not be removed secondary to poor wound healing in these patients. Severe ulceration and complex fistulous disease may ultimately require proctectomy. Galandiuk et al. demonstrated that the presence of colonic disease and anal strictures were predictors of eventual permanent diversion.

Surgical Management

Laparoscopic Surgery for Crohn's Disease

With an elective surgical procedure, laparoscopic surgery is gaining popularity as the procedure of choice for treating Crohn's disease. The benefits of minimally invasive surgery for Crohn's disease have been shown in multiple studies to decrease postoperative pain, reduce length of hospital stay, and hasten recovery. Conversion rates remain low, between 10% and 28%. In one study, laparoscopic ileocolic resections were shown to have significantly decreased rates of small bowel obstruction over 5 years compared with open ileocolic resections. A tour institution, ileocolic resection is the procedure of choice for treating ileocolic Crohn's disease in select cases.

Surgical Management

Crohn's Disease Recurrence

Despite advances in medical and surgical care, Crohn's disease continues to be a complex and vexing condition to treat. Medical management can help maintain remission for some patients, but with a myriad of serious side effects. Surgical intervention, even when used sparingly to treat complications of the disease, results in recurrence of disease. Bernell et al. (2000) retrospectively assessed 1936 patients and found that three of four Crohn's patients will need intestinal resection at some time. In addition, the extent of disease at diagnosis and presence of perianal fistula increase the risk of recurrence after surgery. Yamamoto examined factors affecting Crohn's disease recurrence. Smoking was associated with a significant decrease in postoperative recurrence of disease. In addition, 5-ASA was shown to slightly lower the recurrence rate.

Selected Readings

Bergamaschi R, Pessaux P, Arnaud JP (2003) Comparison of Bernell O, Lapidus A, Hellers G (2000) Risk factors for conventional and laparoscopic ileocolic resection for surgery and postoperative recurrence in Crohn's disease. Crohn's disease. Dis Colon Rectum 46:1129–1133 Ann Surg 231:38–45

Delaney CP, Fazio VW (2001) Crohn's disease of the small bowel. Surg Clin North Am 81:137–158

Fazio VW, Marchetti F, Church JM, et al. (1996) Effect of resection margins on the recurrence of Crohn's disease in the small bowel. A randomized controlled trial. Ann Surg 224:563–573

Fichera A, McCormack R, Rubin MA, et al. (2005) Long term outcome of surgically treated Crohn's disease: a prospective study. Dis Colon Rectum 48:963–969

Galandiuk S, Kimberling J, Al-Mishlab T, et al. (2005) Perianal Crohn's disease predictors of need for permanent diversion. Ann Surg 241:796–802

Joo JS, Weiss EG, Nogueras JJ, et al. (1998) Endorectal advancement flap in perianal Crohn's disease. Am Surg 64:147–150

Wexner SD, Reissman P, Bernstein MA (2001) Surgery of Crohn's disease including strictureplasty. In: Baker RJ, Fischer JE (eds) Mastery of surgery 4th edn. Lippincott, Williams & Wilkins, Philadelphia, pp. 1442–1457

Yamamoto T (2005) Factors affecting recurrence after surgery for Crohn's disease. World J Gastroenterol 11:3971–3979

4
Acute Colonic Pseudo-Obstruction

Raul Martin Bosio and Anthony J. Senagore

Pearls and Pitfalls

- Colonic pseudo-obstruction refers to a clinical syndrome of colonic dilation in the absence of a mechanical obstruction; the presentation may mimic an acute large bowel obstruction.
- Pseudo-obstruction occurs primarily in hospitalized patients, with an incidence as high often >20% after selected surgical procedures or trauma.
- The pathogenesis of this syndrome is not fully elucidated; however, an imbalance in the autonomic regulation of the colon has been suggested.
- Physical findings include a distended, tympanitic abdomen with present but diminished bowel sounds.
- When combined with clinical examination, abdominal x-rays are usually diagnostic or highly suspicious.
- Colon ischemia and subsequent perforation, which occurs in 3–15% of patients, is the most important complication and has a mortality of about 50%.
- The radiographic findings are of marked distention of the proximal colon with the descending and sigmoid colon of normal caliber.
- A water-soluble contrast enema or colonoscopy should be performed to exclude mechanical causes.
- Initial management includes nasogastric tube decompression, replacement of fluid and electrolyte imbalances, and

K.I. Bland et al. (eds.), *Colorectal Surgery*,
DOI 10.1007/978-1-84996-444-9_4,

serial abdominal films; more than 85% of patients recover with conservative management.

- Persistence of symptoms for more than 48 h or a cecal diameter > 12 cm requires intervention, which may include use of neostigmine, colonoscopic decompression, or, rarely, operative intervention. A cecal diameter exceeding 12 cm is associated with an increased risk of ischemia/perforation.
- The use of neostigmine has been associated with a success rate of 90%, leading several groups to advocate its use early in the treatment plan; however, a sustained response is maintained in only 70% of responders.
- Colonoscopic decompression is another effective option, with a primary success rate of about 73–83%; a 4% morbidity has been reported after colonoscopic decompression.
- Colonic resection as opposed to tube cecostomy is indicated after failure of conservative treatment or when clinical findings raise concern of ischemia.

Introduction

First described in 1948 by Sir H. Ogilvie, colonic pseudo-obstruction refers to a clinical situation that resembles an acute large bowel obstruction, with a dilated proximal colon on abdominal films, but in the absence of a mechanical obstruction. Approximately 60% of patients diagnosed with colonic pseudo-obstruction are critically ill in the setting of major trauma or after major surgical procedures. Colonic pseudo-obstruction can also occur in bedridden patients or those on high dose narcotics. The patients are predominantly males in their sixth or seventh decade of life. Both intraperitoneal and extraperitoneal operative procedures have been associated with the development of this syndrome, with urologic, orthopedic (hip, knee, and spinal surgery) and gynecologic procedures (Caesarean section) among the most frequent. As a common feature, in about half of the patients in a postoperative setting, the spine or the retroperitoneum has been traumatized or manipulated. Among 400 non-surgical patients, a retrospective review identified non-operative trauma (11%), systemic infections (10%), and cardiac failure (myocardial infarction, congestive heart failure) (10%) as the most common medical conditions associated with this syndrome. Among a variety of signs and symptoms, the most prominent clinical feature is marked abdominal distention due to massive colonic dilation. Although the pathogenesis of acute colonic pseudo-obstruction is not fully elucidated, autonomic dysregulation of the colon has been implicated (see below). Spontaneous resolution occurs in about 85% of the patients managed by supportive measures; however, patients need to be monitored closely because spontaneous cecal perforation occurs in 15%, with associated mortality of 50%.

Pathophysiology

An imbalance in autonomic regulation of the colon, resulting in dysmotility, has been suggested in the pathogenesis of this syndrome. The parasympathetic nervous system stimulates colonic motility, whereas sympathetic nerves targeting either the myenteric plexus or the smooth muscle inhibit contraction. Vagal innervation of the colon extends up to the splenic flexure, with the distal segments of the colon receiving parasympathetic supply via lumbar nerves from spinal segments S2–S4 (sacral parasympathetic nerves). A transient decrease in the parasympathetic drive, combined with an increased sympathetic input to the colon, has been proposed as the mechanism of this syndrome. Abdominal films usually demonstrate a markedly dilated ascending and transverse colon with the distal colon being of normal caliber. Based on colonic innervation and these radiographic findings, a disruption of parasympathetic input, possibly combined with increased sympathetic inhibitory input to the colon, may be responsible for this functional obstruction. While most investigators believe this disorder to be a dysmotility of the proximal colon, some groups believe that this syndrome represents a disorder of the distal colon with an inhibitory reflex to the proximal colon. In either case, the drugs (i.e., neostigmine, pyridostigmine) that increase parasympathetic activity may produce prompt colonic decompression in patients with acute colonic pseudo-obstruction.

Diagnosis

Prominent abdominal distension is the most characteristic clinical feature of this syndrome. Nausea, vomiting, low-grade fever, and abdominal discomfort or pain may be present. Increasing abdominal pain should be evaluated carefully, because it may imply bowel ischemia or perforation. Physical examination reveals a markedly distended, tympanitic abdomen with mild diffuse tenderness. The presence of bowel sounds and the passage of small amounts of flatus and stool do not exclude the diagnosis. The presence of peritoneal signs usually correlates with ischemia or bowel perforation, requires urgent operative intervention, and is associated with a high mortality.

Abdominal x-rays demonstrate a distended large bowel affecting the ascending colon and, to a variable degree, transverse colon up to the splenic flexure (Fig. 4.1a). A water-soluble contrast enema is usually essential in confirming the diagnosis and excluding a mechanical obstruction. This study

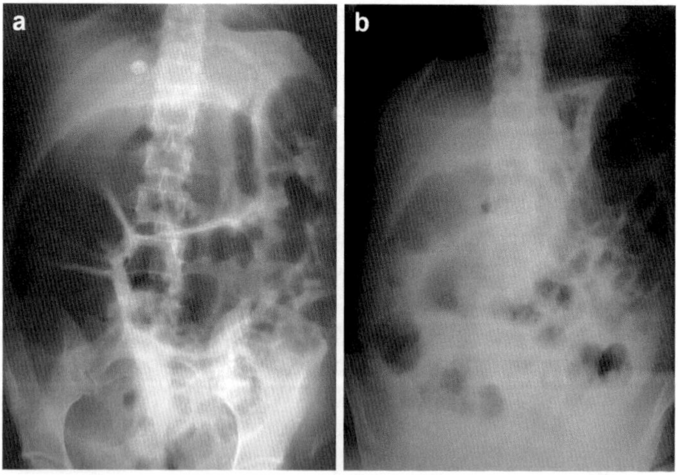

FIGURE 4.1. **a.** Abdominal radiograph showing a distended ascending and transverse colon in a patient with acute colonic pseudo-obstruction. **b.** Abdominal films post treatment with neostigmine.

may induce colonic decompression and contribute to the treatment of the syndrome. If there is concern for ischemia or perforation, the study is contraindicated. Once the diagnosis has been established, plain abdominal films should be obtained every 12 h to monitor colonic diameter closely. A cecal diameter of ≥12 cm or a transverse colon diameter of ≥9 cm are associated with an increased risk of ischemia and may indicate the necessity of more active treatment.

Treatment

As with many medical conditions, early diagnosis and treatment is of great importance in acute colonic pseudo-obstruction. A fivefold increase in the risk of mortality has been reported with prolonged colonic distention (more than 6 days), secondary to ischemia and subsequent bowel perforation. Treatment includes supportive measures, pharmacologic treatment, endoscopic or percutaneous procedures, and operative exploration (Fig. 4.2). Recently, a prospective, randomized, placebo-controlled trial demonstrated that administration of polyethylene glycol upon resolution of symptoms after either neostigmine or endoscopic decompression may decrease the risk of recurrence of this syndrome.

Initial management: Supportive measures refer to placement of a nasogastric tube, suspension of oral intake, discontinuation of medications that may adversely affect gastrointestinal motility, such as opiates and anticholinergics when possible, correction of fluid and electrolyte disorders, and patient mobilization. The efficacy of a rectal tube is questionable, because a rectal tube does not reach the distended segments of the colon. Resolution of acute colonic pseudo-obstruction with the above conservative measures would be expected in about 85% of patients.

Pharmacologic treatment: Persistent or progressive colonic distention after 48–72 h of treatment or a cecal diameter >12 cm usually necessitates a more active approach. Pharmacologic and endoscopic procedures constitute valid treatment options.

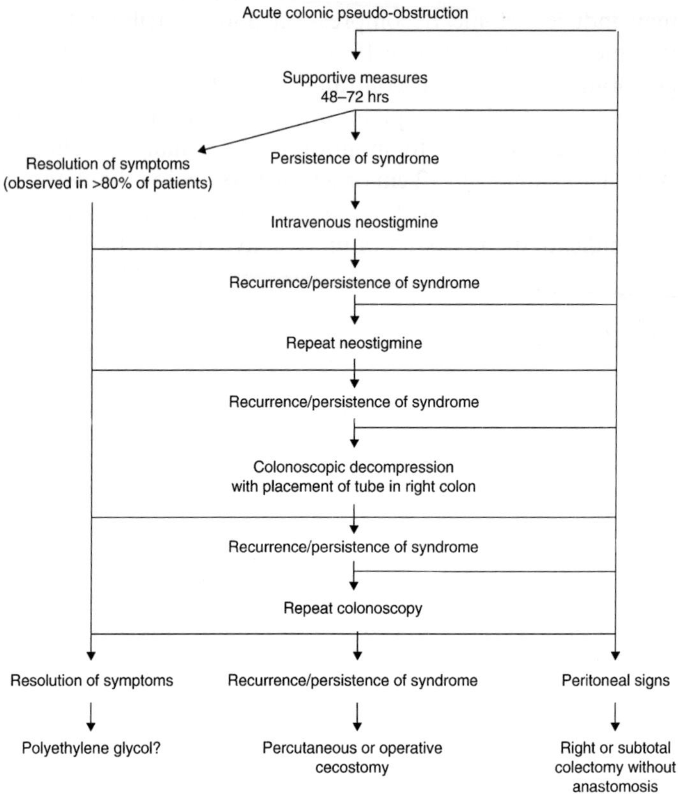

FIGURE 4.2. Suggested treatment algorithm for acute colonic pseudo-obstruction.

Similar success rates with reduced morbidity makes pharmacologic treatment superior to colonoscopic decompression as a second step after failure of conservative management.

Many drugs for the treatment of this syndrome (i.e., erythromycin, cisapride, and metoclopramide, among others), targeting motilin or 5-HT4 receptors among others, have been studied in clinical trials. Most of these reports, however, included only small numbers of patients and failed to show consistent results. More than 30 years ago, Catchpole proposed the combination of a sympathetic blocker (guanethidine) and a parasympathomimetic agent (neostigmine) as a treatment for gastrointestinal motility disorders secondary to autonomic dysfunction. This concept was later applied to acute colonic pseudo-obstruction. Although no clinical improvement was observed after guanethidine, colonic decompression was reported after administration of neostigmine. The first randomized, double-blind, placebo-controlled trial for patients who had not responded to conservative measures with a cecal diameter > 11 cm was published in 1994. Clinical and radiologic response occurred in 91% of patients who received neostigmine, compared with no objective improvement in the placebo group. Cross-over of seven patients from the placebo group to treatment with neostigmine demonstrated success in all but one of these patients.

The rationale behind the use of neostigmine is that it inhibits acetylcholinesterase, an enzyme that hydrolyzes acetylcholine at the neuromuscular junctions. Neostigmine, a reversible competitive inhibitor of acetylcholinesterase, binds to the active site of the enzyme, blocking access to the neurotransmitter and causing a relative increase in acetylcholine, thereby enhancing cholinergic transmission and smooth muscle contraction. Various reversible acetylcholinesterase inhibitors with a short half-life are available, including neostigmine, pyridostigmine, and physostigmine, which can be administered intravenous, orally, and subcutaneously. Most published data, however, support the use of intravenous neostigmine. Oral pyridostigmine has been used in chronic syndromes such us myasthenia gravis. However, erratic absorption and variable bioavailability may occur with oral administration in patients with acute colonic pseudo-obstruction where prolonged fasting and superimposed partial small bowel ileus may negatively affect absorption. Physostigmine crosses the blood-brain barrier and affects the central nervous system, and therefore, is usually not considered in the treatment of this syndrome.

Neostigmine is usually administered in a 2.5 mg dose intravenously over a period of 1–3 min or as an infusion over a period of 30–60 min; the latter is associated with a lower risk of bradycardia. Patients should be under cardiac monitoring for a period of 30–60 min after injection with atropine available for brachycardia. Mechanical obstruction of the colon must be ruled out before initiation of treatment. Side-effects associated with the use of this drug include bradycardia, salivation, sweating, restlessness, nausea, abdominal pain, hypotension, and bronchoconstriction. Relative contraindications to its use involve heart rate < 60 beats/min, systolic blood pressure < 90 mmHg, use of beta-blockers, severe bronchospasm, or known hypersensitivity to this drug, recent myocardial infarction, acidosis, or a serum creatinine > 3 mg/dl due to the renal excretion of the drug.

Colonic decompression is observed usually within minutes after neostigmine administration; evacuation of flatus and stool occurs in about 90% of patients within 30 min (Fig. 4.1b). A sustained response, however, generally drops to 61–80%. In one study, six patients who recurred and the three nonresponders received a second dose of neostigmine. Five out of the six patients that recurred had a sustained response, with no clinical improvement among the other three patients.

Endoscopic treatment: Colonoscopic decompression is usually the next step after failure of neostigmine or when the use of neostigmine is contraindicated or associated with severe side-effects. The presence of peritoneal signs or pneumoperitoneum is obviously a contraindication to its use. Colonoscopy is usually challenging and should be performed with extreme caution by experienced colonoscopists.

Sedation and analgesia is generally administered, although use of opiates should be minimized. Dual channel colonoscopes or colonoscopes with accessory channels of large diameter may contribute to suctioning of gas and stool; air insufflation should be kept to a minimum. The mucosal appearance and viability should be evaluated to determine the presence of ischemia or indirect signs of necrosis, such as a dusky mucosa. These findings generally indicate the need to terminate the procedure and proceed to operative intervention.

Complete colonoscopy, though preferable because it allows assessment of cecal mucosa, is not always necessary, provided right colon decompression is successful at the end of the procedure. Strong consideration should be given to leaving a large bore transanal decompression tube in the proximal colon. Geller et al. reported an overall success rate of 88% after colonic decompression, but found that sustained decompression was maintained in only 25% of patients in whom a decompression tube was not placed. Using a guide wire and, if possible, under fluoroscopy control minimizes loop formation and confirms that the tube has reached the right colon. The tube is usually left in place for 72 h, and should drain by gravity, but needs to be flushed every 6–8 h to prevent clogging.

In a review analyzing outcomes of endoscopic decompression in 292 patients, a 69% rate of initial decompression, including patients with and without decompression tube insertion, was observed. Recurrence was about 25%, but was greater when a decompression tube was not left in the right colon. Overall success rate, including patients who required more than one colonoscopy, varied between 73% and 88%. Morbidity after endoscopic treatment, primarily colonic perforation, has been observed in about 5% of patients.

Operative treatment: Operative intervention is indicated after failure of the above-mentioned treatments or in patients with peritoneal signs or free air. Intraoperative options include creation of a cecostomy in the absence of perforation or a right or a subtotal colectomy when there are findings of ischemia or colonic perforation. Cecostomy can be accomplished percutaneously under fluoroscopic control, as a combined endoscopic-radiologic procedure, by laparotomy (even under local anesthesia), or by laparoscopy. Percutaneous cecostomy may avoid the risk associated with a laparotomy or laparoscopic procedure. Mortality secondary to leakage and abdominal wall cellulitis has been reported after this procedure and needs to be considered; therefore, most surgeons have abandoned cecostomy as definitive therapy in most patients and especially those with ischemia. Diverting ileostomies or transverse colostomies do not always resolve colonic distention and should not be considered as viable options. Colonic resection with end ileostomy and either closure of the distal colon or mucous fistula formation should be considered the gold standard. No matter what operative procedure is used, the operative mortality is about 50%.

In summary, colonic pseudo-obstruction can masquerade as an acute large bowel obstruction, but occurs in the absence of a mechanical obstruction. The etiology appears to be a dysmotility related to an imbalance in the autonomic regulation of colonic motility. A markedly distended abdomen, secondary to massive colonic distension, constitutes the most prominent clinical feature. Abdominal x-rays contribute to the diagnosis and will show a markedly distended proximal colon. Initial supportive therapy leads to resolution in about 85% of patients. Neostigmine and colonoscopic decompression constitute treatment options after failure of supportive measures. Operative treatment is indicated after failure of pharmacologic and endoscopic procedures or when clinical findings raise concern of ischemia or colonic perforation, but has an associated mortality of 50%. The operative procedure usually involves a proximal colectomy, but a tube cecostomy may be utilized in select patients.

Selected Readings

Chevallier P, Marcy PY, Francois E, et al. (2002) Controlled transperitoneal percutaneous cecostomy as a therapeutic alternative to the endoscopic decompression for Ogilvie's syndrome. Am J Gastroenterol 97:471–474

De Giorgio R, Barbara G, Stanghellini V, et al. (2001) Review article: the pharmacological treatment of acute colonic pseudo-obstruction. Aliment Pharmacol Ther 15:1717–1727

Eisen GM, Baron TH, Dominitz JA, et al. (2002) Acute colonic pseudo-obstruction. Gastrointest Endosc 56:789–792

Mehta R, John A, Nair P, et al. (2006) Factors predicting successful outcome following neostigmine therapy in acute colonic pseudo-obstruction: a prospective study. J Gastroenterol Hepatol 21:459–461

Ponec RJ, Saunders MD, Kimmey MB (1999) Neostigmine for the treatment of acute colonic pseudo-obstruction. N Engl J Med 341:137–141

Saunders MD, Cappell MS (2005) Endoscopic management of acute colonic pseudo-obstruction. Endoscopy 37:760–763

Saunders MD, Kimmey MB (2005) Systematic review: acute colonic pseudo-obstruction. Aliment Pharmacol Ther 22:917–925

Sgouros SN, Vlachogiannakos J, Vassiliadis K, et al. (2006) Effect of polyethylene glycol electrolyte balanced solution on patients with acute colonic pseudo obstruction after resolution of colonic dilation: a prospective, randomised, placebo controlled trial. Gut 55:638–642

Tenofsky PL, Beamer L, Smith RS (2000) Ogilvie syndrome as a postoperative complication. Arch Surg 135:682–686; discussion 686–687

5 Surgical Therapy of Constipation

Joe J. Tjandra and Henry Yeh

Pearls and Pitfalls

- The definition of constipation includes fewer than three bowel movements per week, straining at defecation, and/or hard pellet-like stools.
- Constipation includes a constellation of symptoms influenced by local culture, geography, socioeconomic background, and the patient's personality.
- Coexistence of weight loss and rectal bleeding suggests colorectal cancer.
- Diagnosis should attempt to differentiate an extra-colonic or systemic cause from a mechanical or functional colonic cause.
- The key to treatment is appropriate diagnosis.
- Mechanical causes include diverticular stricture, colonic neoplasm, occult rectal prolapse, and rectocele.
- Functional causes include slow transit constipation, irritable bowel disease, psychologic disorders, and pelvic floor dysfunction.
- Diagnosis may involve combinations of colonoscopy, scintigraphic transit studies, anorectal physiologic testing, and defecating proctography.
- Medical therapy for simple constipation involves a high liquid intake and increased dietary fiber.

K.I. Bland et al. (eds.), *Colorectal Surgery*,
DOI 10.1007/978-1-84996-444-9_5,

- Pelvic floor dysfunction is best managed by biofeedback therapy with a regular, structured program that includes a planned process of re-learning.
- Operative therapy can be effective in patients with slow transit constipation (total abdominal colectomy/ileorectostomy) and rectocele (transvaginal or transanal).

Constipation

Constipation is a symptom or a constellation of symptoms influenced by a myriad of factors. These etiologies are as varied as culture, geographic, and socio-economic background, as well as the personality of the individual. A full dietary history and appraisal of the symptoms is important. If the symptoms are of new onset and in the presence of other associated abdominal symptoms, especially weight loss and rectal bleeding, then appropriate investigations should be instituted to exclude a colorectal cancer, diverticular disease and other less common conditions (Table 5.1).

Due to the wide variation in the interpretation of constipation, it is defined commonly as passing fewer than three bowel movements per week, inordinate straining during defecation, incomplete evacuation more than 25% of the time, or hard pellet-like stools more than 25% of the time, with the symptoms lasting more than 12 months. Constipation is common, with a prevalence of 10% in Western societies. Most patients seek help from pharmacists, general practitioners, and naturopaths, while only about 5% are ever referred to gastrointestinal specialists.

The key in management is to identify the underlying etiology of constipation, which can be quite complex. It is important to exclude mechanical bowel obstruction due to a neoplasm or stricture (Table 5.1), which would mandate operative intervention. The focus of this chapter is on functional disorders of the bowel and pelvic floor, which can affect the lifestyle of the affected individuals severely. A systematic workup is extremely important. The first order of evaluation is to differentiate between an extracolonic or systemic cause from a colonic or

TABLE 5.1. Causes of constipation (Adapted from Seow-Choen and Tjandra, 2001).

Mechanical colonic causes
Neoplastic
Benign stricture (ischemic or anastomotic)
Colonic volvulus
Diverticular disease (stricture)
Dietary
Poor fiber intake
Inadequate fluid intake
Medications
Neuropsychiatric medications, e.g. anticonvulsants, anti- Parkinsonian drugs, antidepressants, antipsychotics
Narcotics and opiates
Calcium channel blockers
Antacids
Barium sulfate
Iron tablets
Functional
Irritable bowel syndrome
Psychologic disorders
Slow transit constipation
Ogilvie's syndrome
Anorectal/pelvic disorders
Mucosal prolapse syndrome
Paradoxic puborectalis contraction (anismus)
Rectocele

(continued)

TABLE 5.1. (continued)

Metabolic and endocrine
Diabetes mellitus
Hypercalcemia
Hyperparathyroidism
Hypokalemia
Hypopituitarism
Hypothyroidism
Scleroderma
Neurogenic
Peripheral
Hirschsprung's disease
Autonomic neuropathy
Chagas' disease
Spinal
Cauda equina tumor
Multiple sclerosis
Paraplegia
Central
Cerebrovascular accidents
Parkinson's disease
Cerebral neoplasms

intestinal cause, and then to differentiate between a mechanical colonic cause and a functional bowel disorder, and finally, to assess the relative role of slow gastrointestinal transit, pelvic floor dysfunction and irritable bowel syndrome. A full anorectal examination is mandatory in most patients. A colonoscopy is generally indicated in patients over the age of 40–45 with clinically significant symptoms.

Diagnosis

The diagnosis of constipation should be established. The severity of the symptoms would dictate the extent of investigations. Past treatment(s) should be documented, and may provide insight into the severity of the disorder. Documenting the nature of constipation might also help determine the underlying pathogenesis (Table 5.1). Difficult evacuation requiring digital evacuation of stool would suggest pelvic floor disorder, while a chronic history of abdominal bloating and/or infrequent bowel movement would suggest a delayed intestinal transit. In contrast, a short history of changes in bowel pattern, especially if accompanied by rectal bleeding, a family history of colorectal neoplasm, and/or weight loss, would suggest a more sinister cause, such as a colorectal neoplasm. A mechanical cause such as a neoplasm usually produces a change in bowel habit rather than chronic constipation. With severe symptoms, special investigations are required (see below).

A full physical examination may determine whether a more systemic cause of constipation exists (Table 5.1). Abdominal examination might identify abnormal masses. Anorectal examination would determine whether there is a rectocele present, mucosal rectal prolapse, megarectum, or inappropriate pelvic floor contraction or excessive perineal descent on straining. Proctoscopy will help identify a rectal neoplasm, occult rectal prolapse on straining, or presence of solitary rectal ulcer syndrome.

Pelvic floor disorders such as a rectocele may be corrected by biofeedback therapy, and occasionally, by operative intervention. Abdominal surgery such as a colectomy for slow colonic transit is rarely indicated. Most patients will respond to dietary changes that include an increased intake of liquid and fiber. Simple bulk-forming laxatives might suffice (Table 5.2). For patients persistently troubled by constipation, further investigations are indicated as below.

TABLE 5.2. Common laxatives.

Bulking agents
Bran
Methylcellulose
Lubricants
Liquid paraffin
Osmotics
Lactulose
Magnesium citrate
Epsom salts
Sodium phosphate
Picosulfate
Stimulants
Herbal laxatives
Senna
Biscodyl
Castor oil
Rectal preparations
Enemas
Suppositories

Intestinal Versus Extra-Intestinal or Systemic Cause

Most extra-intestinal or systemic causes (Table 5.1) can be excluded by a careful medical history, review of medications used or tried in the past, and physical examination. Systemic causes such as hypothyroidism or Parkinson's disease should be entertained and can be identified readily. In some patients, despite the presence of or correction of extra-intestinal causes, the constipation may be so severe that its presence mandates further gastrointestinal investigations.

Intestinal Causes: Mechanical Versus Functional

The diagnosis of a functional cause of constipation is made only after exclusion of mechanical causes (Table 5.1). It is most important to exclude a colorectal neoplasm by a detailed history and physical examination, anorectal examination, proctoscopy, and, if indicated, colonoscopy. Recurrent diverticulitis might suggest a diverticular stricture. Double contrast barium enema (Fig. 5.2), combined with a sigmoidoscopy, might be an alternative to a colonoscopy and provides a good image of the topography of the colon and its redundancy. In addition, this contrast radiograph technique provides better definition of diverticular disease than a colonoscopy. A pelvic floor dysfunction can be recognized by digital rectal and perineal examination. Occult rectal prolapse, solitary rectal ulcer syndrome, and rectocele all suggest pelvic floor dysfunction, which might occur in isolation or in conjunction with gastrointestinal dysmotility. Symptomatic rectocele presents as a bulge into the vagina during defecation, and the patient often needs to digitate to help with fecal evacuation.

Treatments of various mechanical colonic disorders are covered in other chapters.

Functional Bowel Disorder

When a mechanical cause of constipation has been excluded, a functional bowel disorder is likely responsible for the chronic constipation.

A gastrointestinal transit study will help delineate the "motility" and emptying of the stomach, small bowel, and colon. The transit studies can be performed by radio-opaque

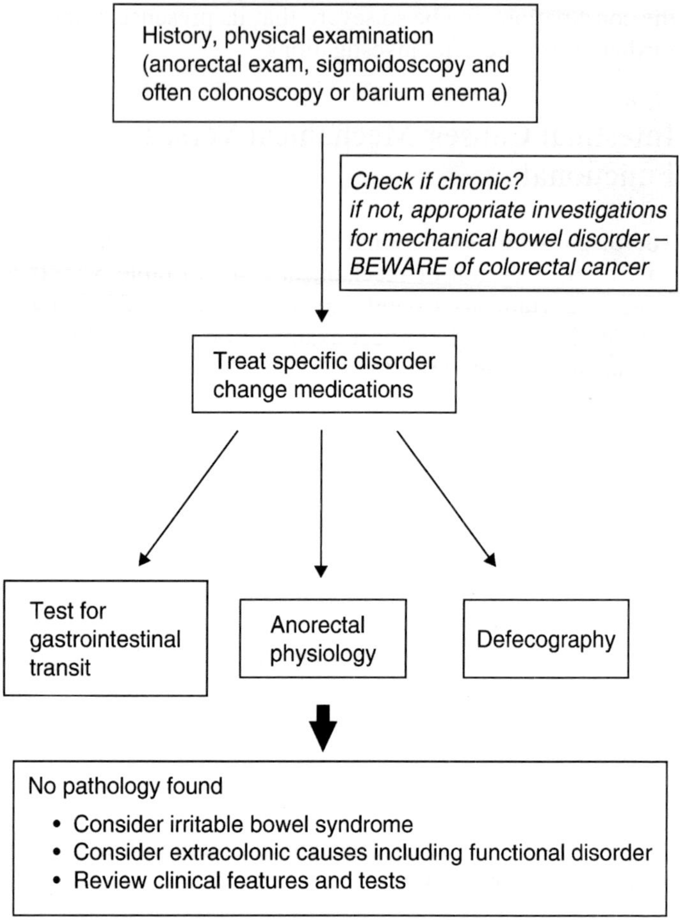

FIGURE 5.1. Overall approach to the patient with constipation.

markers or by scintigraphy. Marker studies evaluate primarily colonic transit and involve ingestion of 20 markers followed by serial plain radiographs of the abdomen. The test takes 7 days to complete or less if the markers are fully eliminated before 7 days. A transit time of greater than 72 h is considered to be "delayed transit," compared with a mean transit time of 36 h in normal subjects.

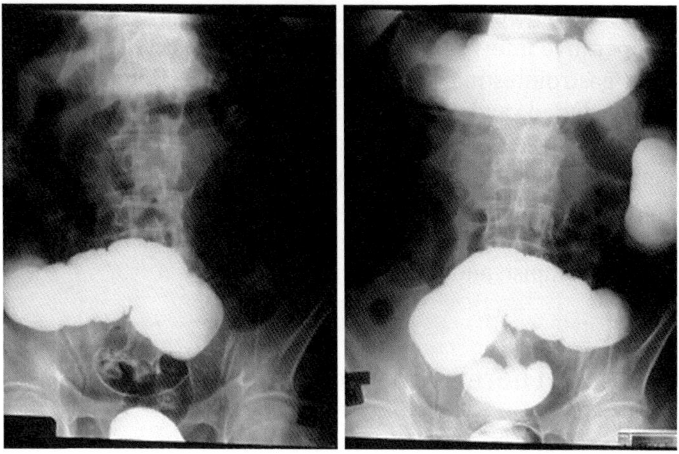

FIGURE 5.2. Barium enema showing a stenosing cancer in rectosigmoid junction of the colon.

Scintigraphic transit studies require the ingestion of a meal mixed with technetium-99m and indium-111 in a delayed-release capsule. The capsules containing technetium-99m are used to assess gastric and small bowel transit, while the cap- [illegible] ium-111, which dissolve in the ileocolic [illegible] [illegible] assess colonic transit.

Pelvic floor function is best evaluated using anorectal physiologic testing. Resting and squeeze anal canal pressures are measured, as well as the rectal compliance and the balloon expulsion test. Surface electromyography will help determine if there is anismus or paradoxic function of pelvic floor. These tests together, rather than individually, provide a global assessment of whether there is any pelvic floor disorder. If identified, pelvic floor biofeedback therapy can be helpful. Absence of a recto-anal inhibitory reflex could suggest the rare adult presentation of Hirschsprung's disease. A definitive diagnosis requires a full-thickness rectal biopsy from the posterior anorectal junction.

Defecating proctography may allow the identification of pelvic floor disorders, such as occult rectal intussusception, rectoceles, and enteroceles. These disorders may respond well to operative intervention in appropriately selected situations.

If gastrointestinal dysmotility and pelvic floor disorders are excluded, and there has been no mechanical cause or systemic cause to the constipation, some patients have constipation related to irritable bowel syndrome or other psychosomatic syndromes. Multi-disciplinary management should then involve a gastroenterologist, psychologist, dietician, physiotherapist, and social worker (Fig. 5.1).

Medical Therapy for Constipation

The vast majority of patients with constipation have "simple" constipation, which can be identified with a careful history and physical examination. Dietary manipulation, a high liquid intake, and physical activity are the backbone of management of chronic constipation. Increased dietary fiber, up to 20 g/day, is helpful. Prudent use of laxatives (Table 5.2) such as oral sodium phosphate might improve the quality of life, but the use of oral or transanal laxatives should be monitored closely.

Slow Transit Constipation

About 10% of patients with severe constipation who present to our specialized center have slow transit constipation; it should be acknowledged, however, that this is a referral practice of highly screened patients. In such patients, excess dietary fiber actually accentuates the bloating and abdominal discomfort. A multi-disciplinary approach, as indicated earlier, is adopted. These patients have often used most laxatives by the time they present to a specialized center. A coordinated prescription of osmotic laxative (lactulose, magnesium citrate) and sodium phosphate enema may be helpful. Due to the chronicity of the problem, stimulant laxatives, such as senna or bisacodyl, are less favored. Newer 5-HT uptake inhibitors have shown some success. These patients often have severe constipation that substantially affects their lifestyle. Ultimately, many patients need a more vigorous laxative such as polyethylene glycol, oral sodium phosphate, or pico sulphate preparation. Even these vigorous laxative tend to become less effective with time, and many patients require repeated hospital admissions for relief of pain and fecal impaction. Finally, operative intervention is considered as an alternative.

Pelvic Floor Disorders

Pelvic floor retraining involves biofeedback but requires a strong commitment of the patient. A multidisciplinary approach, involving physiotherapist, dietician, surgeon, gastroenterologist, and psychologist, is likely to be the most effective therapy. Pelvic floor biofeedback therapy enhances the appropriate pelvic floor function with pushing and fecal evacuation. The duration of pelvic floor training varies, but a regular structured program with a process of planned, repeated relearning is best.

Surgical Therapy for Functional Bowel Disorder

Slow Colonic Transit Constipation

A highly selected group of patients with slow colonic transit will benefit from abdominal colectomy and ileorectal anastomosis. In one series, patients were evaluated extensively with a firm diagnosis of slow transit constipation and good results were obtained. Of 74 patients who underwent operation, 97% were satisfied with the results of colectomy, and all patients were able to pass a stool spontaneously. The morbidity includes the future possibility of small bowel obstruction (9%) and a prolonged ileus (12%). In patients with combined slow colonic transit and pelvic floor dysfunction, pelvic floor retraining should precede operative intervention. Preoperative bowel preparation is often more complex, requiring a protracted bowel cleansing, often with a 48 h liquid.

The operation of choice is a total abdominal colectomy, removing the colon from the terminal ileum to the rectosigmoid junction and constructing an ileorectal anastomosis. This procedure can now be performed laparoscopically. A less extensive procedure, such as a segmental colectomy or less extensive colectomy with an ileosigmoid anastomosis, produces much inferior functional results and should be avoided. It is essential that the anastomosis is to the rectum itself. Prior to definitive colectomy, it is sometimes helpful, as a bridge, to provide a diverting ileostomy for 6 months or so, to ensure that there is a good response when the colon is bypassed. Presence of a concomitant disorder of slow small bowel transit or gastroparesis is an absolute contraindication to abdominal colectomy with ileorectostomy.

In the early postoperative period, the stools are loose and may be frequent, though incontinence is rare. More than 90% of patients have semisolid stools by 4 months, and approximately 30% of patients use some form of antidiarrheal medications to control stool frequency in the first 6 months after operation. With time, the stool tends to become more solid and the frequency of bowel movements decreases.

Rectocele

Rectocele, defined as herniation of the anterior rectal and posterior vaginal wall into the vaginal lumen, can be treated by operative repair. While a rectocele can be asymptomatic, it may also contribute substantially to obstructed defecation and is often associated with mucosal rectal prolapse. Various operative techniques using transvaginal, transanal, transperineal, or transabdominal approaches with or without prosthetic mesh have been described to repair the rectocele. The operative results are variable between studies due to variability in patient selection and operative techniques. Repair of rectocele is performed commonly by the gynecologist via the vaginal route, especially if there is a significant enterocele.

Transanal repair of rectocele is equally effective for smaller rectocele, and especially when there is associated mucosal-rectal prolapse. Transanal resection of the rectal wall, the STARR procedure (stapled trans-anal rectal resection), is currently under study as the operative procedure to treat obstructed defecation syndrome, which is commonly associated with mucosal rectal prolapse and rectocele. With meticulous protection of the posterior wall of the vagina, an approximately 5 × 7cm rectal mucosal flap is resected using the circular stapler. In principle, the rectovaginal septum is strengthened, and the redundant rectal mucosal tissue is resected.

Hirschsprung's Disease

Adult presentation of Hirschsprung's disease is quite rare and usually involves short-segment disease. Ultrashort segment disease in an adult will respond to anorectal strip myectomy where a posterior strip of anal sphincter is resected, which also allows for a histologic diagnosis.

Sacral Nerve Stimulation

Sacral nerve stimulation has been used to treat fecal incontinence since 1995. The same technique suggests that it might help to modulate the sensory responses in the rectum and pelvic floor, and thereby, help with fecal evacuation. There are two active trials, in Melbourne and in Europe, to evaluate this approach. Results are encouraging, but investigators await Level 1 evidence of efficacy.

Selected Readings

Fazio VW, Tjandra JJ, Church JM, et al. (1992) Clinical conundrum of solitary rectal ulcer. Dis Colon Rectum 35:227–234

Nyam D, Pemberton J, Ilstrup D, Rath D (1997) Long-term results of surgery for chronic constipation. Dis Colon Rectum 40:273–279

Ommer A, Albrecht K, Wenger F, Walz MK (2006) Stapled transanal rectal resection: a new option in the treatment of obstructive defecation syndrome. Langenbecks Arch Surg 391:32–37

Seow-Choen F, Tjandra JJ (2001) Chronic constipation. In: Tjandra JJ, Clunie GA, Thomas RJS (eds) Textbook of surgery, 2nd edn. Blackwell, Oxford, pp 628–632

Tjandra JJ, Fazio VW, Petras RE (1993) Clinical and pathological factors associated with delayed diagnosis in solitary rectal ulcer syndrome. Dis Colon Rectum 36:146–153

Tjandra JJ, Ooi BS, Tang CL, et al. (1999) Transanal repair of rectocele corrects obstructed defecation if it is not associated with anismus. Dis Colon Rectum 42:1544–1550

6 Diverticulitis

Daniel L. Feingold and Richard L. Whelan

Pearls and Pitfalls

- The proximal margin of resection is determined by visualizing and palpating healthy descending colon.
- The distal margin of resection is the most proximal healthy rectum such that a true colorectal anastomosis is performed.
- During sigmoid resection, the left ureter is in jeopardy and must be identified accurately and preserved.
- Minimal access surgery offers substantial benefits over traditional open surgery in the setting of diverticulitis.
- In cases where a mucosal-based neoplasm has not been ruled out, a cancer-type operation should be performed.
- Three-stage operations (drainage, resection, reconstruction) are of historic interest only and should be avoided.
- Laparoscopic-assisted operations for complicated "benign" diverticular disease can be more challenging than resections for malignant disease.
- In the vast majority of cases, full mobilization of the splenic flexure is necessary if a full sigmoid resection is to be carried out.
- When presented with an acutely inflamed sigmoid colon or in the presence of a phlegmon or severe fibrotic reaction, initiate the mobilization in an uninvolved area, identify the critical structures and then work towards the disease.

K.I. Bland et al. (eds.), *Colorectal Surgery*,
DOI 10.1007/978-1-84996-444-9_6,

- Consider ureteral stenting when operating on a patient with a phlegmon, severe fibrotic reaction, or colovesical fistula.
- When performing laparoscopic-assisted resection, if the inflammatory phlegmon is large or if the pelvic dissection proves very difficult, use of a hand-assist technique is advised.

Diverticulitis is an inflammatory process that will eventually affect 10–25% of patients with diverticulosis of the colon. Most likely due to the distribution of acquired diverticula in patients in the Western world, the vast majority of episodes of diverticulitis occur in the sigmoid colon. In contrast, in Africa and Asia where the incidence of diverticula in the left colon is much less common, the distribution of diverticular disease favors the right colon. Not only has the incidence of sigmoid diverticulitis increased over the past century, due to the age-related nature of the disease, the prevalence has increased with the aging population as well.

Pathophysiology, Clinical Presentation, and Evaluation

The pathophysiology of diverticulitis has been described through anatomic and histologic studies demonstrating the formation of false, pulsion diverticula within the colon wall where vasa rectae penetrate the inner, circular muscle layer, resulting in points of structural weakness through which mucosa can herniate. Lack of dietary fiber and the relatively high intraluminal pressure associated with the narrow sigmoid colon are thought to predispose to the formation of diverticula at these points of compromised, structural integrity.

The inflammatory process of diverticulitis is the consequence of microperforation caused by "impacted," inspissated stool within a diverticulum; the range of clinical manifestations and presentations varies considerably. Acute, uncomplicated diverticulitis is characterized by localized inflammation, while complicated diverticulitis includes abscess or phlegmons, gross perforation, and generalized peritonitis. Sub-acute and chronic sequelae of complicated diverticular inflammation include fistula formation and large bowel obstruction due to fibrosis of the diseased sigmoid colon resulting in a stricture.

The clinical presentation of diverticulitis depends on the acuity and severity of the inflammation. The triad of left lower quadrant pain, fever, and leukocytosis is the most common manifestation of acute, uncomplicated disease. The redundancy and course of the sigmoid colon may result in right-sided symptoms, making the diagnosis potentially more difficult. Patients with complicated disease may also have a palpable phlegmon, evidence of large bowel obstruction, symptoms of fistulization, or manifestations of sepsis caused by perforation and peritonitis. The differential diagnosis includes inflammatory bowel disease, ischemic or infectious colitis, colon neoplasia, and a variety of genitourinary and gynecologic processes. Successful initial non-operative treatment allows for a thorough diagnostic workup that, in the majority of patients, can exclude other potential diagnoses.

At presentation, patients are evaluated typically with abdominopelvic computed tomography (CT) utilizing oral and intravenous contrast (Fig. 6.1). Whereas this imaging modality can demonstrate reliably the inflammatory changes of the colon and surrounding tissues suggestive of diverticulitis, the clinician should consider other diagnoses as well that can present with similar findings, because the medical and operative treatment for these alternative diagnoses can be substantially different. CT is most helpful in identifying localized intra-abdominal abscesses and other complicated disease; this finding will enable percutaneous drainage of these collections, thus preventing the need for emergent or urgent operation in the acute setting (which usually requires a colostomy) and allows a more elective, one-stage resection and primary anastomosis in the near future after further evaluation. Once the acute inflammatory process has resolved, colonoscopy can be performed to evaluate the colon to rule out malignancy and confirm the diagnosis. Sigmoidoscopy and colonoscopy are usually contraindicated in the acute

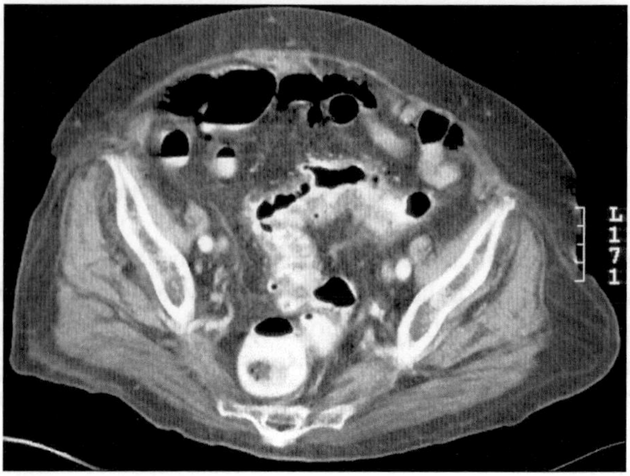

FIGURE 6.1. CT with contrast demonstrating uncomplicated diverticulitis with fat stranding of the mesentery and thickening of the sigmoid colon.

setting, owing to concerns that air insufflation or endoscope insertion may exacerbate the infection. Another complimentary study that may be useful in certain situations is a water-soluble contrast enema. Clearly, care must be taken in the acute setting when instilling the contrast during an enema study.

Treatment

The majority of patients with uncomplicated diverticulitis may be treated on an outpatient basis with oral antibiotics; recurrences can be anticipated in approximately one third of patients. Medical therapy (often referred to by the misnomer "conservative" treatment) utilizes any of a number of single or multi-drug regimens covering gram-negative rods and anaerobic bacteria. Typically, patients with recurrent episodes of uncomplicated inflammation and many patients with exacerbations of chronic complicated disease can be managed medically in anticipation of a planned, elective operation. Of course, acute septic complications (such as free perforation with generalized peritonitis) mandate emergent operation.

According to the most recent consensus statement on the management of diverticulitis by the American Society of Colon and Rectal Surgeons, operative intervention is indicated after two documented episodes of uncomplicated disease or after a single bout of complicated disease. These recommendations are based on thorough review of the data addressing the recurrence, morbidity, and mortality from published series with long-term follow up and take into consideration the purported increasing risks incurred with successive episodes of inflammation and the coincident decreased response rates to non-operative management. Review of the literature, however, demonstrates continuing controversy over operative indications in the setting of diverticulitis and hinges on the considerations of risk of recurrence and failure rates of non-operative, medical management.

The recommendations regarding operative therapy for young patients with diverticulitis are based, for the most part, on anecdotal or limited retrospective reviews and remain controversial. Early reports described a more virulent form of the disease in young patients with substantially increased rates of recurrence and complications; thus, sigmoid resection was advised after resolution of the first episode of uncomplicated diverticulitis. Taking into consideration the more effective, non-operative therapies available currently and the marginal quality of the literature in support of early operate therapy, the treatment algorithm utilized by the authors and most surgical societies no longer discriminates therapeutic decisions based on age at presentation.

Otherwise healthy patients with a clear diagnosis of uncomplicated diverticulitis may be evaluated and treated on an outpatient basis with oral antibiotics and a liquid diet. Those who fail to improve with outpatient therapy, who have a questionable diagnosis, or who have medical comorbidities precluding outpatient treatment require admission. Excluding the minority of patients who present with feculent peritonitis or complete bowel obstruction who require emergent intervention, the management of patients with acute diverticulitis who require hospitalization consists of bowel rest, broad-spectrum intravenous antibiotics, fluid resuscitation, and pain control. The majority of these patients will respond to non-operative care and should undergo further evaluation and treatment in the near future in an elective situation as outlined above. In general, once the decision is made to proceed with elective resection, it may be helpful to consider delaying operation for approximately 6 weeks. Although this practice has not been assessed objectively, proponents believe this waiting period may permit improvement, or even resolution, of the acute inflammatory response and, in addition, allow for nutritional recovery and an easier operation.

Although there has been intense debate about which surgical approach is preferred for diverticulitis, the surgical literature is now replete with studies documenting the feasibility, safety, improved short term outcome, and comparable long-term outcomes of elective, laparoscopic-assisted colectomy when compared with traditional open resection provided the surgeon has mastered techniques requiring advances laparoscopic skills. Thus, presently, minimal-access sigmoid resection with colorectal anastomosis appears to be the operative method of choice in the elective setting. When feasible and practical, it is the preference of the authors to utilize the laparoscopic-assisted method, whereby patients undergo a mobilization, devascularization, and distal bowel transection laparoscopically, followed by specimen extraction and anastomosis via as small an incision as possible.

For obese patients, patients with a bulky specimen, or those in whom the pelvic dissection proves very difficult, a hand-assisted approach is preferred. The rationale for this choice is that in these situations, using standard laparoscopic methods to their fullest, the majority of these patients, in the end, will require an incision 8 cm or larger. The hand-assisted approach facilitates dissection, is easier to teach and learn, and, in the authors' opinion, shortens the operation. Thus, it seems logical to employ a hand-assisted technique once it is clear that an incision as large as your glove size will be needed in the end or if it is evident that completion of the operation via purely laparoscopic means is unlikely.

Operative Techniques

The technical challenges, added degree of difficulty, a need for advanced laparoscopic skills and training associated with minimal-access approaches have limited their use in the general surgical community, thus far, such that the majority of sigmoid colectomies are still accomplished via open technique. Of note, certain fundamental principles regarding colectomy for diverticulitis apply regardless of the operative approach utilized. Pre-operatively, it is advised that patients undergo bowel preparation, per routine, and that an appropriate intravenous antibiotic be administered peri-operatively. Once the abdomen is accessed, the sigmoid colon is mobilized from its lateral and retroperitoneal attachments, and the left ureter is identified and preserved. Confidently visualizing the course of the ureter prior to transecting the mesenteric vascular pedicle is critical to avoid technical misadventure. Intense retroperitoneal inflammation can obscure the ureter and make dissection quite difficult. In this situation, we recommend identifying the ureter in a more cephalad location, away from the inflammation, to establish the plane between the uretogonadal bundle and the mesentery and then to follow the plane into the pelvis. In this fashion, the ureter may be dissected away safely from the disease. In selected patients when a hostile retroperitoneum is anticipated based on review of the clinical history or the preoperative CT, the surgeon should consider strongly the placement of bilateral ureteral stents.

Traditionally, for sigmoid resection, proximal vascular transection is carried out at the level of the main sigmoidal artery after the take-off of the left colic artery from the inferior mesenteric artery (Fig. 6.2). An alternative method calls for mid-mesenteric dissection and transection of the individual sigmoidal branches, thereby preserving the main sigmoidal

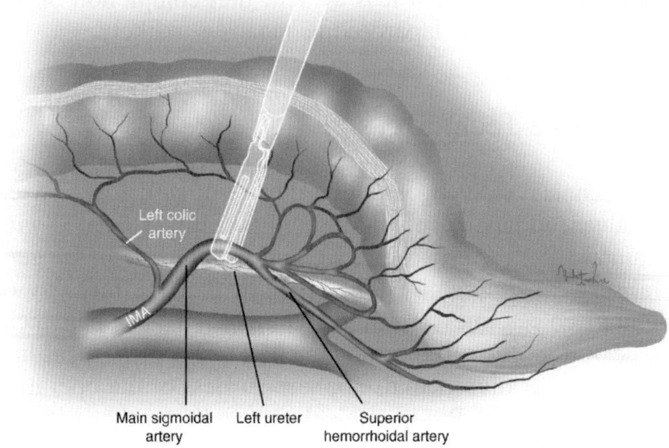

FIGURE 6.2. The anatomy of the inferior mesenteric artery (IMA).

and superior hemorrhoidal arteries. This latter method differs from the conventional approach only with regard to the level of the vascular transection. The colon must still be fully mobilized with the left uretogonadal bundle well visualized and dissected away from the mesentery. This approach is not feasible when the colonic inflammatory process involves the entire mesentery or when the pelvic anatomy is unclear. The purported advantages of a mid-mesenteric transection are that the blood supply to the rectum is preserved, and the hypogastric nerves are protected, because the plane dorsal to the superior hemorrhoidal vessels is not violated. This dissection has not been well studied in an objective manner, but, theoretically, it may decrease colorectal anastomotic leak rates (due to the preserved rectal blood supply), and it may decrease the risk of sexual or bladder dysfunction as compared with conventional dissection.

Mid-mesenteric division can be tedious and is facilitated by using several ancillary devices such as a bipolar diathermy and tissue division device, an ultrasonic scissors, hemostatic clips, and/or a linear stapler. One of the shortcomings of the mid-mesentery transection method is that the rectum is not mobilized posteriorly, because the presacral plane is not dissected. Therefore, there may be a tendency to perform the distal transection of the bowel more proximally than would be the case if the rectum were mobilized partially. Care must be taken to ensure that the entire sigmoid colon is resected and that a true colorectal anastomosis is constructed to avoid leaving any diverticula-bearing sigmoid colon.

Another ramification of avoiding the posterior rectal mobilization is that it can, on occasion, be quite difficult to pass the circular stapler trans-anally up to the proximal limit of the Hartmann pouch because of the curve of the rectum. It is advised that the feasibility of insertion of the circular stapler be assessed by passing trans-anally the metal stapler sizing instruments. There are two options if full insertion of the stapler proves problematic: resect more rectum or carry out a limited posterior mobilization, beginning well caudal to the sacral promontory (so as to avoid the hypogastric nerves).

It is important to recognize that diverticular resection can be very difficult if the inflammatory process or the resulting fibrotic reaction obliterates the usual anatomic planes. Therefore, if minimally invasive methods are being used, conversion may be necessary if the pelvic dissection proves too difficult. In this situation, we recommend strongly that the splenic flexure be mobilized fully and the mesentery divided proximally using laparoscopic methods, if feasible, prior to conversion. If these steps of the operation are performed using minimally invasive methods, then, in almost all situations, the operation can be completed using open methods via a limited, infra-umbilical incision.

Depending on the redundancy of the bowel and the length of colon to be resected, splenic flexure mobilization is performed to allow an adequate tension-free reach of the remaining descending colon to the level of the anastomosis. Adequate resection requires flexure takedown in the vast majority of patients. Once the bowel is mobilized completely and the relevant vasculature addressed, the next step is to determine the appropriate margins of resection. Failing to resect distally to the level of the rectum increases the recurrence rate of diverticulitis considerably, whereas retaining diseased proximal colon jeopardizes anastomotic integrity and may also lead to recurrence. The rectosigmoid junction, described as the confluence of the taenia, usually occurs below the level of the sacral promontory. It is important to appreciate that although the rectum is devoid of diverticula, it may be inflamed secondarily, and the distal margin of resection must be made through healthy rectum as determined by intra-operative inspection and palpation.

Using the laparoscopic-assisted approach, the specimen is delivered via an enlarged port incision, an additional low Pfannenstiel incision, or, in the case of hand-assisted cases, via the hand-port incision. Next, a functional end-to-end circular stapled colorectal anastomosis is carried out using the largest diameter stapler that proves feasible. After tying down the pursestring of the proximal bowel around the stapler anvil, it is important to assess whether any retained diverticula fall directly across the projected path of the circular staple line. If so, the diverticula should be displaced in towards the central rod or outwards, away from the position of the anticipated staple line.

Colovesical fistula: The presence of a colovesical fistula requires specific consideration with regard to the operative plan. Whereas ureteral stents are not required for the vast majority of resections for uncomplicated diverticular disease, these stents are used often for patients with a colovesical fistula, especially if there is evidence on CT of inflammatory changes in the retroperitoneum or at the level of the pelvic inlet. The fistula most often can be taken down bluntly using a finger-fracture type technique, although sharp dissection may be required sometimes to separate the tissues. In the event that a bladder wall defect is identified, it is repaired with absorbable suture; most often, however, no defect is demonstrated. Rarely, if ever, is a partial bladder resection required. To allow the bladder to heal, the urinary catheter is left in place for approximately 5 days and, in those patients in whom bladder repair was carried out, a cystogram is obtained. To reduce the risk of fistula recurrence, it is helpful, when feasible, to interpose healthy tissue between the bladder and the colorectal anastomosis. If a robust greater omentum is available, a pedicle based on the left gastroepiploic artery is mobilized. In the absence of an adequate omentum, if deemed necessary, a rectus sheath flap can be mobilized, preserving the caudal blood supply.

Perforated acute diverticulitis with diffuse peritonitis: While there is general consensus regarding the management of recurrent uncomplicated diverticulitis, associated localized collections, and colovesical fistulas, the optimal management of perforated diverticulitis with diffuse peritonitis still remains somewhat controversial. This controversy is due, in part, to the rarity of the entity (it accounts for 1–2% of patients with acute diverticulitis) and, therefore, a paucity of data. In addition, the morbidity and mortality associated with emergent operative intervention in this setting make it difficult to reach a uniform consensus regarding the most appropriate operation. Hinchey developed a classification of diverticulitis to aid the description of intraoperative findings (Table 6.1).

Through the mid-1970s, the standard operation for Hinchey class 3 or 4 diverticulitis, corresponding to purulent and feculent peritonitis, respectively, was a three-stage approach, with the initial washout of the abdomen and diversion of the fecal stream with a transverse loop colostomy. Subsequently, a second operation for sigmoid resection, performed after the patient recovered, was followed by a third operation for colostomy reversal. The justification for this three-stage approach was to perform as minimal of an operation as possible during

TABLE 6.1. Hinchey classification of complicated acute diverticulitis.

Stage	Characteristics
I	Pericolic or mesenteric abscess
II	Walled-off pelvic abscess
III	Generalized purulent peritonitis
IV	Generalized fecal peritonitis

the acute phase of the illness when patients were often clinically unstable and in critical condition. This three-stage approach has been abandoned due to the unreasonably high complication rates associated with leaving the septic source in place.

Currently, recommended treatment of choice for Hinchey class 3 or 4 diverticulitis is open sigmoid resection with end-colostomy and formation of a Hartmann pouch. In this setting, it is beneficial to resect the sigmoid down to the most proximal healthy rectum in anticipation of future colostomy reversal. Given the potential operative difficulties and morbidity associated with end-colostomy reversal in this setting, a reasonable alternative to the Hartmann procedure is on-table lavage and primary anastomosis with or without diverting loop ileostomy. Clearly, this approach is contingent on the patient's status and ability to tolerate a more extensive operation. The purpose of the lavage is to evacuate as much of the stool column from the colon as possible so as to decrease the contamination from the fecal load in the event of a leak at this high-risk colorectal anastomosis.

Colonic obstruction secondary to diverticulitis: Patients with a critical diverticular stricture of the sigmoid colon often present with a large bowel obstruction indistinguishable from an obstructing sigmoid colon cancer. Often, despite attempts to carry out colonoscopy or contrast enema, a definitive diagnosis cannot be made, and an urgent intervention is required. Prior to operation, an attempt at endoluminal stenting should be considered. In situations where stenting is not available or an attempt at decompression is not successful, operation is required. Laparotomy in this situation is facilitated by decompressing the large bowel early in the operation through a colotomy in the proximal sigmoid or transverse colon. Alternatively, early transection of the sigmoid colon with on-table lavage may be performed. Whereas sparing of the superior hemorrhoidal artery may be advocated in the setting of known diverticular disease, if malignancy has not been excluded, a formal oncologic resection must be performed, with mobilization of the rectum via the presacral plane and division of the main sigmoidal vessel.

Summary

Sigmoid diverticulitis encompasses a spectrum of disease that can be challenging to manage both medically and operatively. The laparoscopic-assisted approach to sigmoid colectomy has marked clinical benefits over the traditional open operation and should be considered in patients with uncomplicated disease as well as in selected patients with complicated disease provided the surgeon has the advanced laparoscopic skills necessary for this approach. Successful operation requires an advanced understanding of the anatomy, as post-inflammatory changes can obliterate tissue planes and make for difficult dissection.

Selected Readings

Benn PL, Wolff BG, Ilstrup DM (1986) Level of anastomosis and recurrent colonic diverticulitis. Am J Surg 151:269–271

Chapman JR, Dozois EJ, Wolff BG, et al. (2006) Diverticulitis: a progressive disease? Do multiple recurrences predict less favorable outcomes? Ann Surg 243:876–883

Milsom JW, Bohm B, Nakajima K (eds) (2006) Laparoscopic colorectal surgery. 2nd edn. Springer, New York

Welch JP, Cohen JL, Sardella WV, Vignati PV (eds) (1998) Diverticular disease: management of the difficult surgical case. Williams & Wilkins, Baltimore, MD

7 Polyposis Syndromes of the Colon

Andrew Latchford, Sue Clark, and Robin K.S. Phillips

Pearls and Pitfalls

- Management of individuals with polyposis syndromes and at-risk family members within organized registries reduces mortality.
- Meticulous colonoscopy technique, with dye spray, polyp count and biopsy is important in clinical diagnosis.
- Failure to identify a mutation in a causative gene does not exclude the diagnosis of a polyposis syndrome.
- It is important to distinguish familial adenomatous polyposis (FAP) arising as a new mutation (with no background family history) from mutY human homolog (MYH) associated polyposis as the different modes of inheritance (autosomal dominant vs. recessive) fundamentally affect management of the family.
- In FAP there are several options for prophylactic surgery, but the aim is to prevent rather than treat cancer, and surgery should be performed usually during teenage years.
- With advances in the management of the large bowel, duodenal and periampullary cancers and desmoid tumors have become the commonest causes of death in FAP.
- 90% of patients with FAP develop duodenal and ampullary adenomas, but just 5–10% develop cancer at these sites.

K.I. Bland et al. (eds.), *Colorectal Surgery*,
DOI 10.1007/978-1-84996-444-9_7,

- Surgery for intra-abdominal desmoid tumor is hazardous and associated with high recurrence rates; it should be avoided if possible, and if necessary be performed in specialist centers.
- In Peutz-Jeghers syndrome (PJS) failure to perform enteroscopy and polyp clearance at laparotomy results in a high re-laparotomy rate.
- PJS is associated with a high risk of gastrointestinal and a number of extra-intestinal malignancies; clinical suspicion should be high.
- Most cases of juvenile polyposis can be managed endoscopically.

Colonic polyposis syndromes have been recognized for many years and have been characterized clinically and pathologically to varying degrees (Table 7.1). These syndromes are associated with increased risk of colorectal and other cancers and are inherited. Their study has not only improved the understanding and management of these conditions, but has also been influential in elucidating the underlying mechanisms of colorectal cancer, in general.

TABLE 7.1. Summary of polyposis syndromes of the colon.

Syndrome	Polyp type	Inheritance	Extracolonic cancer	Management of colon
FAP	Adenoma	AD	Yes	Surgery
MAP	Adenoma	AR	Yes	Surgery/ colonoscopy
JP	Hamartoma	AD	Yes	Colonoscopy/ surgery
PJS	Hamartoma	AD	Yes	Colonoscopy
CS	Hamartoma	AD	Yes	Colonoscopy
BRRS	Hamartoma	AD	No	Colonoscopy
HP	Hyperplastic	Not known	No	Colonoscopy

Adenomatous Polyposis Syndromes

Familial Adenomatous Polyposis

Familial adenomatous polyposis (FAP) was one of the first recognized polyposis syndromes and is the best characterized.

It is also the most common, with an estimated incidence of approximately 1:10,000.

Genetics

FAP is a highly penetrant, autosomal dominant disorder caused by a germline mutation in the adenomatous polyposis coli (APC) gene. This tumor suppressor gene is located on chromosome 5q21, and encodes a 312-kDa protein, the function of which remains to be fully characterized. It has a role in cell adhesion and is involved in regulating the Wnt pathway. When APC is mutated, this pathway is activated causing altered expression of genes that affect proliferation, migration and apoptosis. APC has a role in controlling the cell cycle, thus suppressing tumorigenesis. Finally, by stabilizing microtubules, APC maintains chromosomal stability; when mutated defects in mitotic spindles and chromosomal missegregation lead to aneuploidy.

Clinical Features

The development of adenomatous colorectal polyps is the hallmark of FAP. Polyps usually develop in late childhood and adolescence. Attenuated FAP refers to those cases where less than 100 polyps are present and classical FAP where greater than 100 polyps are observed. In the absence of an identified APC/mutY human homolog mutation, FAP is diagnosed on clinical grounds if >100 adenomatous polyps are found in the large bowel. Polyps are more numerous on the left side of the colon. Although colorectal polyps may present with diarrhea, gastrointestinal (GI) bleeding or pain, the majority of cases remain asymptomatic until cancer develops.

Although FAP is typified by the development of large bowel polyps, a generalized disorganization of tissue regulation is present, resulting in adenomas elsewhere in the GI tract and the extra-colonic manifestations associated with the syndrome. Some have little clinical significance (such as gastric fundic gland polyps, osteomas, sebaceous cysts, congenital hypertrophy of the retinal pigment epithelium (CHRPE), supernumerary teeth), whereas other extra-colonic manifestations represent a significant cause of morbidity and mortality. Desmoid tumors affect around 15% of patients with FAP and are benign tumors of myofibroblastic origin. Desmoid disease and duodenal cancer are the most important causes of mortality in patients with FAP who have undergone colectomy.

Several genotype–phenotype correlations have been observed consistently (Fig. 7.1).Mutations at codon 1309 are associated with a more severe colonic phenotype and increased risk of colorectal cancer, which develops at an earlier age. Far 5´ and 3´ mutations are associated with a more attenuated colonic phenotype, and 3´ mutations have been shown consistently to be associated with an increased risk of desmoid disease.

Cancer Risk

Unless prophylactic surgery is performed, there is a nearly 100% progression to colorectal cancer by 35–40 years of age. Isolated reports exist in the literature of cancer developing in childhood.

About 90%of patients will develop duodenal adenomas by 70 years of age and of these, duodenal cancer develops in 5–10%. The risk of duodenal cancer varies according to the stage of duodenal disease, as might be expected (Table 7.2). For those with stage 4 disease there is a 36% risk of developing duodenal cancer by 10 years.

A number of extra-gastrointestinal neoplasms are associated with FAP, including adrenal adenomas, a variant of papillary thyroid cancer, hepatoblastomas and medulloblastoma. Although patients with

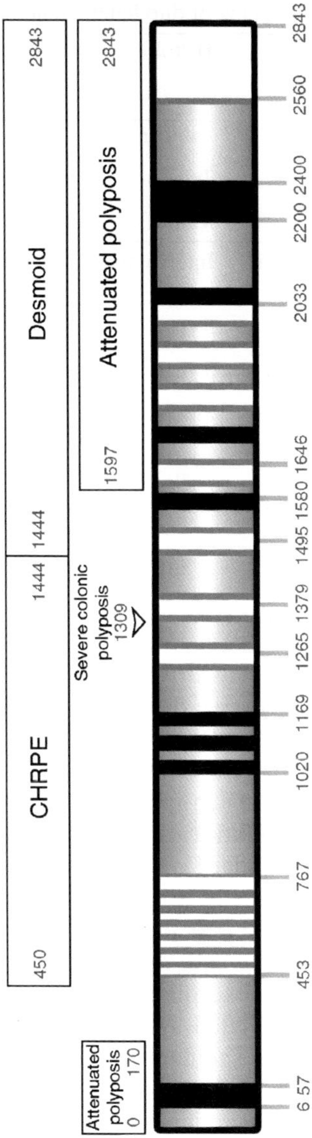

FIGURE 7.1. Genotype–phenotype correlation in FAP.

TABLE 7.2. Spigelman staging of duodenal adenomas in FAP.

No of polyps	Size of polyps (mm)	Histology	Dysplasia	Points
1–4	1–4	Tubular	Mild	1
5–20	5–10	Tubulovillous	Moderate	2
>20	>10	Villous	Severe	3

Total points	Spigelman stage	Interval to next duodenoscopy
0	0	5 years
1–4	I	5 years
5–6	II	3 years
7–8	III	1 year
9–12	IV	6 months

Diagnosis

Management of families with FAP in a specialized registry allows gathering of pedigree data to identify at-risk individuals. Current techniques allow identification of the causative APC mutation in 70% of clinically affected individuals. Once the mutation has been identified predictive testing in at-risk relatives is straightforward and reliable.

In the UK, the standard practice is to offer predictive testing around the age of 12–14 years. There is rarely a need to perform testing sooner, as polyps do not usually start to develop before this age, and an earlier diagnosis does not alter management. An exception to this is an at-risk child who develops bowel-related symptoms or anemia; genetic testing and colonoscopy should be performed promptly.

After a positive predictive test, colonoscopy is performed to assess polyp burden—an important factor in deciding the timing and type of prophylactic surgery. Surgery can usually be delayed until a socially and educationally convenient time in the teens.

In a family in which no mutation has been identified, clinical screening by annual flexible sigmoidoscopy is started at 14 years. Additional colonoscopy at 5-yearly intervals is added from 20 years.

About 20% of cases of FAP have no family history and are due to a new mutation. The diagnosis is initially made clinically if over 100 large bowel adenomas are present.

Management

There is no doubt that prophylactic colectomy before the age of 20 should be recommended in virtually all patients with FAP and extends life expectancy by 30 years. The main issue is what operation should be performed (Clark and Phillips, 1996).

The choice is between colectomy and ileorectal anastomosis (IRA) and proctocolectomy with ileoanal pouch anastomosis(IPAA). Colectomy and IRA is an operation with low morbidity and good functional outcome. The main drawback is the risk of developing rectal cancer in the future. Surveillance of the rectal remnant by flexible sigmoidoscopy should be performed every 6 months and larger lesions removed. If rectal polyps become too numerous then therapy with an non-steroidal anti-inflammatory drug (NSAID; sulindac or celecoxib) may be used or consideration should be given to completion proctectomy and ileoanal pouch. Cancer risk in the rectal remnant is related to age and polyp density.

IPAA surgery seems an attractive alternative in that it theoretically obviates future colorectal cancer risk. However a cuff or small islands of at-risk rectal mucosa may be retained; it is also becoming increasingly clear that there is a risk of developing pouch adenomas and cancer. Thus annual surveillance of the pouch and rectal cuff with flexible sigmoidoscopy is recommended. In addition, pouch surgery is associated with a higher surgical complication rate and less satisfactory function than an IRA, risk of male sexual dysfunction, reduced female fertility and the need for a temporary ileostomy.

These risks are sometimes difficult to accept in the context of an essentially healthy adolescent facing prophylactic surgery.

For those over 25 years, high density of rectal polyposis or the presence of a codon 1309 mutation predict high risk of rectal cancer, and IPAA is recommended. For most others IRA is a reasonable option. Both procedures are increasingly being performed laparoscopically, which make them more acceptable. In very exceptional cases with high risk of desmoid development and a low polyp burden, endoscopic surveillance with NSAID therapy may be considered to delay or avoid surgery.

Patients with a rectal cancer sufficiently low to preclude a sphincter preserving procedure will require abdomino-perineal excision combined with total colectomy and ileostomy. IPAA may be an option in a higher rectal cancer, but the stage of disease and need for radiotherapy may preclude this. Colectomy should be performed if a colonic cancer is present, but a proctectomy is not always necessary. The factors guiding decision making in this scenario are the same as in prophylactic surgery.

The management of the duodenum remains a challenge. Patients should undergo regular upper GI tract surveillance from the age of 25, with frequency determined by the Spigelman stage (Table 7.2). Surveillance should be performed with a side-viewing endoscope (due to the distribution of polyps and the need to assess the ampulla) and by an endoscopist experienced at assessing the duodenum in FAP. Endoscopic therapy may be considered for lesions greater than 1 cm or those with worrying histological features. For those with stage 3 disease, celecoxib may reduce polyp burden (Phillips et al. 2002) but patients need to be counseled adequately regarding the potential cardiovascular and cerebrovascular risks. For those with disease that is not manageable endoscopically or who have stage 4 disease, prophylactic duodenectomy should be considered. After surgical or endoscopic intervention in the duodenum/ampulla there is a risk of recurrent disease and continued endoscopic surveillance is required.

MYH Associated Polyposis

MYH associated polyposis (MAP) was first described in 2002 and its genetic and clinical features are yet to be fully characterized. The true incidence of MAP is not known but it is thought to account for 10–30% of patients who appear to have FAP clinically but in whom no germline APC mutation can be identified.

Genetics

MAP is inherited in an autosomal recessive manner, with high penetrance, and is caused by biallelic mutations in the MYH gene, which codes for a protein involved in the repair of DNA that has been damaged by reactive oxygen species generated during aerobic metabolism.

Homozygous or compound heterozygous germline mutations are required to develop the MAP phenotype. Patients who are heterozygotes for germline MYH mutations do not display polyposis but may have an elevated cancer risk. The heterozygous carrier frequency in the UK population is estimated to be around 1%.

Clinical Features

As with FAP, the hallmark of MAP is the development of colorectal adenomas. Although initially it was thought to be similar to an attenuated FAP phenotype, it is now clear that there may be wide variation, with up to thousands of colonic adenomas being present in some cases. Both duodenal adenomas and cancers have been reported but seem to occur less frequently than in FAP. Osteomas and CHRPE have both been observed but there are no reports of desmoid tumors in MAP.

A number of series have confirmed an increased risk of colorectal cancer associated with biallelic MYH mutations, with a risk up to 50-fold that of those with no MYH mutations.

In the largest reported cohort of MAP, 65% of patients developed colorectal cancer at a median age of 45 years.

There is much debate regarding the cancer risk in heterozygotes. Initially it was felt that they did not carry an increased cancer risk and did not develop polyposis, as one would expect with a classical autosomal recessive pattern of inheritance. However,it has now been reported that heterozygotes may have an increased colorectal cancer risk (odds ratio 1.5–3).

Management

Currently there are no standard guidelines on how these patients should be managed. There is a wide variation in colonic phenotype and management should be tailored to the individual patient. For those who have been confirmed by genetic testing to have biallelic mutations, annual colonoscopy is recommended. Many of these patients will undergo surgery, the type of operation performed depending on tumor burden and site of disease, as for FAP. Some patients with a sparse colonic phenotype may prefer to opt for colonoscopic surveillance, but need to be counseled appropriately on long-term cancer risk. In view of the reports of increased cancer risk in heterozygotes current recommendation is a baseline colonoscopy at the time of diagnosis, and then 5-yearly until 80 years of age.

There are no data to confirm whether duodenal surveillance is effective in patients with MAP, however, it is recommended that bi-allelic carriers undergo duodenal surveillance identical to that of patients with FAP.

Other Polyposis Syndromes

A number of other polyposis syndromes have been described. Peutz-Jeghers syndrome (PJS) and juvenile polyposis (JP) are the commonest, while Cowden syndrome (CS) and Bannayan-Riley-Ruvalcaba Syndrome (BRRS) are very rare. Hyperplastic polyposis (HP) is increasingly recognized, but remains poorly understood.

Peutz-Jeghers Syndrome

Genetics

PJS is genetically heterogeneous. Germline mutation in the LKB1 gene (also called STK11), has been identified as the cause of PJS but is detected in only 50% of patients. LKB1 is involved in regulation of cell polarity and proliferation and also has a role in inhibiting the Wnt signaling pathway.

The reported incidence of PJS varies widely but is likely to be around 1:100,000. The association of mucocutaneous pigmentation with intestinal polyposis typifies PJS. Traditional diagnostic criteria are histological confirmation of characteristic gastrointestinal polyps and two out of three of the following:

- Small bowel polyps
- Family history of PJS
- Pigmented macules on the buccal mucosa, lips or digits

The polyps of PJS have a typical histopathological appearance and may occur throughout the GI tract but are most commonly found in the jejunum, where they cause bleeding and anemia or obstruction, either directly or by intussusception. They may be found at extra-intestinal sites, such as the kidney, ureter, gallbladder, nasal passages and bronchus. Pigmented lesions occur in over 90% of patients and vary in size, number and color. These lesions generally develop in infancy and may fade after puberty. Although most frequently observed on the buccal mucosa, lips and digits, these lesions may also be seen in the rectum, vulva and conjunctiva.

Cancer Risk

It is now firmly established that there is an increased cancer risk in PJS. In the largest analysis of 419 individuals there was an 85% risk of developing a cancer by the age of 70. The most common cancers were gastrointestinal in origin and the risk of colorectal cancer was 3%, 5%, 15%, and 39% at ages 40, 50, 60, and 70, respectively. An increased risk of all GI tract, pancreatic, breast and gynecological cancers has been observed with reported risks at 70 years of 57%, 11%, 45%, and 18%, respectively. Adenomatous foci may be seen within PJS which may progress to cancer along the adenoma-dysplasia-carcinoma pathway. However it is not clear whether in fact most GI cancers arise in polyps or in the "normal" mucosa, which may be unstable due to mutated LKB1.

Management

The two main problems facing the clinician caring for individuals with PJS are the lifetime risk of cancer and the management of small bowel polyps, particularly the need to prevent repeated emergency laparotomies and subsequent loss of small bowel.

Panenteric examination is recommended every 3 years (more frequently for those with a particularly dense phenotype), with removal of any significant lesions at the time of upper GI and lower GI examinations. Video capsule endoscopy is used for small bowel imaging and removal of small bowel polyps when they reach 1–2 cm in size (earlier if associated with symptoms), is recommended (Fig. 7.2). Removing significant polyps reduces the future rate of intussusception/obstruction and the need for emergency surgery (Edwards, 2003); it may reduce occult GI blood loss and may alter the risk of developing cancer. In most patients, prophylactic colonic surgery is not required and endoscopic surveillance and treatment will suffice.

Cervical and breast screening is recommended as per national guidelines, unless there is a family history of breast cancer when screening by MRI at a younger age should be considered. Self-examination of the breasts/testes is to be encouraged.

Juvenile Polyposis

This is a clinically and genetically heterogeneous condition that affects 1 in 100,000–160,000 people. It is distinct from

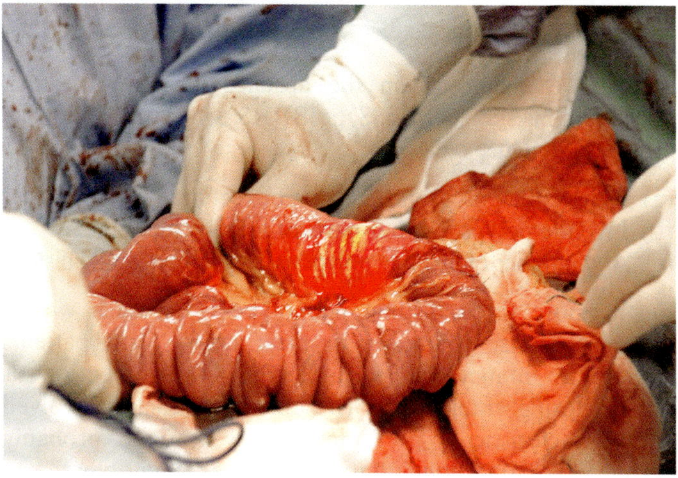

FIGURE 7.2. PJS on table enteroscopy.

solitary juvenile polyps, which develop in 1–2% of children and adolescents. Although cases of carcinomatous change have been described in a solitary juvenile polyp, it is accepted that patients with such solitary lesions are at no increased relative risk of colorectal carcinoma or death compared with the general population.

Genetics

JP is an autosomal dominant condition with incomplete penetrance. Two genes have been implicated, with some families having mutation identified in SMAD4 and others in BMPR1A.

The remaining 60% of cases of JP are termed mutation negative. Both SMAD4 and BMPR1A mutations cause disruption of the transforming growth factor b (TGF b) signal transduction pathway, which regulates apoptosis and growth inhibition responses.

Clinical Features

JP can be diagnosed, in the absence of extra-intestinal features consistent with CS or BRRS, when the following criteria are met:

(a) >5 juvenile polyps of the colon or rectum
(b) Juvenile polyps in other parts of the GI tract
(c) Any number of juvenile polyps and a positive family history

Furthermore three distinct phenotypes exist each with a different disease course. In its most severe form, patients present in infancy with GI bleeding, intussusception or protein losing enteropathy. The entire GI tract is involved and characteristically no family history is found, probably because the condition is fatal. The other phenotypes may present at a later age (5–15 years) and affect either the colon and rectum alone or the entire GI tract. Both these phenotypes may present as acute or chronic GI bleeding, anemia or abdominal pain. In a review of 272 patients with JP, the colorectum was involved in 98%, the stomach in 14%, duodenum in 2% and jejunum/ileum in 7%.

Cancer Risk

JP is associated with a significant malignant potential, predominantly affecting the GI tract. St Mark's Polyposis Registry data have shown that the cumulative risk of cancer was 68% by 60 years of age. The largest review assessed reports on 271 patients with JP and found that the overall incidence of carcinomas was 17% (47 patients). The large bowel was the site at which most of these developed, but gastric, duodenal and pancreatic cancers were also reported. The risk of malignancy appears to start when patients are in their 20s.

Management

The mainstay of management for those with JP is regular GI tract surveillance. Patients and at-risk family members should undergo colonoscopy and esophagogastroduodenoscopy at 1–3-yearly intervals depending on polyp number and symptoms. Colonic polyps can usually be managed by endoscopic polypectomy. If severe dysplasia or invasive cancer is found, or if polyps are too numerous or causing symptoms (especially anemia or protein losing enteropathy), then colectomy is recommended. In the majority of cases IRA is sufficient, but if there is carpeting of the rectum or rectal cancer then IPAA will be necessary. Long term endoscopic surveillance of the rectal stump or pouch is required for those who have undergone surgery.

Similarly, the management of the upper GI tract is dependent on disease severity and symptoms. In most cases endoscopic polypectomy suffices, however with diffuse gastric disease subtotal or total gastrectomy may be required. Small bowel polyps may require removal by enteroscopy or surgery.

In addition to GI tract surveillance, patients should annually undergo review and check hemo-globin concentration, as long-term studies suggest that symptoms or anemia usually precede the development of malignancy.

These very rare syndromes have considerable clinical and genetic overlap, and may represent different ends of the spectrum of a single disorder. Up to 60% of patients with CS will develop gastrointestinal polyps, which are indistinguishable from the JPS polyp. However, it is the extraintestinal manifestations that are most striking, especially the mucocutaneous lesions which affect 80–90% of patients. Of these, facial trichilemmomas, acral keratosis, palmoplantar keratoses and oral papillomas are the most common. In addition, breast and thyroid cancers are particularly common, but the risk of gastrointestinal malignancy is unclear.

Intestinal polyposis affects 45% of patients with BRRS. Other features include multiple hemangiomas, macrocephaly, developmental delay, pseudopapilledema, lipomas and pigmented papules on the penis. There are no reports of increased risk of malignancy in patients with BRRS.

Both CS and BRRS are inherited in an autosomal dominant manner but with incomplete penetrance. Germline PTEN mutations are found in up to 80% of patients with CS and also in BRRS. PTEN acts as a tumor suppressor gene and is associated with a number of malignant tumors.

We would suggest an initial upper GI endoscopy and colonoscopy at 25 years of age, and thereafter as guided by polyp burden or if symptoms develop. Regular breast and thyroid screening is recommended in CS.

Hyperplastic Polyposis

Hyperplastic polyps are the most frequently observed colorectal polyps. The incidence of such polyps increases with age, occurring in 70–80% of individuals over 60 years of age. These lesions have been considered to be an inconsequential finding, with no malignant potential. However, recent literature supports the concept that there is a morphologically and genetically distinct type of hyperplastic polyp, which may be pre-malignant.

Clinical Features

HP, sometimes called metaplastic polyposis, has no extracolonic features. Various definitions have been used but the WHO definition is widely accepted:

1. At least 5 histologically proven hyperplastic polyps proximal to the sigmoid colon, of which 2 are greater than 10 mm
2. Any number of hyperplastic polyps occurring proximal to the sigmoid colon in an individual with a first degree relative with HP
3. More than 30 hyperplastic polyps distributed throughout the colon

HP is a heterogeneous condition, most commonly diagnosed in the 6th and 7th decades of life.

Genetics

The WHO definition of HP includes familial aggregation, thus intimating that this maybe an inherited disorder. However, only few cases with familial clustering have been reported and it is still not clear whether this truly is an inherited disorder.

Cancer Risk

An increased risk of colorectal cancer in patients with HP is supported by a number of published series. The reported risk has been between 50–70%. Cancers may arise through a serrated neoplasia pathway, leading to microsatellite-unstable and typically right-sided colon cancer.

Management

Given the rarity of this condition and the conflicting literature, it remains unclear how best to manage these patients. Colonoscopic surveillance is advocated 1–3-yearly depending on the number and size of hyperplastic polyps identified. Given the WHO definition it is reasonable to offer screening colonoscopy to first degree relatives of affected patients.

Selected Readings

Agnifili A, Verzaro R, Gola P, et al. (1999) Juvenile polyposis: case report and assessment of the neoplastic risk in 271 patients reported in the literature. Dig Surg 16:161–166

Al Tassan N, Chmiel NH, Maynard J, et al. (2002) Inherited variants of MYH associated with somatic G:C to T:A mutations in colorectal tumours. Nat Genet 30:227–232

Clark SK, Phillips RKS (1996) Desmoids in familial adenomatous polyposis. Brit J Surg 83:1494–1504

Edwards DP, Khosraviani K, Stafferton R, et al. (2003) Long-term results of polyp clearance by intraoperative enteroscopy in the Peutz-Jeghers syndrome. Dis Colon Rectum 46:48–50

Groves CJ, Saunders BP, Spigelman AD, Phillips RKS (2002) Duodenal cancer in patients with familial adenomatous polyposis (FAP): results of a 10 year prospective study. Gut 50:636–641

Hearle N, Schumacher V, Menko FH, et al. (2006) Frequency and spectrum of cancers in the Peutz-Jeghers syndrome. Clin Cancer Res 12:3209–3215

Nielsen M, Franken PF, Reinards THCM, et al. (2005) Multiplicity in polyp count and extracolonic manifestations in 40 Dutch patients with MYH associated polyposis coli (MAP). J Med Genet 42:e54
Phillips RKS (1995) Familial adenomatous polyposis: the surgical treatment of the colorectrum. Semin Colon Rectal Surg 6:33–37
Phillips RKS, Wallace MH, Lynch PM (2002) A randomised, double blind, placebo controlled study of celecoxib, a selective cyclooxygenase 2 inhibitor, on duodenal polyposis in familial adenomatous polyposis. Gut 50:857–60

8 Clinical Management of Patients with Fecal Incontinence

Ian G. Finlay

Pearls and Pitfalls

- Fecal incontinence usually has a multifactorial etiology; consequently, all patients having surgery should be fully investigated.
- Irritable bowel syndrome is a common cause of incontinence.
- Obstetric anal sphincter injuries during child birth should be repaired under good light sources with anesthetic facilities by an experienced surgeon soon after the delivery.
- Sacral nerve stimulation is an exciting new development but the mechanism is an yet unclear are unknown.
- Many patients respond to treatment with amitriptyline or biofeedback.
- Less than 10% of patients referred for surgery require an operation.
- Do not offer surgery to patients in whom the principal symptom is incontinence for liquid stool.
- Patients who undergo surgery should be warned that all recognized operations have the potential to make the symptoms worse.
- Patients with irritable bowel syndrome have a poor outcome after surgery.

K.I. Bland et al. (eds.), *Colorectal Surgery*,
DOI 10.1007/978-1-84996-444-9_8,

- Beware of performing a hemorrhoidectomy in patients with perineal descent.
- Avoid anal stretch operations, since they risk producing diffuse disruption of the internal anal sphincter.

Introduction

Fecal incontinence is a disabling and distressing condition that affects all age groups. It is more common in women than men with the highest prevalence in the elderly. It has been estimated to affect 1–2% of the population over 40 years of age.

Mechanism of Continence

Fecal control is maintained by an extraordinary and complex sphincter mechanism that is not fully understood. It is, however, recognized as comprising of the following components—an internal anal sphincter, an external anal sphincter, pelvic floor muscles and a sensory and motor nerve supply.

The internal anal sphincter (IAS) is an involuntary smooth muscle under autonomic control (sympathetic innervation is excitatory, whereas parasympathetic supply is inhibitory). The function of the IAS is to keep the anal canal closed. Injury to the IAS leads to leakage of mucous and fecal staining rather than incontinence.

The external anal sphincter (EAS) encircles the IAS and is continuous with the puborectalis muscle and other muscles of the pelvic floor. It is of note that during surgical dissection, there is no visible separation between the EAS and the puborectalis. The EAS is under voluntary control as a consequence of innervation from the pudendal nerve with connections to the ventral horn of S2 (Onuf's nucleus) and the corticospinal pathways. The motor neurons of Onuf's nucleus are unusual since they are tonically active during sleep. The integrity of the nerve supply to the EAS may be determined on clinical examination by either stroking the perianal skin or asking the patient to cough; both should cause spontaneous contraction of the EAS. The EAS (in conjunction with the pelvic floor) may be contracted voluntarily by the patient to avert the call to stool but this can only be maintained for less than a minute. Consequently, the principal symptom in patients with an EAS defect is the inability to avert the call to stool leading to urgency.

The muscles of the pelvic floor provide a "sling support" for the rectum and pelvic organs and are composed of a sheet of striated muscle. Four component parts of the muscle have been identified; the puborectalis, pubococcygeus, iliococcygeus and ischiococcygeus. The nerve supply is uncertain but includes ventral fibers from S2 and S3, which enter the muscle posteriorly where they may be vulnerable to stretch-injury during childbirth. When contracted, the puborectalis causes an angle of approximately 90° to develop between the anal canal and the rectum. This is probably the most important single factor contributing to the continence of solid stool, but has no beneficial effect in controlling liquids, since in contrast to solids they flow easily around bends.

It would appear therefore, that the control of loose stool or diarrhea is provided by voluntary contraction of the striated muscles (EAS and pelvic floor muscles) explaining the observation that the control of liquid stool is precarious even in normal subjects. This is important in clinical practice since many patients who seek advice regarding symptoms of incontinence are only symptomatic when they have loose stool. Such patients are unlikely to respond to surgical intervention and treatment should be directed towards alleviating the cause of the diarrhea.

It is an extraordinary fact that the anorectum in conjunction with the sphincter muscles can function such that it is possible for humans to expel gas in a downward direction while maintaining control of solids. The probable explanation for this phenomenon is that the puborectalis contracts vigorously producing an acute angle of less than 90° between the anal canal and rectum. The external anal sphincter also contracts resulting in "a retort shape". Air is then pushed from the rectal chamber by transiently raising intra-abdominal pressure above sphincter pressure. This process is aided by the abundance of sensory fibers at the mucocutaneous junction in the anal canal that have been considered to contribute to the mechanism of continence.

The exact mechanism, whereby rectal filling is detected and results in the call to stool is poorly understood but can be sensed by both the stretch receptors of the pelvic floor and "sampling" in the anal canal. This would explain why patients who have undergone a restorative proctectomy with anal canal mucosectomy have a near normal perception of pouch filling.

Etiology of Fecal Incontinence

There are numerous causes of fecal incontinence; the most important are given in Table 8.1. Patients rarely have a single abnormality and the cause of symptoms is invariably multifactorial necessitating careful clinical examination and investigation. In addition, it has been the author's experience that

TABLE 8.1. Causes of fecal incontinence.

Congenital
Congenital anomalies including agenesis of the anorectum
Acquired
Fecal impaction and spurious diarrhea
Anorectal cancer and villous adenoma
Conditions causing autonomic neuropathy, e.g. diabetes
Irritable bowel syndrome
Inflammatory bowel disease
Rectal prolapse
Fistula in ano
Sphincter injury to internal or external anal sphincters (childbirth, anorectal surgery or trauma)
Sphincter and pelvic floor neuropathy (childbirth, demyelinating spinal injury cerebral vascular injury)

patients who have had episodes of incontinence suffer from anxiety and apprehension that it may occur again, thereby complicating both clinical assessment and the efficacy of treatment.

IAS defects or weakness leading to symptoms of fecal staining may be associated with autonomic neuropathy secondary to conditions such as diabetes or excessive alcohol consumption. The internal anal sphincter may also be deliberately divided at surgery in the operation of internal sphincterotomy or inadvertently during hemorrhoidectomy producing a "gutter deformity". Diffuse disruption of the IAS may occur after an anal stretch operation but fortunately this procedure is now used rarely.

The EAS may be subject to trauma but the most frequent and important cause of injury occurs during childbirth. Post partum perineal injuries that involve the EAS are defined as third degree tears while those that also involve the rectal mucosa are classified as fourth degree tears. The risk of sustaining a tear is increased if the birth is complicated or prolonged; risk factors include multiparity, prolonged second stage of labor (more common with the routine use of epidural anesthesia), large babies and the use of forceps. Severe perineal tears have been reported to occur in 0.6–0.9% of deliveries.

The attendant at the delivery has a duty of care to identify the presence of a sphincter tear. When a tear is found it should be repaired in good light under appropriate anesthesia by trained personnel. Evidence suggests that if patients have an immediate repair of a third or fourth degree tear then subsequent incontinence to solid stool is infrequent(<5%) but leakage of liquid stool or gas has been reported in up to one third of patients. This contrasts with the poor results reported for delayed repairs by Hajivassiliou and others. Missing a sphincter injury at the time of delivery, therefore, has serious consequences probably because the divided muscle ends retract and are difficult to identify in scar tissue during a later operation.

Despite guidelines highlighting the need for careful post partum examination, it is now recognized that minor sphincter tears are missed frequently. Several studies using ultrasound have reported occult internal and external sphincter injuries in over a third of all women who have had a vaginal delivery. Most of these patients, however, are asymptomatic.

Childbirth also causes a neuropathic injury to the pelvic floor. Electromyographic studies have shown that all vaginal deliveries cause a degree of injury to the pelvic floor muscles but this is more extensive in complicated deliveries and is cumulative with multiple births. Patients who suffer severe neuropathy have features of perineal descent leading to an obtuse anorectal angle. This condition is often named idiopathic fecal incontinence (IFI) but there is now sufficient evidence to attribute it to childbirth. IFI is associated with prolonged pudendal nerve conduction time leading to weakness of the EAS and reduced squeeze pressures in the anal canal. Paradoxically, as a consequence of the pelvic floor weakness, patients with IFI may also have difficulty emptying the rectum necessitating straining; this in turn causes further damage to the pudendal nerve. It is not uncommon, therefore, for these patients to complain of both "incontinence and difficulty in emptying". Since the neuropathy affects the entire pelvic floor, the patient may also have incontinence of urine with a vaginal/ uterine prolapse.

Loss of rectal support may cause a rectal intussusception or even an overt rectal prolapse. The exact cause of rectal prolapse is unknown but many of the features observed in IFI are also found in patients with rectal prolapse. Rectal prolapse is a common cause of incontinence that merits surgical treatment. In contrast, there is debate regarding the significance of the presence of a midrectal intussusception if diagnosed by proctography, since it is unlikely to be the cause of incontinence.

Congenital abnormalities are an unusual but important cause of incontinence since they affect young adults who often seek a surgical solution. The severity of the abnormality varies but pelvic MRI may help to define whether there is any evidence of either the IAS or EAS (usually absent) or evidence of the pelvic floor musculature (usually present). It is extraordinary and important for our understanding of the physiology of continence that these patients, who have no IAS or EAS may have relatively few symptoms thereby confirming the importance of the pelvic floor in the mechanism of continence.

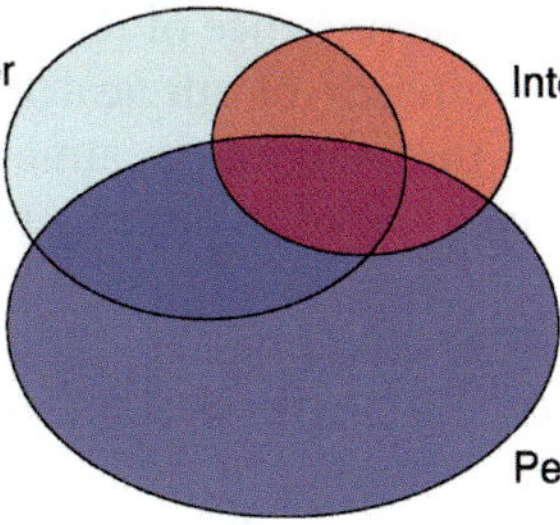

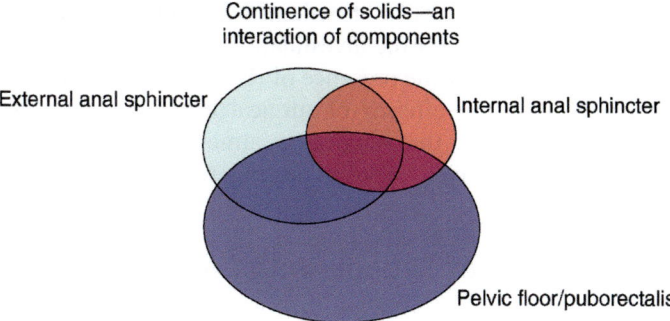

FIGURE 8.1. Continence of solids is dependent on the interaction of various components, including the internal/external anal sphincter, pelvic floor and an intact neurological supply. Since their functions overlap, some loss of a component may occur without the development of clinical incontinence.

It is the "way of nature" that human organs have considerable reserve function and are able to sustain a considerable degree of deterioration before symptoms develop. So it is in the anorectum; substantial loss of a component of continence may occur before the patient becomes symptomatic (see Fig. 8.1). For example, the anal sphincter (IAS and EAS) may be divided partially at a fistula operation in the majority of cases with few consequences. The exception is the female patient who already has a pelvic floor neuropathy from previous childbirth and in whom even a minor sphincter division may cause symptoms. It is for this reason that all patients with anorectal pathology require experienced and careful assessment.

It has been shown recently that up to 50% of patients with incontinence presenting for assessment have an abnormality of both rectal sensation and colonic motility. These patients have a hypersensitive rectum with low maximum tolerated volumes on balloon distension. This gives rise to symptoms of severe urgency. These patients also have evidence of colonic hypermotility in response to standard stimuli such as ingestion of food or the injection of neostigmine. In brief, they have irritable bowel syndrome fulfilling the Rome criteria. It has been shown that IBS was either the principal cause or a major contributing factor in 50% of patients who had been referred to a colorectal clinic for the investigation of incontinence. It is important to identify the presence of IBS since it has a deleterious effect on the efficacy of surgical treatment. It is the author's experience that surgical treatment of incontinence should, if possible, be avoided in patients with IBS.

Investigation of Patients with Incontinence

All patients with fecal incontinence for whom surgery is being considered should be investigated. Patients who have had a change of bowel habit require a colonoscopy to exclude neoplastic conditions such as villous adenoma, carcinoma and inflammatory bowel disease.

Ano-rectal physiology studies may identify pudendal nerve neuropathy and abnormalities of rectal sensation. Hyper and hyposensitivity of the rectum are both recognized to lead to incontinence. Anal canal pressures are recorded frequently, but their value in clinical decision making has been questioned. Complex studies of rectal compliance are principally research tools but can be helpful in cases of megarectum.

Evacuating proctography is less useful in investigating patients with incontinence than in those with outlet obstruction disorders but may show an unexpected rectal intussusception or prolapse. It also provides objective evidence for perineal descent. It is the author's practice to proceed to an examination under anesthesia in patients in whom occult prolapse is suspected. Only those patients in whom the rectum may be easily drawn through the anus are then considered for surgical correction.

Anorectal ultrasound examination is an indispensable investigation in patients with incontinence. In experienced hands, a clear image of the integrity of the IAS and EAS may be obtained. This may include a spectrum of abnormality from minor atrophy to complete disruption.

MRI can be useful in selected patients including those with congenital abnormalities when it aids in defining the anatomy. It also has an important role in assessing patients with complex fistula in ano who may have residual sepsis contributing to their symptoms of leakage.

Treatment

Treatment is based upon careful clinical assessment. It is important to identify the cause or in most cases, causes, for the incontinence.

Medial Management of Incontinence

Many patients with minor incontinence only require reassurance and will respond to the judicious use of anti-diarrheal agents. Patients with spurious diarrhea secondary to fecal impaction should be treated with enemas or bowel washouts. This is an important group to diagnose since patients with incontinence secondary to impaction are often reluctant to accept that the cause is "constipation". Clinicians should be aware that although most common in the elderly, this condition can occur at any age.

It is especially important to identify those patients with IBS since they are numerous and often respond to a small dose of amitriptyline. It is unknown whether the efficacy of this treatment is due to a central or peripheral effect. It is the author's practice, however, to prescribe treatment even in cases of doubt because of the beneficial effects observed. Indeed, amitriptyline has been shown to be efficacious in the treatment of incontinence in the absence of irritable bowel symptoms. This observation merits further investigation.

Symptom improvement has also been reported by post menopausal women when they commence hormonal replacement therapy. Female patients who have evidence of a pelvic floor neuropathy may attribute the onset or exacerbation of their symptoms to the menopause. It has been postulated that symptoms develop as muscle tone diminishes due to fall in estrogen levels.

In addition to oral medicines, there are a variety of commercial products available including anal plugs that may be used to treat patients with minor leakage.

The technique of biofeedback has been reported to improve symptoms but the mechanism of action is unknown. It is of note in this respect that physiotherapy has been shown to be ineffective in treating fecal incontinence but is of benefit in patients with urinary incontinence. Since biofeedback is relatively simple and non invasive, it should be used before more invasive techniques.

Surgical Management

Surgery is indicated in less than 10% of patients who undergo investigation for fecal incontinence. It is important that patients are carefully apprised before surgery with regard to the risks as well as the potential benefits of the operation. In particular, all patients should be warned that there is a risk that surgical intervention could make the symptoms worse.

Internal Anal Sphincter Repair and Correction of an Anal Canal Deformity

Internal anal sphincter disruption in isolation most commonly results from surgical intervention such as internal sphincterotomy or hemorrhoidectomy (gutter defect).

Repair of the IAS after sphincterotomy has been reported to be effective. This, however, has not been the experience of the author who has found the results of surgery disappointing. Furthermore, there is a high risk that surgery to the IAS may make the symptoms worse. In contrast, surgical correction of a gutter or key-hole deformity after hemorrhoidectomy is often highly successful. Although defects may be directly repaired, a cutaneous advancement flap is usually required.

Generalized disintegration of the IAS after manual dilatation of the anus does not have a surgical solution and it for this reason that anal stretch should be avoided.

External Anal Sphincter Repair

The availability of endoanal ultra-sonography has led to the identification of increasing numbers of patients with an external anal sphincter defect. Although these can occur as a consequence of anal trauma, the majority are secondary to perineal tears during childbirth. The resulting defect may be partial or complete. Since the sphincter is under tension, a complete division allows retraction of the muscle ends and may lead to a defect that is half the circumference of the anal canal in size. In such circumstances, the ends become embedded in scar tissue making mobilization to facilitate an adequate repair difficult.

EAS defects often occur in association with IAS defects, pelvic floor weakness, pudendal nerve neuropathy and symptoms of irritable bowel syndrome. Although these associated abnormalities are not necessarily a contraindication to attempting a sphincter repair, they may contribute to a poor outcome. It is the author's preference to repair an IAS defect en-bloc with the EAS. The literature has produced conflicting reports regarding the effect of pudendal nerve neuropathy on outcome. Some studies have suggested no detrimental effect; others have suggested a profound effect. Consequently, the presence of a pudendal nerve neuropathy should not prevent the surgeon from attempting a repair. However, in the author's experience, the presence of diarrhea-predominant IBS will limit the results of a repair and should be treated before attempting surgery.

Several techniques have been reported for EAS repair. In the first instance, it is necessary to identify the scar tissue within the defect and dissect laterally until pliable and mobile muscle is identified. Care must be taken in large defects to avoid injury to the pudendal nerves that enter in the 3 and 9 o'clock positions. The presence of nerves limits the extent of the dissection. Indeed it has been shown that injudicious dissection may cause pudendal nerve neuropathy leading to a poor long-term outcome. For this reason, some surgeons use a nerve stimulator to identify the exact site of the pudendal nerves.

Having identified the muscle ends (see Fig. 8.2), it is necessary to reconstitute the anal sphincter. The author usually uses an overlap repair but on occasion, a "keel" type repair may be employed. The type of suture material used varies between surgeons; the author now uses PDS since non-absorbable sutures such as prolene often need to be removed at a later stage. Fast-absorbing sutures are also avoided because early disruption of the repair has been observed. The author recommends the frequent use of a defunctioning colostomy if a

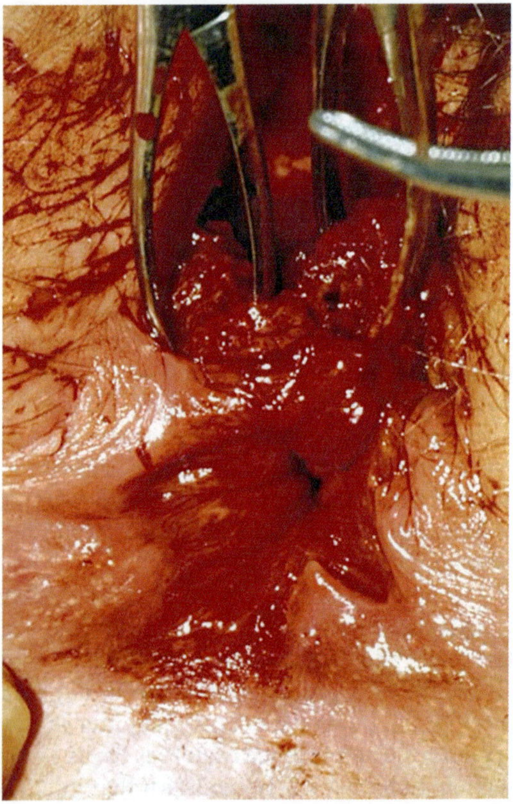

FIGURE 8.2. An example of an anterior anal sphincter repair for trauma after childbirth (showing the ends of muscle after mobilization that will be brought together).

major repair is undertaken. This prevents fecal impaction with disruption of the repair and is more comfortable for patients. It should be noted that the only randomized trial, albeit including only small numbers of patients, showed no benefit with the use of a stoma. However, that study included patients who had undergone only limited repairs.

Early reports suggested that the efficacy of surgery for EAS repair was excellent with continence restored in approximately 70% of patients. Unfortunately, these results are not maintained and after 10 years of follow up, only 10–30% of patients remain continent. Sometimes, it is evident that the failure is due to disruption of the repair. Although repeat repairs may be attempted, the surgery is technically difficult and the outcome likely to be poorer than those obtained after primary repairs.

Post Anal Repair

Patients with pelvic floor neuropathy present evidence of perineal descent and an obtuse ano-rectal angle. The operation of posterior anal repair, devised by Parks, aims to recreate an acute anorectal angle by plication of the pelvic floor muscles behind the anus after an intersphincteric dissection. Early reports suggested that the procedure was highly efficacious in restoring continence with success rates of over 70% but later reports were less favorable and the procedure is now rarely used.

Rectal Prolapse Surgery

Rectal prolapse is a relatively common cause of fecal incontinence although it produces other distressing and compelling symptoms. Consequently, surgical repair is usually recommended for patients who are otherwise fit. The condition is characterized by a neuropathy of the pelvic floor muscles, diastases of the levator ani muscles and a patulous anal sphincter.

Although over 100 different operations for rectal prolapse have been described they share common principals. Surgery may be undertaken by either the abdominal or perineal route.

The former involves dissection of the rectum followed by fixation and in some cases excision of the redundant bowel. These operations are highly effective in correcting the prolapse but often produce a poor functional outcome with approximately 50% of patients suffering from severe constipation. Indeed this may be the mechanism whereby incontinence is corrected. In an attempt to avoid constipation, sigmoid colectomy has been advocated but this can increase the risk of postoperative incontinence. It is the author's practice to avoid colectomy in patients undergoing surgery for rectal prolapse when incontinence is the predominant symptom. Despite this selective approach, approximately one-third of patients who have undergone abdominal rectal prolapse surgery will suffer from incontinence.

Perineal operations are usually reserved for patients who are unfit for abdominal surgery since they are less effective at correcting the prolapse. There is however, evidence that the functional results are superior with less constipation and incontinence.

Stoma

Since fecal incontinence is such a socially devastating symptom, the option of creating a stoma should not be overlooked. Used in conjunction with techniques such as colonic irrigation a stoma may greatly improve the quality of life for these patients.

Artificial Bowel Sphincters

At present, there are two artificial bowel sphincters available for use in patients with fecal incontinence. The first is the artificial bowel sphincter or ABS; an ingenious design first used in urinary incontinence. The device has three component parts: a cuff that encircles the anus, a constant pressure balloon and a hydraulic control pump. For evacuation, the patient depresses the pump thereby transferring fluid from the cuff to the balloon. This fluid then "bleeds" back slowly closing the device.

The ABS has been shown to be highly effective in restoring continence; indeed such is the efficacy that patients often report difficulty with emptying. Unfortunately, the reported complication rate including infection and erosion has been high. Despite this, some surgeons have reported success. It has been suggested that serious complications of infection and erosion may occur because the device is implanted in the perineum. Further, the cuff can create localized areas of high pressure when wrapped around the bowel.

A new artificial sphincter known as the PAS (prosthetic anal sphincter) has been designed by the author and colleagues that aims to overcome the difficulties encountered with the ABS. The device utilizes a constant pressure balloon like the ABS, but the cuff component is implanted in the pelvis where it reproduces the action of the puborectalis (see Fig. 8.3). The cuff of the PAS differs from the ABS having been designed specifically to avoid localized areas of high pressure. Early clinical studies have been encouraging and the product has only recently come on the market.

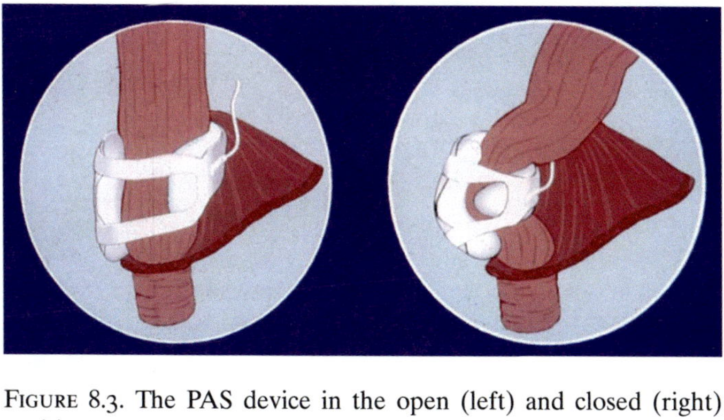

FIGURE 8.3. The PAS device in the open (left) and closed (right) positions.

Dynamic Gracilis Muscle Transposition

Attempts have been made to improve continence in patients with deficient anal sphincters by using the gracilis muscle to wrap around the anal canal. One or both muscles may be used (see Fig. 8.4). Although initial reports were promising the technique proved to be disappointing with longer follow up. In particular, patients either lacked control or were unable to empty the rectum because the muscle produced adynamic constriction.

In an attempt to improve the outcome, the gracilis muscle was electrically stimulated, to change the characteristics of the muscle from "fast to slow twitch" fibers that were less likely to fatigue. The operation performed in expert hands can be highly effective in restoring continence. Unfortunately the operation has high complication rates limiting the value of the procedure. Since the advent of sacral nerve stimulation, it is rarely used.

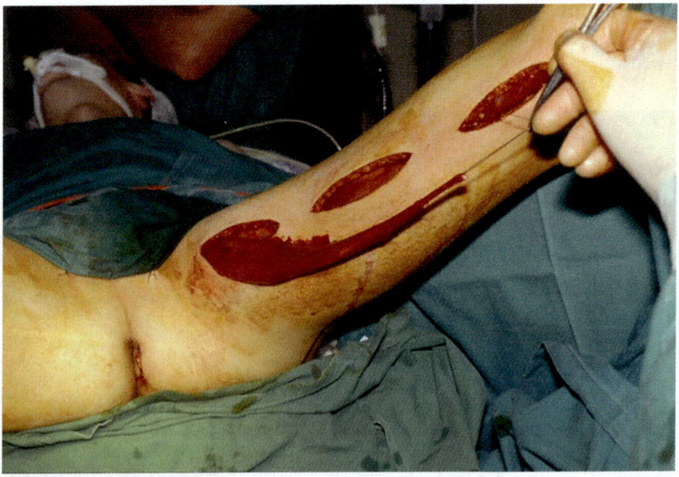

FIGURE 8.4. The gracilis muscle is first mobilized from the thigh, carefully preserving the neuro-vascular bundle.

Sacral Nerve Stimulation

Of all the treatments for fecal incontinence to emerge over the past 25 years, sacral nerve stimulation (SNS) is perhaps the most promising.

Sacral nerve stimulators were first used in the early 1980s to treat urge incontinence of urine. It was noted that there was also an improvement in bowel function in these patients. SNS was first reported to have been used in patients with fecal incontinence in 1995. Since then it has been used and reported to be successful in patients who have suffered incontinence from a variety of causes including spinal cord injury, idiopathic degeneration, post rectal prolapse repair, after low anterior resection and even in patients with a sphincter defect. Although the numbers of patients in these studies was small, improved continence for liquid and solid stool was reported in 50–75% of patients.

SNS has the advantage that patients may have a trial of treatment using a temporary electrode before being subjected to the surgical procedure of placing a permanent electrode. It is usual to attempt to place the electrode through the third sacral foramen, although both the second and fourth have also been used successfully. Open implantation has recently been superseded by percutaneous techniques but it remains necessary to make a subcutaneous pocket for the stimulator. Currently, work is being undertaken to compare unilateral with bilateral stimulation and to define the optimal settings for the stimulator.

It is important to note that at present the mode of action of SNS is unknown. In particular it is unknown whether it has a peripheral or central action. There is some evidence, however, that it may modify rectal motility and sensation. This would be especially interesting given the high number of patients with fecal incontinence who have IBS. Studies have suggested that SNS does not work as a placebo although it would be interesting to compare SNS with traditional treatment such as amitriptyline in a randomized crossover trial.

SNS is arguably the most promising treatment available at present for the treatment of fecal incontinence but it should be remembered that many treatment options have previously been reported as demonstrating potential only to disappoint with long term follow up. Given current knowledge, SNS should be tried first after failed medical management with implantation of artificial sphincters reserved for SNS failures.

Selected Readings

Chapman AE, Geerdes P, Hewett P, et al. (2002) Systematic review of dynamic graciloplastyin the treatment of faecal incontinence. Br J Surg 89:138–153

Donnelly V, Fynes M, Campbell D, et al. (1998) Obstetric events leading to anal sphincter damage. Obstet Gynaecol 92:955–961

Finlay IG, Richardson W, Hajivassiliou CA (2004) Outcome after implantation of a novel prosthetic anal sphincter in humans. Br J Surg 91:1485–1492

Fitzpatrick M, Behan M, O'Connell PR, O'Herlihy C (2000) A randomised clinical trial comparing primary overlap with approximation repair of third degree tears. Am J Obstet Gynecol 183:1220–1224

Ganio E, Masin A, Ratto C, et al. (2001) Short term sacral nerve stimulation for functional anorectal and urinary disturbances: results in 40 patients: evaluation of a new option for anorectal functional disorders. Dis Colon Rectum 44:1261–1267

Hajivassiliou CA, Carter KB, Finlay IG (1996) Anorectal angle enhances faecal incontinence. Br J Surg 83:53–56

Jarrett MED, Varma J, Duthie G, et al. (2004) Sacral nerve stimulation for faecal incontinence in the United Kingdom. Br J Surg 91:755–761

Lehur PA, Zerbib F, Neunlist M, et al. (2002) Comparison of quality of life and anorectal function after artificial sphincter implantation. Dis Colon Rectum 45:508–513

Malouf AJ, Norton CS, Engel AF, et al. (2000) Long term results of overlapping anterior anal sphincter repair for obstetric trauma. Lancet 355:260–265

Perry S, Shaw C, McGrother C, et al. (2002) Prevalence of faecal incontinence in adults aged 40 years or more living in the community. Gut 50:480–484

Poen AC, Felt-Bersma RJ, Strijers RL, et al. (1998) Third degree obstetric perineal tear: long term clinical and functional results after primary repair. Br J Surg 85:1433–1438

Sultan AH, Monga AK, Kumar D, Stanton SL (1999) Primary repair of obstetric anal sphincter rupture using the overlap technique. Br J Obstet Gynaecol 106:318–323

Swash M (1993) Faecal incontinence; childbirth is responsible for most cases. BMJ 307:636–637

9
Pruritus Ani

Santhat Nivatvongs

Pearls and Pitfalls

- Idiopathic pruritus ani can be intractable.
- Hand washing with mild soap (best with glycerine soap) is the optimal way to clean the perianal area (unless the patient is allergic to soap which is rare).
- Applying Capsaicin cream is a novel treatment, start with 0.025%.
- Proper use of methylene blue injection should be considered as a last resort.
- Soaking in water is not cleaning.
- All anal wipes contain chemicals and do not help.
- Traditional washing with a soapy wash cloth without washing it off with water is a bad practice which gives soap a bad name.
- There is no evidence that eating or drinking certain kinds of food or liquid is the cause of pruritus ani.

Pruritus ani is not a disease but a symptom of itching of the perianal skin. It is estimated to occur in approximately 1–5% of the population, with a male-to-female ratio of about 4:1. The onset of the condition is most commonly in the fifth and sixth decades of life. Most patients have only a mild form of the condition and respond quickly to proper treatment. To treat pruritus ani rationally, one must have a clear-cut concept of the etiologic factors involved in its production.

K.I. Bland et al. (eds.), *Colorectal Surgery*,
DOI 10.1007/978-1-84996-444-9_9,

Clinical Manifestation

Itching, usually combined with burning, is the prominent complaint. The itching may occur any time of the day or during sleep. Anything that keeps the anal skin moist causes itching. The itch-scratch cycle usually creates abrasions of the perianal skin, resulting in seepage of serum which further irritates the perianal skin.

Careful history taking usually uncovers clues of the problem. Often, the patient has more problems at night or in hot, humid weather, although this is not always the case. The itching may also be exacerbated by friction from clothing, wool, and nylon. With time, the condition may progress to an unrelenting itching and burning with an insurmountable urge to scratch. Poor anal hygiene is often a major contributing factor. Questions about the patient's cleaning habits and how the perianal skin is cleansed are important to ask. Wiping with toilet paper only spreads and smears feces to the perianal skin. All cleaning wipes contain chemicals that also damage the sensitive perianal skin. Specific dietary ingredients and neurogenic, psychogenic, and idiosyncratic reactions with pruritus should be suspected whenever another factor is not identified readily. Because the diagnosis is made by exclusion, inquiries about diabetes, antibiotic use, and vaginal and anal discharge may establish the factors responsible for the symptoms. Stress and anxiety often exacerbate pruritus ani. Common complaints revolve around family, work, and finances.

Physical Findings

In the early stage, examination of the perianal skin reveals minimal erythema and excoriation. As the symptoms progress, the perianal skin becomes friable, inflamed, and weeps from excoriation. Poor anal hygiene may be apparent with staining of stool or mucus and a wet anal area. In the later stages, the typical findings of long-standing idiopathic pruritus ani include thickened, whitish, ulcerated, or abraded perianal skin from scratching, with deep furrows with radial ridges of perianal skin.

Flexible sigmoidoscopy or colonoscopy should be performed to rule out associated diseases, particularly in patients with chronic pruritus ani who are older than 50 years of age. Daniel and coworkers found associated colorectal disease in 35% of patients with chronic pruritus ani, including rectal cancer in 11%, proctitis in 5%, squamous cell carcinoma of anus in 5%, inflammatory bowel disease in 5%, adenomatous polyp in 4%, anal diseases in 2%, and colon cancer in 2%.

Etiologic Factors

Pruritus ani can be divided into secondary type and idiopathic type. With proper history, examination, and patch tests, the causes of the itching will be discovered eventually. The idiopathic type is diagnosed by means of exclusion.

Secondary Pruritus Ani

From Within Anorectum

Prolapsing hemorrhoids (grade 3 or 4) cause a mucous discharge which, if not washed off, irritates the perianal skin. Treatment with rubber band ligation or hemorrhoidectomy is indicated. Anal fissures cause seepage of serum from the ulcer and thus should be treated conservatively with bulk agents and warm sitz baths, nitroglycerin or nifedipine paste, or if unresponsive to these measures, lateral internal sphincterotomy. Discharge from an anal fistula is also caustic to the anal skin. Fistulotomy usually cures the problem. Other surgically correctable conditions include anal skin tags and prolapsed hypertrophied anal papillae.

Fecal incontinence, especially of liquid stool, can be a major problem. Radiation proctitis may cause leakage of mucus and liquid stool. Patients with pruritus ani have an abnormal rectal inhibitory reflex and abnormal, transient, internal sphincter relaxation. Whether these abnormalities are the cause or the effect remains unknown. Heavy coffee drinking causes relaxation of the internal sphincter, which may cause seepage of mucus and liquid stool. The main management of these problems is to eliminate the cause.

Anal hygiene is important in these situations. Patients should be discouraged from sitting in water to relieve itching, because it causes maceration of the skin. Instead, washing with water by hand with or without glycerine soap is the best way to clean and relieve the irritation. In patients who have incomplete evacuation of the stool, irrigation of the anal canal with bulb syringe to wash away stool from the anorectum after each bowel movement is helpful to prevent seepage of stool. Dietary measures to firm the stool should be initiated. For radiation proctitis, cortisone retention enemas may be helpful.

From Outside the Anorectum

Sweating, particularly in overweight patients and in patients with a deep natal cleft, causes maceration of skin with potentially bacterial or fungal invasion. Wearing tight or non-porous underwear also traps the moisture. An irritating vaginal discharge should also be excluded. Proper washing with mild soap and water by hand will improve the condition.

From Perianal Skin Disease

In a study of patients with pruritus ani, Dasan and co-workers found 34 of 40 patients to have an underlying dermatosis which accounted for their symptoms, the most common form being psoriasis. Many of these patients also have a high incidence of sensitization to previously used topical preparations on patch testing. These patients should be referred to a dermatologist for proper tests and management.

Anal condyloma acuminata can be diagnosed easily and should be treated with excision and/or electrocautery. Perianal Paget's disease and Bowen's disease can cause intense itching and mimic a dermatitis; a biopsy should often be performed to confirm or exclude the diagnosis. Treatment consists of a wide local excision; in the case of Bowen's disease, electrocoagulation has become the treatment of choice.

Radiation to perianal area, such as for carcinoma of the prostate and cervix, damages the skin causing erythema, ulceration, and seepage. The problem is usually temporary and improves with time. The area should be kept clean by hand washing. Cortisone cream often helps as well.

Idiopathic Pruritus Ani

This category includes all patients with no known cause of the condition. Typically, the patients have long-standing disease. The appearance of the perianal area varies from pale but otherwise normal looking, to ulcerated and seepy, to thickened with deep furrows. Many of these patients are excessively clean and have tried all kinds of topical preparations including over-the-counter cream and steroid preparations. All these agents should be stopped.

Oztas and co-workers showed that washing with a liquid cleanser (Protex liquid cleanser; Colgate-Palmolive) was as effective as topical steroids. Using a liquid cleanser, however, is unnecessary; proper hand-washing with soap (preferably glycerine soap) and water is excellent treatment. The patients should be instructed not to use a wash cloth. This regime should be done after each bowel movement and whenever there is discharge or sweat in the perianal area. Also any psychologic aspect should not be overlooked. In some patients, the anal itching may be the primary behavior, and this eventually perpetuates to the itch-scratch cycle. Dietary measures are helpful for many patients with pruritus ani with the goal to achieve a bulky, formed stool. Fungus infection of the perianal skin is usually a secondary involvement from the moist and poor hygiene and is aggravated by antibiotic usage for this and other conditions.

Topical Capsaicin

This approach is a novel treatment for idiopathic intractable pruritus ani. Capsaicin is a natural alkaloid extracted from red chili peppers. There is an over-the-counter topical analgesic cream (0.075% and 0.025%) commonly used for arthritis pain relief. Topical application of Capsaicin in therapeutic dose (0.075%) to pruritus ani produces profound loss of intraepidermal fibers within 24 h. Nerve terminals regenerate and reinnervate if Capsaicin application is discontinued; repeated application is often required.

The perianal area should be washed clean. Initially, the lower concentration of the cream should be tried first, applying a thin film to the itching area three to four times a day.

The Last Resort

When all etiologic factors have been excluded and other treatments have failed, one should consider injection of the perianal skin with methylene blue as the last resort. The solution for injection is prepared as follows:

10 ml of 1% methylene blue
5 ml normal saline
15 ml 0.25% bupivacaine with 1:200,000 epinephrine

The mixture is injected subdermally and subcutaneously in the anoderm and perianal skin. In their preliminary experience with 23 patients, Eusebio and colleagues found that cellulitis developed in three patients, and full thickness skin necrosis developed in three others when a 0.5% methylene blue solution alone was used; nevertheless, 21 of 23 patients had relief of their itching. Methylene blue causes necrosis of nerve endings, and the injected area becomes numb for about 1 month. This temporary denervation breaks the itch-scratch cycle and allows the skin to heal and return to normal. Because the methylene blue solution alone can cause tissue necrosis, it should be mixed and diluted as described above. The patient should be warned that his or her urine will turn blue for a few days. The skin in pruritus ani appears to have a low resistance to infection. The injected area should be cleansed with antiseptic before the injection. In some patients, prophylactic antibiotics should be considered as well.

Selected Readings

Anand P (2003) Capsaicin and menthol in the treatment of itch and pain: Recently cloned receptors provide the key. GUT 52:1233–1235

Daniel GL, Longo WE, Vernava AM (1994) Pruritus ani. Causes and concerns. Dis Colon Rectum 37:670–674

Dasan S, Neill SM, Donaldson DR, Scott HJ (1999) Treatment of persistent pruritus ani in a combined colorectal and dermatological clinic. Br J Surg 86:1337–1340

Eusebio EB (1991) New treatment of intractable pruritus ani (Letter). Dis Colon Rectum 34:289

Eusebio EB, Graham J, Mody N (1990) Treatment of intractable pruritus ani. Dis Colon Rectum 33:770–772

Lysy L, Sistiery-Ittah M, Israelit Y, et al. (2003) Topical capsaicin – a novel and effective treatment for idiopathic intractable pruritus ani: a randomized, placebo controlled, crossover study. GUT 52:1323–1326

Oztas MO, Oztas P, Onder M (2004) Idiopathic perianal pruritus: washing compared with topical corticosteroids. Postgrad Med J 80:295–297

10
Rectovaginal Fistulas

**Richard Cohen, Alastair Windsor,
and Kumaran Thiruppathy**

Pearls and Pitfalls

- Rectovaginal fistulas cause an underappreciated morbidity to affected women.
- The incidence of these fistulas in underdeveloped countries is underappreciated.
- The most common causes are traumatic obstetrical injuries during childbirth, postoperative causes, radiation therapy, invasive malignancies, and diverticulitis.
- Rectovaginal fistulas are classified as simple or complex and involve either the upper, middle, or lower third of the rectovaginal septum.
- Etiology and techniques of repair depend on location of the fistula.
- Lower third rectovaginal fistulas are usually repaired by a perineal approach, either transanal or transvaginal.
- Upper third rectovaginal fistulas are approached trans-abdominally.
- Approach to middle third rectovaginal fistulas depends on etiology; some can be repaired via a perineal approach, others require a trans-abdominal approach.
- Complex rectovaginal fistulas often require temporary or permanent proximal colonic diversion.

K.I. Bland et al. (eds.), *Colorectal Surgery*,
DOI 10.1007/978-1-84996-444-9_10,

- Techniques of repair may involve resection, flap advancement, or primary repair.
- The function of the anal sphincter should be evaluated preoperatively in all patients.

Introduction and Etiology

There are few afflictions, unattended with danger to life, which give rise to greater anxiety or produce more disagreeable results than cases of rectovaginal fistula. Tanner 1855.

A rectovaginal (RV) fistula is an abnormal communication between the epithelial surfaces of the vagina and the anal canal or rectum. These fistulas cause considerable morbidity to afflicted individuals and a severe headache to the treating surgeons, because recurrence with the need for perseverance and multiple procedures is often required. Although these fistulas are believed to be a rare condition, they are hugely underestimated worldwide.

The management of RV fistulas depends on the etiology as well as the anatomic configuration. RV fistula due to underlying pathology (Crohn's disease, tuberculosis, postradiotherapy) are much more difficult to manage, because there is an inherent resistance to healing within the tissue. This chapter will not, however, address pouch-vaginal fistulas after ileopouch anal procedures.

Most rectovaginal fistulas are acquired, although congenital RV fistulas do occur (Table 10.1). Obstetric trauma is the leading cause of RV fistulas worldwide. The incidence increases dramatically across developing countries where obstetric care is sparse. Risk factors include the use of forceps or other assisted methods of delivery, perineal tears, or an episiotomy that extends into the rectum. Long and difficult labor can cause weakness, necrosis, or tearing, which result in fistulas with the adjacent structures, such as the bladder, urethra, rectum, or perineum. These complex/difficult labors are most frequent in primiparous and young women and can result in low RV fistulas.

Other traumatic causes include blunt or penetrating perineal trauma. Traumatic fistulas respond well to treatment. If the RV fistula is secondary to a foreign body, removal of the foreign body usually results in spontaneous healing.

TABLE 10.1. Etiology of RV fistula.

Congenital causes
Acquired causes
Inflammatory bowel disease
Ulcerative colitis
Crohn's disease
Postoperative causes
Colorectal procedures (anastomoses near vaginal vault)
Gynecologic surgery
Traumatic
Obstetric trauma
Foreign bodies
Penetrating injuries
Infection and inflammation
Diverticular disease
TB
Cryptoglandular sepsis
Pelvic irradiation
Neoplasms
Idiopathic
Miscellaneous
Coital injury
Fecal impaction

Diverticular disease is a disease of an aging population; 30% of people ≥60 years old suffer with the condition, of whom some will develop fistulas. As 40–60% of diverticula are found in the sigmoid, which is also the most mobile part of the colon, it is this site which is most associated with colovaginal fistulas. In contrast to colovaginal fistulas which occur in women who have undergone a previous hysterectomy or some other form of pelvic surgery, RV fistulas secondary to diverticulitis are much less common, but when they occur, they cause high vaginal lesions.

Inflammatory bowel disease (ulcerative colitis and Crohn's disease) is associated with formation of external and internal fistulas. The incidence is far greater in Crohn's disease where the disease is transmural and abscess formation is more common. It is estimated that 80% of patients with Crohn's disease will develop some form of internal fistula, but less than 10% will develop RV fistulas. This discrepancy is due to the low incidence of Crohn's disease involving the rectum. The incidence of RV fistula in ulcerative colitis is about 4%. These fistulas arise primarily or, more often, in relation to a peri-rectal abscess and/or fistula and manifest most commonly as complicated peri-anal sepsis.

Malignancies are a rare cause of RV fistulas and may be due to primary, recurrent, or metastatic disease. The most common offending cancers are rectal, cervical, vaginal, and uterine. A history of any of these or other perineal cancers in the presence of a RV fistula requires a biopsy of the fistula.

With more liberal use of pelvic radiation therapy for adjuvant and neoadjuvant treatment of advanced rectal and gynecologic malignancies, there is an increasing incidence of radiation injury in the rectum with a high incidence of progression to fistula formation. The incidence of radiation-induced RV fistulas had varied between 1% and 6%. These RV fistulas are usually in the mid or upper vagina and occur within 2 years of the radiation treatment. Radiotherapy causes irreversible tissue and vascular damage resulting in poor tissue quality, poor healing, and inflammation. Radionecrotic ulceration occurs, inducing fistula formation. The degree of radiation damage is dependent on patient and treatment factor. The incidence of RV fistulas increases with radiation-related parameters such as total dose and overlapping radiation portals, patient factors (radiation effects are worse in thin patients and children), patient co-morbidities, especially diabetes and malnutrition, and iatrogenic factors, including chemotherapy and previous pelvic or abdominal surgery.

A variety of infectious conditions can lead to RV fistulas. Commonly implicated are peri-rectal abscess or fistula and peri-anal abscesses. Less common conditions are tuberculosis, lymphogranuloma venereum, and Bartholin gland abscess.

Classification

Anatomy

The rectovaginal septum is the thin septum separating the anterior rectal wall and the posterior vaginal wall (Fig. 10.1). The caudal portion of the septum comprises the perineal body, an important supporting structure linking muscles that extend across the pelvic outlet and providing support to the

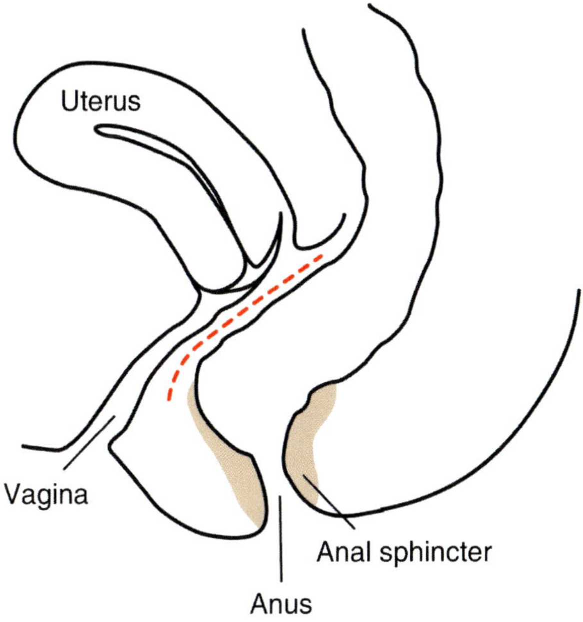

FIGURE 10.1. Rectovaginal fascia.

pelvic floor and pelvic diaphragm. Disruption or attenuation of this structure can lead to prolapse of pelvic viscera and formation of cystocele and rectocele. The anal sphincters are located in the posterior portion of the perineal body and can be compromised by an initial insult or during treatment.

Proximal to the perineal body, the septum is of variable thickness, often with a cephalic extension. The septum consists of three separate layers, including the posterior vaginal wall, the anterior rectal wall and mesorectum, and, in between, a thin, dense fascial layer consisting of collagen, smooth muscle, and coarse elastin. This inner layer helps provide the RV septum with durability and strength.

Classification

RV fistulas have been classified in many different ways, according to their etiology, size, anatomic location, or indeed, the various surgical approaches. Alternatively, they can be classified into simple or complex fistulas, depending on the ease with which treatment can be given (see Table 10.2).

TABLE 10.2. Classification of rectovaginal fistulas.

Simple fistula
<2.5 cm
Lower or middle third
Infective or traumatic origin
Complex fistula
>2.5cm
Upper third lesion
Neoplastic, inflammatory, radiation
Congenital fistulas
Other organ involvement
Multiply recurrent fistulas

The rectovaginal septum can be divided conveniently into thirds. The lower third anterior to anal sphincter complex and perineal body, the middle third involving the thin fascial layer, and the upper third covered posteriorly with peritoneum. Simple RV fistulas include small (<2.5 cm in diameter), lower third (Fig. 10.2), or middle third (Fig. 10.3) fistulas resulting from infection or trauma. Large (>2.5 cm), high fistulas involving the upper third of the septum (Fig. 10.4) are considered complex, as well as those caused by inflammatory bowel disease, cancer, or radiation, congenital fistulas, or those involving other organs. RV fistulas that have failed multiple prior repairs are also classified as complex.

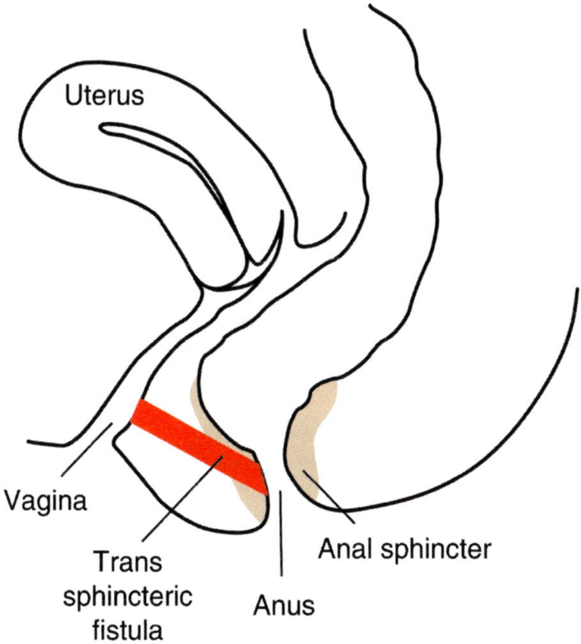

FIGURE 10.2. Low rectovaginal fistula.

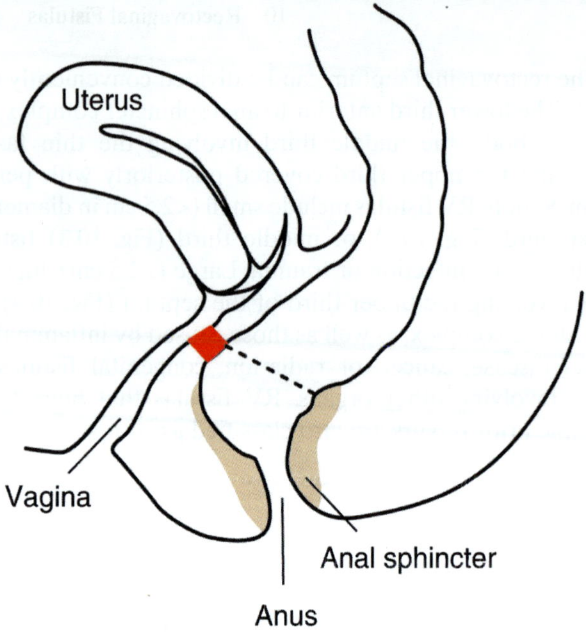

FIGURE 10.3. Mid rectovaginal fistula.

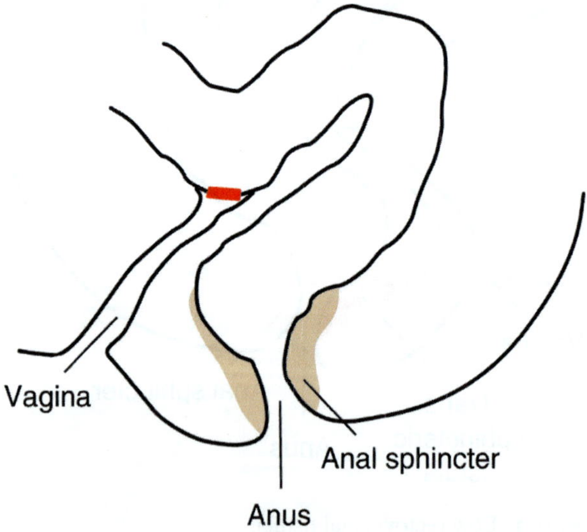

FIGURE 10.4. High rectovaginal fistula.

Presentation

The symptoms of RV fistula range between minimal egress of flatus and vaginal discharge to the passage of feces per vagina. The volume and character of the discharge varies and depends on the size, site, and etiology of the fistula. Patients may present with nonspecific signs. Acute exacerbation of inflammatory conditions (diverticulitis or inflammatory bowel disease) or abscesses may present with abdominal pain, low grade fever, nausea and vomiting, or diarrhea. On examination, a pelvic mass may be palpable and can be inflammatory or caused by a neoplasm.

Management

For successful management of these patients, it is essential to address several important principles. First is to confirm the presence of the fistula. Second is to define the anatomy, size, site, and complexity of the fistula, especially addressing the presence of multiple fistulas and other organ involvement. Third, it is crucial to determine etiology and other underlying pathology. And finally, involvement and functional capacity of the anal sphincter is of vital importance.

Diagnosis

The diagnosis is made invariably on the history taken from the patient. Examination and investigations may be used to confirm the diagnosis and delineate the anatomy of the problem. The most useful investigation may be a careful examination under anesthesia. Imaging with retrograde contrast radiographs, computed tomography (CT), and magnetic resonance imaging (MRI) helps to further define local anatomy.

Clinical Examination

Careful examination in the clinic can be helpful, bearing in mind that the area can be very excoriated and sore. Digital rectal examination complemented with bimanual pelvic examination may reveal scars, defects, or masses on the anterior rectal wall and posterior vaginal wall. Proctosigmoidoscopy may demonstrate the fistula itself or underlying inflammatory bowel disease or malignancy. Insufflation of air into the rectum at proctosigmoidoscopy can produce audible air escaping from the vagina through a fistula. When indicated, colonoscopy is a useful tool in evaluating the proximal colon looking for related colonic pathology (e.g., Crohn's disease).

Examination under anesthetic (EUA) may be the most useful examination available to the surgeon faced with a RV fistula. Careful, comprehensive, and painless assessment of the lower anorectum and entire vagina can be carried out without embarrassment or discomfort to the patient. Fistula probes and hydrogen peroxide may help to delineate tracks and locate internal openings. Rectocele can be assessed, and a catheter can be left in high tracks to allow targeted fistulography.

Retrograde barium enema radiographs can be useful in the study of rectovaginal fistulas. Although the usual barium contrast can be too thick for many fistulas to fill, the other findings add valuable information in the diagnosis of other GI pathologies such as inflammatory bowel disease, diverticular disease, or malignancies. Vaginograms may prove successful in identifying small and multiple RV fistulas. The technique is performed by placing a Foley catheter into the vagina, inflating the catheter to form a seal, and instilling contrast into the vagina. As contrast flows into the vagina, the fistula and involved bowel can then be imaged.

High-resolution CT and MRI have come to play an invaluable role in the delineation of complex fistulas. Cross-sectional imaging is employed routinely when underlying pathology or other organ involvement is suspected. These non-invasive imaging techniques allow a quick and effective way of assessing GI and extra-gastrointestinal structures. MRI of the pelvis is particularly useful for evaluating the elusive mid and upper third fistula, because the inflammatory reaction shows up as a bright white signal on a black background.

Anal Sphincter

Before planning operative correction of an RV fistula, it is crucial to know the state and function of the anal sphincter complex. The sphincter can be assessed on digital examination in the awake patient, but a more formal evaluation by endorectal ultrasonography and/or anorectal physiology is usually indicated.

Treatment

Medical therapy: While operative therapy is usually required to treat an RV fistula, it is important to ensure maximal medical therapy of any underlying inflammatory bowel disease or unusual infection such as tuberculosis. It is best to adopt a multidisciplinary approach in these patients involving gastroenterologist and, if necessary, other colleagues in gynecology, infectious diseases, etc., depending on the ctiology of the RV fistula.

Surgical therapy: Operative treatment of RV fistula is approached differently according to the etiology. For infections, the treatment involves drainage of the site with appropriate antibiotic coverage. For certain non-reconstructible RV fistulas, proximal colonic diversion is most appropriate. For lower third RV fistulas that are repairable, the fistula can be closed by a perineal approach using a transvaginal repair, a transperineal repair with sphincter reconstruction, transanal repair, or an interposition graft (Martius graft). For upper third RV fistulas, an abdominal approach is best using either resection, mucosectomy, and coloanal sleeve anastomosis or an anterior resection and omental interposition. On rare occasions, an ablative excision (abdominoperineal excision) is required. Mid third RV fistulas can be approached from the perineum, but when they involve a previous anastomosis or radiotherapy sites, they are often managed via an abdominal approach.

Lower third RV fistula: Most of these fistulas are either post-obstetric or cryptoglandular in origin and can be managed from a perineal approach. The operative plan depends on the competence of the anal sphincter. If the anal sphincter requires a concomitant repair, a perineal operation is advocated, with excision of the fistula and laying open the sphincter muscles anteriorly. The anorectal mucosa is then repaired, and an overlapping anterior sphincter repair is carried out before closing the vagina. This approach has the added advantage of providing the bulky sphincter repair to sit between the anorectal and vaginal repairs. It is also a useful procedure when simple transanal or transvaginal flaps have failed.

If the anal sphincter complex is intact, a transvaginal or transanal flap repair can be performed. The authors prefer the transvaginal route, because the access is far greater than struggling through the anal canal. An incision is made in the posterior fourchette of the vagina, and the rectovaginal septum is carefully dissected out well above the level of the fistula. Care is taken to avoid the vaginal veins, which need to be oversewn if injured. The fistula-bearing vaginal mucosa is then excised and the fistula into the anorectum cored out. The rectal defect is repaired as per any bowel anastomosis; the authors prefer interrupted 3/0 polyglactin suture material. The rectovaginal septum can be plicated with 2-0 polydiaxone and the vaginal flap brought down to the vaginal skin with polyglactin sutures. The vagina can be packed for 24 h if dissection is difficult, in which case bladder catheterization is required.

In patients who have had previous attempts at repair, a useful modification is the use of a labial fat pad graft (Martius graft). The dissection is as above, but the left hand labia is also incised allowing dissection of the labial fat pad. This fat pad has both proximal and distal blood supply but will survive on its distal vessels, thereby allowing full mobilization. The fat pad can then be swung to interpose in the rectovaginal septum between the anorectal and vaginal repairs.

It is possible and occasionally necessary to perform repeat attempts at closure until success is achieved. The authors have seen successful closure of RV fistula after multiple transanal and transvaginal failures. In a recent series of 17 patients with RV fistula, of which 13 were a postsurgical complication, 16 (94%) were treated successfully by these approaches.

The role of a defunctioning stoma in the management of RV fistula is debated and unproven. The authors believe that it is not necessary to suggest a defunctioning stoma in a first time attempt at closure if there is no underlying bowel pathology. In contrast, after previous attempts at repair and in the presence of diseases such as Crohn's disease or post radiation, we advocate the use of a defunctioning stoma. Our approach is based on the empiric assumption that the chance of success would be greater if fecal flow were taken out of the equation. The luminal pressures of a patient straining at stool after a complex fistula closure can only put strain on a delicate situation.

In very symptomatic patients where all else has failed, ablative excision via abdominoperineal excision of the anorectum using an intersphincteric technique can be employed. In the presence of Crohn's disease, the perineal wound can cause continuing trouble, and the authors advocate the use of myocutaneous flaps in difficult cases.

Upper third and middle third RV fistula: These types of RV fistulas require an abdominal approach. The abdomen is opened via a midline laparotomy, and a full assessment of the peritoneal cavity is made, looking for evidence of an otherwise unappreciated inciting cause. The required operation usually falls into one of two categories, either a colovaginal fistulation from diverticular disease or invasive malignancies into the vault of the vagina after a previous hysterectomy, or fistulation from the rectum into vagina, either from an anastomosis or after prior therapy. In the former circumstances, traditional resection of the diseased segment of colon with a sigmoid colectomy or high anterior resection is advocated. Care must be taken to separate the newly formed anastomosis from the repaired vaginal vault to minimize risk of re-fistulation. Interposition of omentum is a useful trick. In the latter situation, the key is to ensure maximum separation of the vaginal repair from any anastomosis using the technique of a coloanal pull-through. The rectum is transected below the level of the fistula, and the remaining rectal remnant mucosa is excised either from above or below as appropriate. The proximal, undiseased colon "pulled through" the rectal muscle cuff is anastomosed by hand from below to the dentate line. A defunctioning ileostomy is often prudent.

Selected Readings

Bahadursingh AM, Longo WE (2003) Colovaginal fistulas. Aetiology and management. J Reprod Med 48:489–495

Bangser M (2006) Obstetric fistula and stigma. Lancet 367:535–536

Casadesus D, Villasana L, Sanchez IM, Diaz H, Chavez M, Diaz A (2006) Treatment of rectovaginal fistula: a 5-year Review review. Aust N Z J Obstet Gynaecol 46:49–51

Grissom R, Snyder TE (1991) Colovaginal fistula secondary to diverticular disease. Dis Colon Rectum 34:1043–1049

Hudson CN (1970) Acquired fistulae between the intestine and the vagina. Ann R Coll Surg Engl 46:20–40

Lindsey I, Guy RJ, Warren BF, et al. (2000) Anatomy of Denonvilliers' fascia and pelvic nerves, impotence, and implications for the colorectal surgeon. Br J Surg 87:1288–1299. Review

Rahman MS, Al-Suleiman SA, El-Yahia AR, et al. (2003) Treatment of rectovaginal fistula of obstetric origin: a review of 15 years' experience in a teaching hospital. J Obstet Gynaecol 23:607–610

Tahzib F (1983) Epidemiological determinants of vesicovaginal fistulas. Br J Obstet Gynaecol 90:387–391

11 Pseudomembranous Colitis

Lisa M. Colletti

Pearls and Pitfalls

- Antibiotic-associated diarrhea is common; in the outpatient setting, this is most commonly due to the antibiotic. In the inpatient setting, it is most commonly due to *Clostridium difficile*.
- *Clostridium difficile* colitis should be considered in all hospitalized patients with new onset diarrhea; failure to treat this disease can have substantial morbidity and mortality.
- *Clostridium difficile* colitis produces a range of symptoms from minor self-limited diarrhea to colonic perforation and sepsis.
- All antibiotics and many antineoplastic agents can predispose to the development of *Clostridium difficile* colitis.
- Development of *Clostridium difficile* colitis is not associated with duration or dose of antibiotic treatment.
- Diarrhea is the presenting sign in *Clostridium difficile* colitis.
- Risk factors for *Clostridium difficile* colitis include: advanced age, antibiotic therapy, immunocompromised state, ICU stay, burns, uremia, and enteral feeding.
- Diarrhea may be absent in patients with severe *Clostridium difficile* colitis causing ileus or toxic megacolon.
- Toxic megacolon due to *Clostridium difficile* colitis causing hypovolemic shock, cecal perforation, and/or toxic dilation of the colon with secondary sepsis is a surgical emergency with a 10–20% mortality rate.

K.I. Bland et al. (eds.), *Colorectal Surgery*,
DOI 10.1007/978-1-84996-444-9_11,

- Diagnosis of *Clostridium difficile* colitis is made by testing a stool sample for toxin A and B or visualization of pseudomembranes on sigmoidoscopy.
- *Clostridium difficile* can rarely affect the ileum or jejunum in the post-colectomy patient.
- Treatment for *Clostridium difficile* colitis includes fluid resuscitation, discontinuing the offending antibiotic, and administration of metronidazole.
- Antidiarrheal agents should NOT be used in the treatment of *Clostridium difficile* colitis, as they may inhibit clearance of the toxins.
- Oral vancomycin is an alternative treatment for *Clostridium difficile* colitis; the drug of choice is currently metronidazole in an effort to prevent the development of bacteria drug resistance to vancomycin in other enteric bacteria (i.e. enterococcus).
- Operative intervention is necessary for the patient with toxic megacolon due to *Clostridium difficile* colitis; the procedure of choice is total abdominal colectomy with ileostomy.

Introduction

The incidence of antibiotic-associated diarrhea varies from 5% to 39%, depending on the antibiotic used, and most cases in outpatients are due to the antibiotic and not to a specific bacteria. In contrast, most hospital or nursing home outbreaks of antibiotic-associated diarrhea are secondary to *Clostridium difficile*. *Clostridium difficile* causes 300,000–3,000,000 cases of diarrhea and colitis in the United States every year, and its incidence appears to be increasing. In addition, it is the fourth most common nosocomial infection reported to the Centers for Disease Control and Prevention. This disease is associated commonly with the use of antibiotics. Although clindamycin, ampicillin, and cephalosporins are associated most commonly with development of *Clostridium difficile* colitis, any antibiotic can predispose a patient to this infection.

Antibiotics alter the balance of normal gut flora and allow overgrowth of *Clostridium difficile*. The clinical presentation can vary from asymptomatic colonization to a mild diarrhea to fulminant disease, with high fever, severe abdominal pain, and toxic megacolon, sometimes with perforation. The most sensitive and specific test for *Clostridium difficile* infection is a tissue culture assay for the cytotoxicity of toxin B, however, detection of the toxin by ELISA (enzyme-linked immunoassay) is more rapid and inexpensive. Oral metronidazole or oral vancomycin are the drugs of choice for treatment, and most affected patients respond well to medical therapy. Approximately 15–25% of patients will relapse and require repeat treatment. Recurrent disease can be difficult to treat.

Epidemiologic Features

Clostridium difficile is a gram-positive, spore-forming anaerobic bacillus; interestingly, it was not implicated with antibiotic-related diarrhea until the late 1970s. *Clostridium difficile* is the cause of approximately 25% of cases of antibiotic-associated diarrhea and virtually all cases of pseudomembranous colitis. Most cases of *Clostridium difficile*-associated diarrhea occur in hospitals or nursing homes; the incidence of this infection in the outpatient setting is much lower, however, it does occur. Clindamycin is the most common antibiotic associated with this infection, however, it is also associated commonly with use of ampicillin, amoxicillin, and cephalosporins. While these antibiotics are the most common etiologies for *Clostridium difficile*-colitis, this disease can develop with the use of virtually any antibiotic. Other predisposing factors include advanced age, bowel ischemia, recent bowel or abdominal surgery, Cesarean section, burns, uremia, malnutrition, chemotherapy, malignancy in general, shock, and possibly enteral feeding. After controlling for antibiotic use, patients receiving enteral feeding have a 20% chance of testing positive for *Clostridium difficile*, while a control group tested positive only 8% of the time. Patients fed distal to the stomach were at increased risk compared to patients who were fed intragastrically.

The spectrum of disease ranges from an asymptomatic carrier state to diarrhea without colitis, to colitis with or without the presence of pseudomembranes, to toxic megacolon, colonic perforation, and death.

Pathogenesis

In general, *Clostridium difficile* is a non-invasive pathogen, although rare cases of actual tissue invasion have been reported in children with malignancy or a compromised immune system. The first step in development of *Clostridium difficile* colitis is disruption of the normal colonic flora, most commonly by use of antibiotics, although this disrupted intraluminal milieu can be related to use of antineoplastic or immunosuppressive drugs. Colonization occurs via the fecal-oral route. The spores are ingested, are able to survive the acid environment of the stomach, and germinate in the colon; overgrowth of *Clostridium difficile* then occurs with toxin production and development of diarrhea and colitis. Symptoms of colitis may occur as early as the first day of antibiotic use or 6 weeks or longer after the antibiotics are stopped.

Some strains of *Clostridium difficile* do not produce toxins and are therefore do not cause colitis. The strains that cause clinical disease produce both Toxin A and Toxin B; indeed, it is these toxins that are largely responsible for symptomatic disease. Toxin A binds to mucosal receptors and disrupts cytoplasmic microfilaments. Toxin B then enters the damaged mucosa and causes hemorrhage, inflammation, and necrosis. Full tissue damage requires the presence of both toxins. In patients with severe or fulminant disease, inflammation involves the deeper layers of the colonic wall, resulting in toxic megacolon and possible perforation. Severity of associated illness and decreased levels of serum IgG antibody to toxin A increase the severity of colitis. In animal models, antibodies against Toxin A prevent toxin binding, neutralize the secretory and inflammatory effects, and limit or prevent clinical disease. The immune response to Toxin B is less well-understood, but anti-Toxin B antibodies also protect against *Clostridium difficile* colitis. Cellular immunity appears to be less important in this process, however, it has not yet been studied in detail.

Infants and young children commonly have *Clostridium difficile* in their fecal flora but have no symptoms related to *Clostridium difficile* toxin. As an individual ages, the prevalence of *Clostridium difficile* in the fecal flora decreases for unknown reasons. While asymptomatic carriers of *Clostridium difficile* are an important reservoir of the bacteria, clinical symptoms only develop in about one third of colonized patients, and asymptomatic colonization may be associated with a decreased overall risk of developing symptomatic colitis. *Clostridium difficile* spores persist in the environment for years, which explains why contamination by these spores is common in hospitals and long-term care facilities, especially in rooms occupied previously by infected/colonized individuals.

Early histologic changes due to *Clostridium difficile* toxins include patchy epithelial necrosis and exudates of fibrin and neutrophils. Epithelial necrosis with ulceration develops, with associated overlying pseudomembrane containing cellular debris, leukocytes, fibrin, and mucin (gross appearance: Figs. 11.1a and b; microscopic appearance: Figs. 11.2a and b).

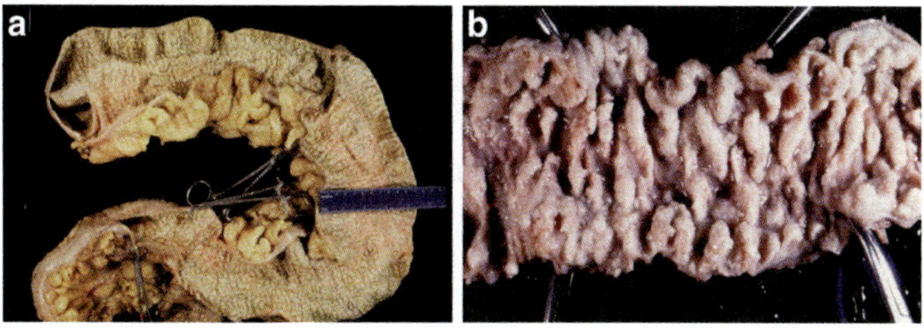

FIGURE 11.1. **a, b.** Gross pathology of florid pseudomembranous colitis due to *Clostridium difficile*.

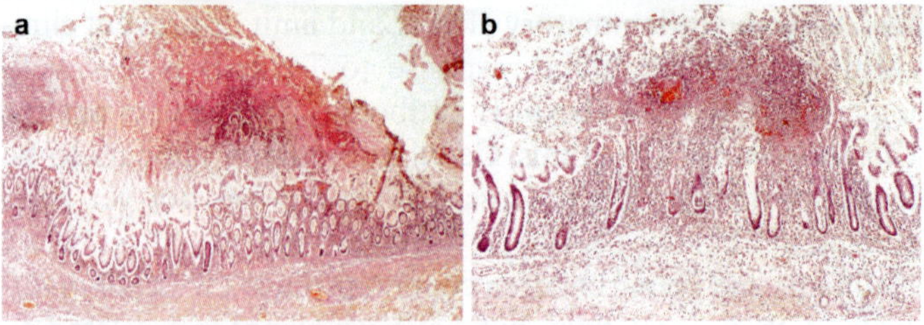

FIGURE 11.2. **a, b.** Microscopic section of severe pseudomembranous colitis due to *Clostridium difficile*. The pseudomembrane of dead leukocytes, mucosal epithelial cells, mucus, and adherent fibrin is obvious in the upper portion of photograph.

Clinical Presentation

Clostridium difficile diarrhea or colitis usually presents within 1–2 weeks of antibiotic treatment, although the presentation can vary from 1 day to 6 weeks. The symptoms can be quite variable and may include abdominal pain, low grade fevers, and diarrhea, which may be watery, mucoid and may contain blood. The spectrum of the colitis varies from colitis without pseudomembranes, pseudomembranous colitis, to fulminant colitis. Some individuals harbor both the bacteria and the two toxins yet never become symptomatic. Mild to moderate disease is usually associated with abdominal cramping, without other systemic manifestations. Moderate to severe colitis presents with profuse diarrhea, abdominal distention, abdominal pain, and occasionally, occult GI bleeding. Dehydration, electrolyte depletion, and hypoproteinemia due to a protein-losing colonopathy may occur with prolonged or severe disease. Systemic symptoms such as fever, malaise, nausea, and anorexia are usually observed. Fulminant colitis occurs in 1–3% of patients and presents with ileus, toxic megacolon, and perforation; death can occur in this form of disease. In addition, because of ileus and loss of colonic muscular tone, there may be a decrease in diarrhea in this form of disease. Other complications can include GI hemorrhage, sepsis, and pneumatosis coli. Overall, mortality is low (2–5%) but is considerably higher in elderly or debilitated patients (10–12%).

For patients with fulminant colitis or toxic megacolon, mortality approaches 30–80%.

In about 10% of patients, the disease is localized to the proximal colon and therefore is more difficult to diagnose. Patients with toxic megacolon typically present with an acute abdomen, localized rebound tenderness or guarding, no diarrhea, and no abnormalities on sigmoidoscopy. Abdominal films should be obtained to exclude free intraperitoneal air. The supine film in patients with toxic megacolon usually demonstrates a dilated transverse colon, thickened bowel wall, loss of haustra, and occasionally pseudopolyps. Contrast enema or endoscopy should not be pursued in patients when perforation or toxic megacolon is suspected.

Occasionally, this clinical picture can develop in neutropenic patients secondary to antineoplastic agents and can occur in the absence of antibiotic use; this presentation is typically ileocecitis or typhilitis caused by *Clostridium difficile*. Another severe form of *Clostridium difficile* colitis can be seen in women undergoing Cesarean section; altered colonic motility associated with pregnancy, in addition to the opiates given for post-operative pain management, well as the pre-operative prophylactic antibiotics contribute to development of *Clostridium difficile* colitis. This form of Clostridium difficile colitis is often associated with toxic megacolon in the absence of diarrhea. Another situation in which *Clostridium difficile* is a common etiologic agent is in the setting of enterocolitis associated with Hirschsprung's disease in infants and children.

Although the vast majority *Clostridium difficile* disease manifests as a colitis, *Clostridium difficile* enteritis is an established entity, albeit rare, that should not be overlooked in the post-colectomy patient. Several reports have documented fatal cases involving enteritis of both ileum and jejunum.

Diagnosis

Staphylococcal enterocolitis is a more uncommon cause of antibiotic-associated diarrhea but should be suspected when tests for *Clostridium difficile* are negative, and gram-positive cocci are seen on a stool smear. Neutropenic enterocolitis or typhilitis is the most common etiology of diarrhea and abdominal pain in patients receiving chemotherapy, particularly in the setting of neutropenia. Crohn's disease and ulcerative colitis can also mimic antibiotic-associated colitis, and an active *Clostridium difficile* infection in these patients can also cause what appears to be a flare of the primary disease. Other disease in the differential diagnosis of antibiotic-associated colitis include chemical colitis, ischemic colitis, and other infections, such as Campylobacter, Salmonella, Shigella, Escherichia coli, Listeria, and cytomegalovirus.

The diagnosis of *Clostridium difficile* colitis is based on a combination of clinical findings, laboratory tests, and occasionally, endoscopy. Fecal leukocytes may be seen on a stool smear, but their absence does not exclude *Clostridium difficile* colitis. Culture of *Clostridium difficile* is difficult and a poor choice for diagnosis, as many people are asymptomatic carriers.

The most sensitive and specific test for diagnosis of *Clostridium difficile* is a tissue culture assay for cytotoxicity of toxin B, using preincubation with neutralizing antibodies to show the specificity of the cytotoxicity. This test is 94–100% sensitive and 99% specific. This test is expensive, requires tissue culture facilities, and takes 1–3 days to run. Enzyme-linked immunosorbent assays (ELISA) are much easier, faster, and cheaper to conduct. These assays detect either toxin and have a sensitivity of 71–94% and a specificity of 92–98%. In 5–20% of patients, more than one stool sample may be required to detect the toxins. If *Clostridium difficile* is suspected and the first ELISA is negative, 1–2 additional stool samples should be sent. If ELISA remains negative, but the clinical index of suspicion is high, then the cytotoxicity test should be performed; this test will detect an additional 5–10% of cases missed by ELISA.

Radiologic imaging may be helpful in suspected cases of fulminant colitis. Plain abdominal x-rays may reveal ileus and/or a dilated colon and should also be obtained to rule out free air (Figs. 11.3a and b). Diffusely thickened or edematous

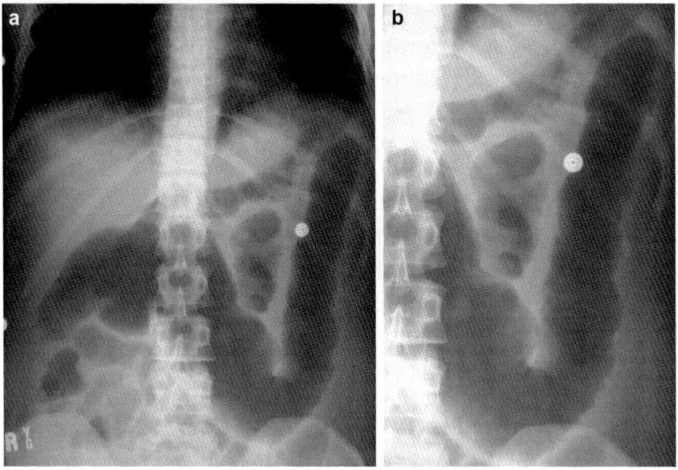

FIGURE 11.3. **a, b.** Plain abdominal radiograph of a patient with toxic megacolon due to severe *Clostridium difficile* enterocolitis; dilation involves primarily transverse colon.

colonic mucosa can sometimes be detected on abdominal computed tomography (CT) or as "thumbprinting" on plain abdominal x-rays. CT may also demonstrate colonic distention, thickening, or pericolonic inflammation and may be most helpful in cases where *Clostridium difficile* is localized to the proximal colon. A barium enema should not be performed because there is a high risk of perforation, especially with megacolon.

Sigmoidoscopy or colonoscopy is reserved for special situations such as the need to exclude another disease, need for rapid diagnosis, or in situations where a stool sample cannot be obtained due to ileus. One should remember, however, that sigmoidoscopy may be normal in patients with mild disease. In more severe colitis, pseudomembranes should be visible, although in 10% of cases, only the right colon may be involved. Most patients have some abnormality of colonic mucosa, ranging from minimal erythema or edema, to ulcerated mucosa, often with nodular exudates, which will eventually coalesce to form yellowish "pseudomembranes". Due to the increased risk of perforation, endoscopy should not be the first diagnostic intervention.

Treatment

Antibiotic treatment should be discontinued if possible and supportive therapy with fluids and electrolyte replacement instituted. Precautions of enteric isolation are recommended. Antiperistaltic and opiate drugs should be avoided, as they may mask symptoms or may worsen the course of the disease. Diarrhea resolves spontaneously, without specific antimicrobial therapy, in 25% of patients.

Antimicrobial treatment is indicated in any patient with other associated illness and in all cases of moderate to severe disease. In the appropriate clinical setting, antimicrobial treatment should be instituted before lab results confirm *Clostridium difficile*. Oral metronidazole or oral vancomycin are the drugs of choice; *Clostridium difficile* is sensitive uniformly to vancomycin. Rare cases of resistance to metronidazole have been reported. Because of the risk of selecting vancomycin-resistant enteric organisms, such as enterococcus, initial therapy with metronidazole is preferred at doses of 250–500 mg three times per day for 10–14 days. Therapy with metronidazole or vancomycin is effective in 95% of patients, although 10–20% of patients relapsed subsequently.

With severe ileus or toxic megacolon, intravenous metronidazole should be used, at doses of 500 mg given every 8h. Although intravenous therapy with vancomycin is not effective, this drug may be given rectally.

Despite successful treatment of the initial episode of *Clostridium difficile* diarrhea, 15–25% of patients will relapse after completing antibiotic therapy. Treatment of recurrent diarrhea includes conservative therapy without antibiotics, re-treatment with specific antibiotics against *Clostridium difficile*, use of anion binding resins, probiotics (therapy with "friendly" microorganisms), or immunoglobulin therapy. Conservative treatment of recurrent diarrhea is preferable to resumption of metronidazole or vancomycin, because these agents perpetuate the disturbance of the normal colonic flora; however, most patients are not able to tolerate ongoing diarrhea and will demand treatment. Persistent or worsening diarrhea, with confirmed *Clostridium difficile* infection, is an indication for more active treatment.

The most common therapy for recurrent *Clostridium difficile* diarrhea is a second course of the same antibiotic used to treat the first episode. Ninety-two percent of patients respond to a single course of repeat therapy. For patients with multiple recurrences, a prolonged course of vancomycin or metronidazole should be successful. Other treatment for persistent or recurrent disease include anion exchange resins such as cholestyramine to bind *Clostridium difficile* toxins, and biotherapy with probiotics aimed at restoring the "normal" colonic flora; these agents may include brewer's or baker's yeast taken by mouth, lactobacillus GG given as a concentrate in skim milk, a mixture of colonic bacteria in saline administered rectally in enema form, oral administration of non-toxigenic *Clostridium difficile*, and Saccharomyces boulardii, given as a capsule. No good, controlled studies have evaluated the efficacy of probiotic therapy.

Evidence now suggests that the immune response to *Clostridium difficile* toxin plays a major role in host susceptibility to this disease. Serum antibodies to *Clostridium difficile* toxin are low in patients with recurrent *Clostridium difficile* diarrhea. For these patients, treatment with normal, pooled, intravenous gamma globulin containing IgG anti-Toxin A was associated with a marked increase in serum antitoxin antibody and resolution of diarrhea. This therapy remains experimental.

Operative intervention is only required for *Clostridium difficile* colitis in about 3% of patients and only in those with more severe disease. More severe colitis is associated with advanced age, malignancy, renal failure, chronic pulmonary disease, immunosuppression, use of anti-peristaltic drugs, hypoalbuminemia, hemoconcentration, and significant increases or decreases in the patient's white blood cell count. Indications for operative intervention include acute abdomen, sepsis, multiorgan failure, hemorrhage, toxic megacolon, perforation, or deterioration despite aggressive medical treatment. Pneumatosis coli does not necessarily mandate operative treatment if it responds to aggressive medical treatment.

At laparotomy, the colon is edematous and distended. The serosa can appear normal despite severe mucosal disease. Segmental resections and diverting ileostomy without colonic resection have been described; however, these operations often fail, and an additional operative intervention is required, and mortality increases. Therefore, the operation of choice is a total abdominal colectomy with end ileostomy and Hartmann's pouch. Mortality for these patients is high, partly due to delay in diagnosis and need for total colectomy. In addition, the risk of local complications, such as perforation, increases substantially in patients with fulminant colitis which does not respond to medical therapy. Therefore, all patients with severe *Clostridium difficile* colitis whose condition does not respond to medical treatment within 48–72 h should be considered for operative intervention.

Selected Readings

Barbut R, Petit JC (2001) Epidemiology of *Clostridium difficile*-associated infections. Clin Microbiol Infect 7:405–410

Fekety R (1997) Guidelines for the diagnosis and management of *Clostridium difficile*-associated diarrhea and coli-tis. American College of Gastroenterology, Practice Parameters Committee. Am J Gastroenterol 92:739–750

Kelly CP, Pothoulakis C, LaMont JT (1994) *Clostridium difficile* colitis. N Engl J Med 330:257–262

Kyne L, Kelly CP (2001) Recurrent *Clostridium difficile* diarrhea. Gut 49:152–153

Lipsett PA, Samantaray DK, Tam MT, et al. (1994) Pseudo-membranous colitis: a surgical disease? Surgery 116:491–496

McFarland LV (1998) Epidemiology, risk factors and treatments for antibiotic-associated diarrhea. Dig Dis 16:292–307

Morris LL, Villalba MR, Glover JL (1994) Management of pseudomembranous colitis. Am Surg 60:548–551

Yassin SF, Young-Fadok TM, Zein NN, Pardi DS (2001) *Clostridium difficile*-associated diarrhea and colitis. Mayo Clinic Proceed 76:725–730

12 Toxic Megacolon

Bruce G. Wolff and Anne Marie Boller

Pearls and Pitfalls

- Initial medical management, in the absence of peritonitis or perforation, is appropriate and consists of supportive care, intravenous fluids, antibiotics, and steroid therapy.
- All narcotic medications (antidiarrheal, anticholinergic, and some antidepressant agents) should be discontinued upon suspicion of toxic megacolon.
- Associated underlying conditions and diseases include:
  - Ulcerative colitis
  - Crohn's disease
  - Bacterial infections such as Clostridium difficile colitis
  - Viral (CMV) and parasitic infections (Entamoeba histolytica, Cryptosporidium)
- CT scan may prove useful in demonstrating subclinical abscesses or perforations.
- Colonoscopic decompression is not recommended.
- Emergent surgical intervention is required for progressive dilatation or increasing systemic toxicity, perforation, peritonitis, hemorrhage, or failure of medical therapy.
- Surgical intervention is recommended with persistent colonic dilatation after 48–72 h of medical therapy.
- Subtotal colectomy with an end-ileostomy is the procedure of choice in the emergent or urgent setting.

K.I. Bland et al. (eds.), *Colorectal Surgery*,
DOI 10.1007/978-1-84996-444-9_12,

- Toxic megacolon which progresses to peritonitis and perforation is associated with an increased mortality rate.
- Delay in surgical intervention is associated with an increased mortality rate.
- Although controversial, toxic megacolon as the initial presentation of inflammatory bowel disease has been associated with a grave prognosis.
- Even "successful" medical management has been associated with recurrent bouts of toxic megacolon and the necessity for subsequent emergent surgical intervention.

Introduction

Toxic megacolon is a potentially fatal complication of inflammatory, ischemic, and infectious colitis. Early recognition, appropriate therapy, and surgical intervention are paramount when this diagnosis is suspected. Classically, toxic megacolon is defined as segmental or total colonic dilation greater than 6 cm, accompanied by signs of systemic toxicity and acute colitis. In 1950, Marshak et al. first described toxic megacolon in the literature as a complication with specific clinical features in relation to ulcerative colitis. Since this time, the diagnosis of toxic megacolon has been recognized in association with multiple different underlying diseases, including ulcerative colitis, Crohn's disease, pseudomembranous colitis, and additional infectious causes of colitis. Toxic megacolon requires immediate surgical consultation, as a delay in its diagnosis and the implementation of appropriate surgical interventions increases the risk of complications and associated mortality. In a study from the Mayo clinic which followed 38 patients with toxic megacolon managed nonoperatively, Grant and Dozois found a 29% incidence of recurrent bouts of toxic megacolon or colitis, which most often required emergent, subsequent surgery. Their results led them to the conclusion that medical management of toxic megacolon should be "regarded almost exclusively as preparation for imminent surgery."

Incidence

Exact estimations of the incidence of toxic megacolon are difficult to determine given the various underlying diseases responsible for the disorder, the lack of prospectively collected data, and the referral bias manifested by centers publishing reports regarding their experience with toxic megacolon. Although traditionally toxic megacolon was associated exclusively with ulcerative colitis, it is now recognized in association with Crohn's disease and most inflammatory causes of colitis. Grieco et al. cited the lifetime incidence of toxic megacolon in patients with ulcerative colitis between 1% to 2.5%, and in Crohn's disease between 1% to 6%. Current incidence rates associated with antibiotic-induced pseudomembranous colitis and subsequent toxic megacolon are estimated in up to 3%, although this number increases accordingly with the rising prevalence of this diagnosis.

Etiology

Although the majority of recognized cases are associated with ulcerative colitis, it is now recognized that a wide array of underlying diseases and causes of colitis may progress to toxic megacolon (Table 12.1). In addition to the diagnoses of inflammatory bowel disease, specifically ulcerative colitis and Crohn's disease, this includes the bacterial and viral causes of colitis such as Clostridium difficile, Salmonella, Shigella, Campylobacter, Cryptosporidium, Entameba histolytica, Yersinia and Cytomegalovirus. In contrast to Clostridium difficile, the remaining etiologies of bacterial colitis are rarely associated with the development of toxic megacolon. In HIV compromised patients, the diagnosis of CMV colitis is most frequently associated with the development of toxic megacolon, although Kaposi's sarcoma has also been implicated in this setting. Cytomegalovirus also has been documented in the development of toxic megacolon in the setting of immunocompromised patients and ulcerative colitis. Ischemic

TABLE 12.1. Causes of toxic megacolon.

Inflammatory bowel disease	Ulcerative Colitis
	Crohn's disease
Bacterial infection	*Clostridium difficile*
	Shigella Salmonella
	Yersinia
	Campylobacter
Viral infection	Cytomegalovirus
Other	Ischemic colitis
	Immunodeficiency
	Kaposi's sarcoma

colitis, especially associated with cancer chemotherapy, has been associated with the development of toxic megacolon.

Several risk factors have been noted in the development of toxic megacolon. In inflammatory bowel disease patients, the major risk factor is the severity of the underlying colitis. While ulcerative colitis typically involves the colonic mucosa, the underlying colitis and inflammation associated with toxic megacolon progresses transmurally in affected patients. Medications associated with toxic megacolon and inflammatory bowel disease include sulfasalazine, 5-aminosalicylic acid (5-ASA) and corticosteroids. Premature discontinuation of these medications, or a decrease in the dosage, may also be associated with toxic megacolon. Additional risk factors include barium enemas, antimotility medications, anticholinergics, and some antidepressants. Colonoscopy in the setting of suspected toxic megacolon is not recommended due to historic reports of its association with the development of the disorder.

Pathogenesis

While the exact mechanism responsible for the development of toxic megacolon is unclear at this time, there are likely several contributory factors. Severe inflammation associated with toxic megacolon progresses transmurally into the smooth muscle. The inflammation causes dysfunction of the associated smooth muscle and subsequent dilatation. It has been postulated that the severity of the dysmotility and dilatation are directly correlated with the degree of transmural inflammation. Metabolic disturbances and hypokalemia, which occur with toxic megacolon, are more commonly thought of as markers of disease progression, rather than inherent to the pathogenesis of the disease.

Nitric oxide (NO), a vasodilator, may contribute to the pathogenesis of toxic megacolon. Mourelle and colleagues studied the activity of nitric oxide synthase in a rat model and in humans affected by ulcerative colitis and toxic megacolon. The rat model revealed a correlation between inducible nitric oxide generation and impaired smooth muscle contractility. The human cohort studied colonic tissue from three different sets of patients: those with active pancolitis, toxic megacolon, and nonocclusive colon neoplasms. Toxic megacolon specimens were associated with inducible nitric oxide synthase in the muscularis propria of the affected colon. Excessive nitric oxide produced by NO synthase may be responsible for the colonic atony and dilatation associated with toxic megacolon.

Clinical History

The clinical picture of toxic megacolon may present as pancolitis or segmental disease. The diagnosis is equally prevalent in both genders and may occur at any stage of inflammatory bowel disease, with a notable portion of patients manifesting toxic megacolon as the initial presentation of their disease.

Toxic megacolon is defined as dilatation of the colon ≥6 cm in the setting of acute colitis, with the concomitant onset of systemic toxicity. Patients will present with clinic findings consistent with acute colitis, including diarrhea which is often bloody, abdominal pain, and cramping. These symptoms may precede colonic dilatation by a week or more. Progression to toxic megacolon may be accompanied by increasing distention, fever, tachycardia, an increased white

TABLE 12.2. Criteria for toxic megacolon (Modified from Sheth and LaMont (1998). Copyright 1998. With permission from Elsevier).

Jalan's criteria	
Fever	>101.5°F (38.6°C)
Heart rate	>120 beat/min
WBC	>10.5 (10^9/l)
Anemia	
Plus one of the following:	
	Dehydration
	Mental status changes
	Electrolyte disturbances
	Hypotension

blood cell count, or anemia. Jalan and colleagues established criteria for the diagnosis of toxic megacolon (Table 12.2). These criteria include the aforementioned clinical criteria with at least one of the following additional criteria: dehydration, mental changes, electrolyte disturbances, or hypotension. In this setting, patients may or may not manifest signs of peritonitis.

Immunocompromised patients, including HIV patients, may have minimal signs or symptoms on clinical examination. Medications should be reviewed for steroid usage and specifically, as possible risk factors, including antidiarrheal medications, narcotics, anticholinergics, and some antidepressants. All such medications, including narcotics, should be discontinued in a setting of suspicion for toxic megacolon.

Electrolyte disturbances are frequently present. Laboratory studies will reveal an elevated white cell count and anemia. Hypokalemia and hypoalbuminemia reflect ongoing diarrhea losses and dehydration. Stool cultures should be sent for Clostridium difficile toxin and blood cultures should be drawn. Endoscopy is indicated in the work up only when pseudomembranous or CMV colitis is suspected, and only on a limited basis. The high risk of perforation precludes the use of colonoscopy.

The clinical picture is supported by radiographic findings. Abdominal radiographs will demonstrate colonic dilatation ≥6 cm. Normal haustra may be absent on evaluation of the plain radiograph. The transverse colon is most frequently affected by the dilatation due to its superior and anterior anatomical position; however, the bowel gas may redistribute with patient position. Small bowel dilatation has been implemented in patients at high-risk for developing toxic megacolon. CT scans are useful in the evaluation of toxic megacolon. The presence of abscess and microperforations are discernible on CT scan but may be indiscernible on plain radiograph. Submucosal edema, wall thickening, ascites, and assessment of colonic and small bowel dilatation may also be accurately assessed with this modality. Toxic megacolon associated with pseudomembranous colitis may be more effectively evaluated with a CT scan, as many of the more subtle abscesses and small perforations have not been shown on plain film.

Management

A high index of suspicion and early intervention are crucial to the successful management of toxic megacolon. Medical management, surgical consultation, and appropriate surgical intervention are all required.

Medical management should be initiated immediately on suspicion of toxic megacolon. Bowel rest, nasogastric and bladder decompression, and intravenous fluid resuscitation are begun simultaneously with a surgical consultation. A long intestinal tube may be placed under fluoroscopic guidance. All narcotic medications, antimotility agents, and anticholinergics are discontinued. Appropriate broad-spectrum antibiotics are initiated and all previously administered antibiotics are halted, especially in bacterial colitis cases such as Clostridium difficile. Stress ulcer therapy and deep venous thrombosis prophylaxis are started at admission. Daily electrolyte values and abdominal films should be ordered and reviewed for signs of improvement or clinical degeneration. Patient repositioning to the prone or knee-elbow position multiple times throughout the day has been advocated to assist in decompressing the bowel. Total parental nutrition has not been shown to affect outcomes in patients with toxic megacolon, but is associated with septic and line-associated complications.

Intravenous corticosteroids should be started in the inflammatory bowel disease patient with toxic megacolon. Jalan and colleagues reviewed and compared ulcerative colitis patients treated with supportive care and those treated with steroids. Their retrospective analysis revealed a higher remission rate and better overall mortality within the group of patients who received steroids.

Patients whose condition does not improve in 48–72 h should proceed to surgery. Signs of perforation, persistent fever, signs of systemic toxicity, or ongoing transfusion requirements would indicate an earlier necessity for surgical intervention. Conversely, some patients who show an improvement in their colonic dilatation, without the onset of systemic complications, may be treated conservatively for as long as 7 days without surgical intervention.

Those requiring surgery due to ongoing dilatation or lack of clinical improvement should receive an elective subtotal colectomy and end ileostomy. Mortality rates decrease significantly when perforation is avoided (2–8% vs. 40%) and surgical intervention is elective (5%) and not emergent (30%). Dozois and Grant recognized that nearly one-third of their patients suffered a second episode of toxic megacolon, strengthening their assertion that "medical management of toxic megacolon should be regarded almost exclusively as a preparation for imminent surgery." Furthermore, their findings highlighted two additional groups who should be considered for surgery after the initial assessment: inflammatory bowel disease patients whose initial presentation occurs in the setting of toxic megacolon, and pregnant patients who present with toxic megacolon.

Conclusion

Toxic megacolon is a devastating manifestation of ischemic, infectious, and inflammatory colitis. Continuous monitoring and surgical surveillance is warranted in order to manage these patients appropriately. Timely surgical intervention decreases the mortality associated with toxic megacolon and improves patient outcomes.

Selected Readings

Caprilli R, Vernia P, Latella G, Torsoli A (1987) Early recognition of toxic megacolon. J Clin Gastroenterol 9:160–164

Dallal RM, Harbrecht BG, Boujoukas AJ, et al. (2002) Fulminant Clostridium difficile: an underappreciated and increasing cause of death and complications. Ann Surg 235:363–372

Gan SI, Beck PL (2003) A new look at toxic megacolon: an update and review of incidence, etiology, pathogenesis, and management. Am J Gastroenterol 98:2363–2371

Grant CS, Dozois RR (1984) Toxic megacolon: ultimate fate of patients after successful medical management. Am J Surg 147:106–110

Greenstein AJ, Sachar DB, Gibas A, et al. (1985) Outcome of toxic dilatation in ulcerative and Crohn's colitis. J Clin Gastroenterol 7:137–143

Grieco MB, Bordan DL, Geiss AC, Beil AR, Jr (1980) Toxic megacolon complicating Crohn's colitis. Ann Surg 191:75–80

Imbriaco M, Balthazar EJ (2001) Toxic megacolon: role of CT in evaluation and detection of complications. Clin Imaging 25:349–354

Jalan KN, Sircus W, Card WI, et al. (1969) An experience of ulcerative colitis. I. Toxic dilation in 55 cases. Gastroen-terology 57:68–82

Latella G, Vernia P, Viscido A, et al. (2002) GI distension in severe ulcerative colitis. Am J Gastroenterol 97:1169–1175

Marshak RH, Lester LJ (1950) Megacolon a complication of ulcerative colitis. Gastroenterology 16:768–772

Mourelle M, Casellas F, Guarner F, et al. (1995) Induction of nitric oxide synthase in colonic smooth muscle from patients with toxic megacolon. Gastroenterology 109:1497–1502

Mourelle M, Vilaseca J, Guarner F, et al. (1996) Toxic dilatation of colon in a rat model of colitis is linked to an inducible form of nitric oxide synthase. Am J Physiol 270:G425–430

Sheth SG, LaMont JT (1998) Toxic megacolon. Lancet 351:509–513

13 Colonic Volvulus

Chrispen D. Mushaya and Yik-Hong Ho

Pearls and Pitfalls

Sigmoid Volvulus

- More common than, appreciated, it represents the third most common cause of large bowel obstruction in the West; however, elsewhere, it may be the most common cause.
- Usually presents in elderly *males*; however, there is a young male predominance in areas with high incidence.
- Presenting signs and symptoms include: gross abdominal distension (may cause cardiac and respiratory embarrassment), colicky abdominal pain, and constipation.
- Plain abdominal x-rays show "omega"/inverted "coffee bean" sign or "Northern exposure" sign.
- Early recognition of imminent gangrene is crucial; non-gangrenous volvulus can be decompressed endoscopically with staged elective sigmoid colectomy.
- Gangrenous colon requires resuscitation and emergent sigmoid colectomy. Primary anastomosis is not recommended; a Hartmann's procedure is the preferred treatment.
- A subtotal colectomy should be considered as the primary procedure if there is concomitant megacolon or megarectum, because this will reduce the risk of recurrence after sigmoid colectomy alone.

K.I. Bland et al. (eds.), *Colorectal Surgery*,
DOI 10.1007/978-1-84996-444-9_13,

Cecal Volvulus

- Much less common! Usually in elderly *female* patients.
- Vomiting is prominent (because of involvement of terminal ileum); colicky abdominal pain and abdominal distension are other features.
- X-ray signs of volvulus on right side may be subtle and require a high index of suspicion.
- The diagnosis is often made only at laparotomy.
- Right hemicolectomy(primary anastomosis or stoma as appropriate) is indicated; reduction alone results in high risk of recurrence.

Sigmoid volvulus was first described as far back as the Ebers Papyrus in 1500. Colonic volvulus usually occurs in the sigmoid colon and less commonly in the cecum, however, volvulus occurs, rarely in the transverse colon and splenic flexure.

Pathogenesis

Anatomic variation involving a freely mobile colonic mesentery and a narrow base allows volvulus to occur. Other risk factors include chronic constipation, megacolon, neurologic diseases, adhesions, Hirschsprung's disease, Chagas' disease, ischemic colitis, ileus, and pregnancy. In areas with a high incidence of sigmoid volvulus, such as Africa, a diet high in fiber and carbohydrates results in large fecal bulk and gas content, which predisposes the sigmoid mesentery to twist, leading to chronic sigmoiditis. This cicatricial reaction further narrows the base of the mesentery, increasing the risk for volvulus. The degree of torsion varies with more than 360 degrees in over 50% of the patients, most commonly in a counterclockwise manner (Fig. 13.1). Cecal volvulus is predisposed by an incomplete embryologic bowel rotation and retroperitoneal fixation, the so called floppy cecum, which occurs in about 10% of adults.

Closed-loop obstruction causes early gangrene with an attendant high morbidity and mortality. Anaerobic bacteria

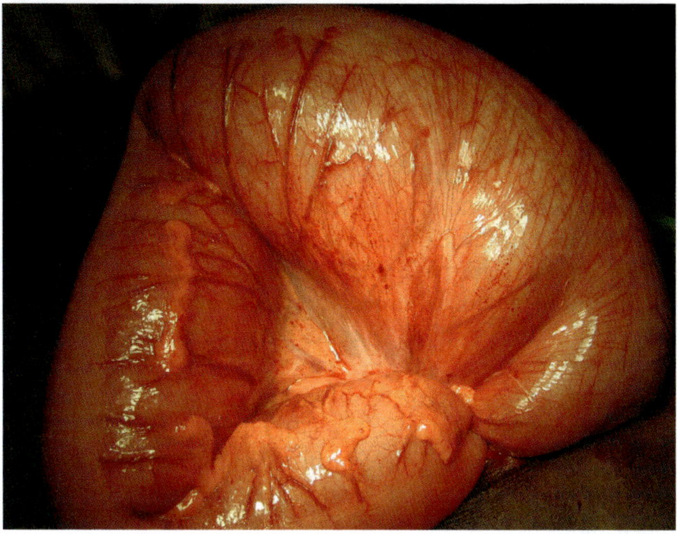

FIGURE 13.1. Sigmoid volvulus with 360° counterclockwise torsion, forming a knot.

produce massive amount of endotoxins which easily traverse the compromised bowel and highly permeable peritoneum to enter the circulation. Progression to perforation and generalized peritonitis in the elderly, frail patient is almost universally fatal.

Sigmoid Volvulus

Clinical presentation: In most Western countries, sigmoid volvulus is the third most common cause of colonic obstruction after cancer and diverticulitis, and accounts for about 5% of all colonic obstructions. In many areas of the developing world, including Africa, Asia, Eastern Europe, South America, and the Middle East, sigmoid volvulus is the most common cause (~50%) of large bowel obstruction. The most common presentation in the West of a frail, elderly, 70- to 80-year-old male (63%) contrasts with the younger 40-year-old male in countries where sigmoid volvulus is more common. This condition is rare in children, occurring predominantly in males (90%) with a mean age of 10 years; in this age group, sigmoid volvulus is often associated with ileosigmoidal knotting in which the small bowel mesentery becomes chronically inflamed from recurrent twisting of the sigmoid mesentery. These children often suffer from worm infestation. Acute, marked, abdominal distension is an important feature, so much so as to cause cardio-respiratory compromise in some patients. Constipation tends to be absolute, but vomiting is unusual unless there is ileosigmoidal knotting. Abdominal pain is initially colicky and centered in the left lower quadrant, but becomes more diffuse as the condition progresses. Emptiness can be seen or felt in the left iliac fossa in as many as 28% of patients. The differential diagnosis involves other causes of large bowel obstruction, including colorectal cancer, diverticulitis, pseudo-obstruction, and constipation with megacolon.

Patients tend to have multiple medical co-morbidities and are often institutionalized for psychiatric conditions, making their clinical condition more desperate. Over 50% of patients have at least one clinically important operative risk factor. It must be emphasized that gangrene occurs in the twisted sigmoid loop in up to 20% of patients and is an ominous factor predisposing to morbidity and mortality. Fever, hemodynamic compromise, or peritonitis should raise suspicion for colonic gangrene. In severe cases, the abdominal distension may cause respiratory compromise (Fig. 13.2).

Diagnosis: A confident diagnosis of sigmoid volvulus can be made on abdominal x-rays in 60–75% of patients. The characteristic "omega" or inverted "coffee bean" sign or shape is formed by grossly dilated and closely opposed sigmoid loops, and the "Northern exposure" sign, formed by dilated sigmoid colon that ascends cephalad to the transverse colon, is virtually pathognomonic (Fig. 13.3). If the diagnosis is in doubt, a water-soluble contrast enema will show a "bird beak" sign from the characteristic obstruction at the rectosigmoid junction. CT of the abdomen is employed rarely and shows a "whirl pattern" of the dilated sigmoid loop around the mesocolon and a "bird beak" shape formed from the

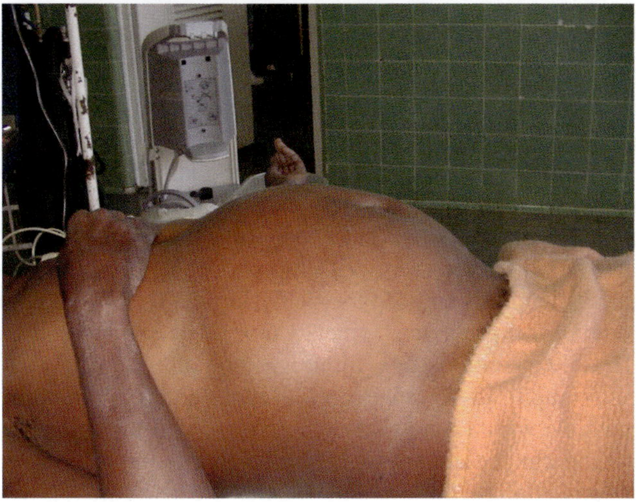

FIGURE 13.2. Sigmoid volvulus with marked abdominal distension causing acute respiratory compromise.

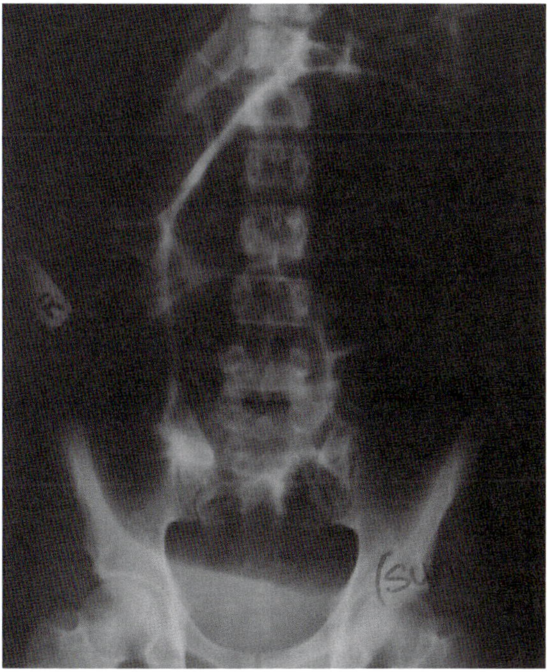

FIGURE 13.3. "Coffee bean" sign of sigmoid volvulus on plain x-ray.

affected segments. In lieu of contrast or complex radiologic investigations, a flexible sigmoidoscopy can be both diagnostic and therapeutic.

Treatment: When the bowel is *not* gangrenous, management involves non-operative relief of obstruction by endoscopic decompression. This approach allows for optimizing the frail, elderly patient with significant co-morbidities so that an elective operation can be performed to prevent recurrence. Decompression is typically more successful with use of a flexible sigmoidoscope, although the colonic twist usually occurs about 15–25 cm from the anal verge and should be accessible with a rigid sigmoidoscope. A well-lubricated rectal tube can be advanced carefully and gently beyond the torsion to deflate the volvulus. If a flexible instrument is used, the endoscope is passed carefully beyond the twist, and the distended bowel is deflated by suction. The deflated bowel will untwist spontaneously, but it is prudent to leave a tube for decompression until the patient is prepared for elective surgery to reduce the risks of early recurrences. In one report, 86% of patients who did not undergo operative intervention developed recurrent volvulus within a median of only 2.8 months.

Elective sigmoid colectomy is advised within the same hospital admission, but only after optimization of co-morbidities. Pre-operative workup should include a complete colonoscopy, as appropriate; a repeated bowel preparation is not necessary if the operation is timed in close proximity, and the patient kept on clear fluid oral intake. Pre-operative antibiotics against Gram negative bacteria and anaerobes are usually given on induction of general anesthesia; regional anesthesia can be employed safely in selected patients if indicated by co-morbidities. A mini-laparotomy with a 4–5 cm, muscle-slitting incision in the left iliac fossa enables the procedure to be performed easily and expediently with similar invasiveness as the laparoscopic approach. Provided that the diagnosis is correct, the redundant sigmoid colon is identified easily and exteriorized fully through the incision. There is no need to ligate the sigmoidal vessels at the base of the sigmoid mesentery. Instead, the latter can be divided effectively at the level of the

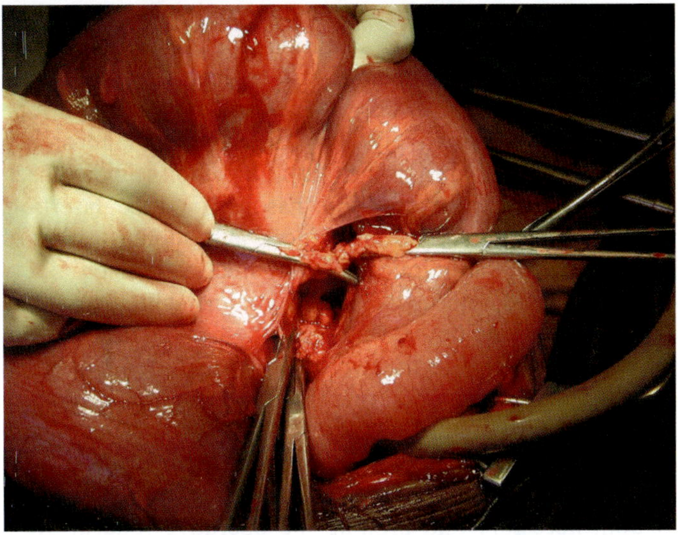

FIGURE 13.4. Thickened sigmoid mesentery in volvulus.

skin incision; the resultant adhesions should then prevent recurrence of volvulus. The sigmoid mesentery is always thickened, and special care must be taken to avoid bleeding from slipped ligatures (Fig. 13.4). A functional, end-to-end anastomosis can then be performed expediently. When performed properly, the entire operation can be completed safely. When there is concomitant megacolon or megarectum, a subtotal colectomy is recommended as the primary procedure to reduce the risk of recurrence after a sigmoid colectomy alone. In such circumstances and when the expertise is available, a laparoscopic approach may be suitable. Other methods to prevent recurrences of sigmoid volvulus after decompression include colopexy, laparoscopic or open sacral fixation, and mesosigmoid plasty. These procedures have not stood the test of time and are not accepted widely.

Emergent operative intervention is indicated if endoscopic decompression fails or is contra-indicated. The latter applies when the obstruction has been present for more than 72 h or when gangrenous bowel is suspected by clinical features described above (often accompanied by an increasing leukocytosis); under these conditions, the risk of perforation from endoscopic manipulation will be high. Delay in treatment is equally detrimental, however, and the patient must be resuscitated aggressively for an urgent laparotomy. Preoperative preparation includes intravenous fluid resuscitation, bladder catheterization, nasogastric tube insertion, correction of electrolyte imbalances, and administration of broad spectrum antibiotics. A lower midline incision is recommended for rapid access with minimal blood loss. The bowel may or may not be viable, but the sigmoid volvulus can be detorsed and a sigmoid resection performed. The fecal load in the colon can be evacuated manually, and a primary anastomosis can still be undertaken in select patients with very good results, even on rare occasions when the bowel is gangrenous. Elaborate measures such as on-table lavage are seldom necessary and prolong the operative time in these sick patients. In most patients, when the patient's general condition remains unstable or when there is gross peritoneal soiling, a Hartmann's procedure is the procedure of choice. A double-barrel or loop colostomy diversion proximal to a primary anastomosis can be an alternate consideration.

Outcomes: The patient should show objective improvement by postoperative day4, otherwise an anastomotic leak should be suspected. The overall hospital mortality is about 6–14%; the greatest mortality occurs in patients undergoing emergent resection and primary anastomosis in the presence of gangrenous sigmoid colon.

Cecal Volvulus

Clinical presentation: Cecal volvulus is a much more uncommon cause of bowel obstruction, being responsible for less than 2% of intestinal obstructions. The patient is usually an elderly lady, although in endemic areas, patients present at a younger age. Clinical features depend on the degree and duration of the twist. The "floppy" or "mobile" cecum syndrome occurs when patients present with acute right lower abdominal pain, which resolves after passing a large gush of flatus. These patients usually have a history of similar attacks in the past. In contrast, if the volvulus is complete, the patient will present with clinical features of small intestinal obstruction with colicky abdominal pain, constipation, abdominal distension, and especially vomiting. When the cecum becomes gangrenous, the clinical presentation is more ominous; findings of peritonitis maybe florid and perforation becomes an imminent risk. The cecal bascule is a different anatomic entity which includes an upward and anterior twist of the cecum. Cecal bascule shares many similarities with cecal volvulus, including a tendency to give rise to intestinal obstruction.

Diagnosis: Because cecal volvulus is uncommon, a high index of suspicion is needed to make the diagnosis. The abdominal x-ray findings include right-sided colonic distension and obstruction or a "coffee bean" sign pointing to the left upper quadrant. Small bowel dilation may be prominent as well. If gangrenous bowel is not suspected, a contrast enema may demonstrate the volvulus with a sharp cut off "beak" sign; this test has a diagnostic sensitivity approaching 90%. The contrast enema may also reduce the volvulus in some patients. An abdominal CT is rapidly becoming the preferred imaging modality, because it shows the characteristic dilated cecum with air fluid levels ("coffee bean" sign) and progressive tapering of bowel loops at the site of the volvulus ("bird beak"). In addition, signs of mural ischemia suggestive of gangrene may be evident as well, although the sensitivity for ischemia is not high.

Treatment: If the diagnosis is suspected preoperatively, which is not always the case, an initial effort at non-operative treatment can be attempted. This approach is suitable only when the patient presents early, and ischemic bowel is not suspected. Reduction by barium enema reportedly been successful, although this approach is not advised as a treatment option in most patients. Endoscopic decompression can be employed, but again, this approach is known to have a limited success rate of less than 30% and requires experienced endoscopists. The risk of perforation is high.

The surgical options in these patients are variable and depend on the patient's condition at presentation, the intra-operative findings, and the surgeon's experience. Because cecal volvulus is not a common condition, no randomized trials are available to guide management. If the bowel is viable, manual detorsion of the volvulus can be performed, but simple detorsion of the volvulus has a recurrence rate of over 70%. Cecopexy is another well-described technique, where the cecum and ascending colon are anchored or pexed broadly to the lateral parietal peritoneum with suture fixation. The recurrence rate after this technique is as great as 40%. Surgeons who favor this approach claim that this is an easy and quick procedure, hence, the patient spends less time under anesthesia. Moreover, preservation of the terminal ileum and ileocecal valve results in less physiologic disturbance. The seromuscular sutures are difficult to place, however, and are poorly retained in edematous tissue. Cecostomy is an option, but carries a high risk of postoperative mortality. Leakage around sutures and cecal necrosis leading to loss of fixation around the cecostomy tube is not uncommon.

When bowel ischemia occurs, resection is necessary, and in most patients a primary anastomosis with well-vascularized bowel is possible. In some patients, however, it may be safer to fashion a stoma because an anastomotic leak will confer disastrous consequences. Where the patient is treated in an elective setting, laparoscopic colectomy can be considered if a skilled laparoscopist is available.

Outcomes: An excessively mobile cecum, together with other factors which include chronic constipation and a high fiber diet, suggest the occurrence of a cecal volvulus. Colonic distension with cecal displacement during pregnancy may also cause this condition in susceptible individuals.

Ideal patient care is largely determined by the particular case merits, and hence, the judgment of the treating physician. Most patients with cecal volvulus are difficult to diagnose preoperatively, and many patients are operated on with the presumptive diagnosis of peritonitis or small bowel obstruction. Adequate preoperative fluid and electrolyte resuscitation is important, especially if there is gangrenous bowel, which adversely affects the outcome of the patient.

Operative options depend largely on the experience of the surgeon, although it is generally agreed that colectomy will avoid recurrence. The ideal operative option remains controversial, but most surgeons favor ascending colectomy. In a series in which a right hemicolectomy was performed, the postoperative mortality was 7% and the morbidity was 20%, mainly attributed to sepsis.

Selected Readings

Atamanalp SS, Yildirgan MI, Basoglu M, et al. (2004) Sigmoid colon volvulus in children: review of 19 cases. Pediatr Surg Int 20:492–495

Ballantyne GH (1982) Review of sigmoid volvulus: history and results of treatment. Dis Colon Rectum 25:494–501 Catalano O (1996) Computed tomographic appearance of sigmoid volvolus. Abdom Imaging 21:314–317

Chung YFA, Eu K-W, Nyam DCNK, et al. (1999) Minimizing recurrence after sigmoid volvulus. Br J Surg 86:231–233

Tuech JJ, Pessaux P, Regenet N, et al. (2002) Results of resection for volvolus of the right colon. Tech Colopoctol 6:97–99

Utpal D, Ghosh S (2003) Single stage primary anastomosis without colonic lavage for left-side colonic obstruction due to acute sigmoidal volvolus: a prospective study of one hundred and ninety-seven cases. ANZ J Surg 73:390–392

14 Rectal Prolapse and Solitary Rectal Ulcer

Susan Galandiuk

Pearls and Pitfalls

- Always examine patients in the upright straining position; prolapse may not be apparent in other positions.
- Full thickness prolapse can be differentiated from hemorrhoidal disease by the concentric rings of mucosa, unlike the "clusters" associated with hemorrhoids.
- In the absence of overt prolapse, but with symptoms suggestive of constipation and straining, a defecating proctogram may be helpful in identifying the source of the problem.
- In the presence of non-relaxing puborectalis syndrome, operative intervention will be doomed to failure if paradox muscle function is not first corrected through biofeedback.
- Failure to reduce and treat overt rectal prolapse may lead to permanent sphincter damage.
- In the majority of patients, one can only assess the restoration of sphincter function to its baseline 6 months following correction of rectal prolapse.

Clinical Presentation

Straining is the common denominator among rectal prolapse, procidentia and solitary rectal ulcer syndrome. Rectal prolapse, while very common in the nursing home population, is

K.I. Bland et al. (eds.), *Colorectal Surgery*,
DOI 10.1007/978-1-84996-444-9_14,

approximately six times more common in women than in men. The highest incidence in women starting in the 5th and subsequent decades. Women who are particularly at high risk are those who have had multiple vaginal deliveries and especially those who have had a hysterectomy. In some studies, more than half of the patients with prolapse have a history of constipation and a history of straining. If not corrected and not reduced, rectal prolapse can lead to permanent injury of the anal sphincter due to stretching. Prolapse should therefore, always be reduced and should be repaired soon after diagnosis. Most patients with prolapse have several common anatomic abnormalities including: (1) relative separation or diastasis of the levator ani muscles; (2) a deep cul-de-sac; (3) redundant sigmoid colon; (4) a narrow small caliber rectum with loosening of the normal posterior and lateral attachments, that allows the rectum to "telescope" out as a prolapse; and (5) a weakened anal sphincter. Prolapse in children is different from that in adults and will be addressed separately at the end of this chapter.

Diagnosis

Symptoms: Other than the obviously prolapsing rectum, loose discharge or incontinence for mucus is a typical symptom in cases of rectal prolapse. Due to trauma to the prolapsing rectal mucosa, rectal bleeding is common. With the close proximity of the bladder, in women, due to pelvic floor laxity, there is often an associated cystocele. In assessing the patient's symptoms, one should therefore inquire regarding difficulty urinating, urinary incontinence and urinary tract infections. In most patients with rectal prolapse, the prolapse acts almost like a "plug" and causes significant constipation. The degree of impairment of fecal continence may therefore be more difficult to ascertain.

Physical examination: Rectal prolapse is an embarrassing situation, and unless the patient is very frail and old and doesn't care, demonstration of rectal prolapse to a physician is typically associated with anxiety and embarrassment on the part of the patient! It is best demonstrated in the upright position while straining and this is best done on a toilet. Unless the prolapse is huge, it may not be apparent in other positions. Almost all patients with rectal prolapse will have a lax anal sphincter. Rectal prolapse can be differentiated from hemorrhoids by the concentric rings characteristic of full thickness prolapse in contrast to hemorrhoids (Fig. 14.1).

Patient evaluation: Evaluation of the patient should assess the colon in order to exclude pathology such as cancer and polyps. Because of the significant constipation and difficulty cleansing the colon, subsequent difficulty clearing barium, and frequently impaired sphincter function, barium enemas are frequently nearly impossible to perform in these patients. The pre-operative evaluation can be performed on 2 different days with two different sets of tests performed: (1) defecating proctography and then at another time;

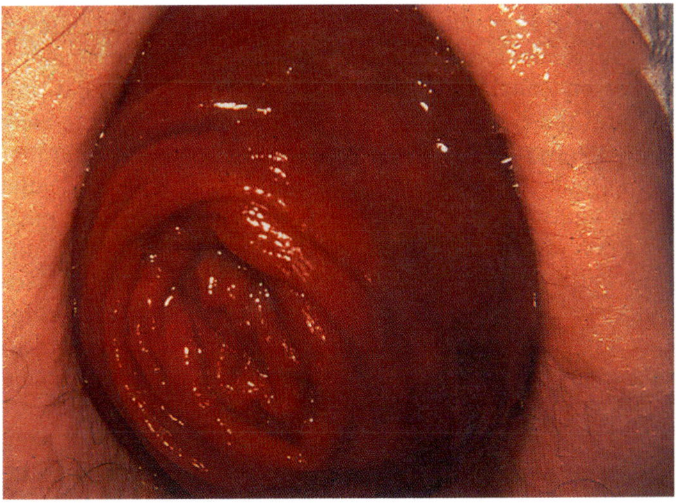

FIGURE 14.1. Full thickness rectal prolapse. Note the concentric folds characteristic of full thickness prolapse, which contrast to the clusters of "bundles" characteristic of prolapsing grade III or IV hemorrhoids.

(2) pudendal nerve terminal motor latency testing, anorectal manometry, endoanal ultrasound and colonoscopy. With a defecating proctogram, thick barium paste is inserted into the rectum. Barium is used to mark the vagina, and contrast is instilled into the bladder. Dynamic views during straining and defecation demonstrate whether there is appropriate puborectalis muscle relaxation. The defecating proctogram allows for assessment of associated vaginal vault prolapse and determination of whether a cystocele is present. With the close proximity of the pelvic organs, failure to correct an associated vaginal prolapse could, for example, act as a lead point for a prompt recurrence of rectal prolapse. Performing a sacrocolpopexy, cystocele repair or bladder suspension in conjunction with a urogynecologist or gynecologist may therefore be important in lessening the risk for postoperative recurrence.

If anorectal physiology testing is not available, only colonoscopy is performed in addition to defecating proctography. This excludes proximal pathology as the cause of constipation. If available, pudendal nerve terminal motor latency testing can demonstrate whether or not there has been injury to the pudendal nerve from chronic stretch injury and prolapse of the rectum. This is very simply assessed by an electrode that is strapped to the index finger of the examiner that allows one to deliver an electrical signal to the pudendal nerve and measure the time delay for an electrode to measure contraction of the anal sphincter. Prolongation of this time indicates nerve injury. Anorectal manometry allows for objective assessment of internal and external anal sphincter function and endoanal ultrasound allows the examiner to document the degree of sphincter atrophy and also any unsuspected anterior obstetrical injury, which is often present. This information is helpful in predicting what anal sphincter function the patient will have after correction of the rectal prolapse. Pudendal nerve terminal motor latency testing, anorectal manometry and endoanal ultrasound, each take about 5 min to perform and are typically done prior to the colonoscopy.

Treatment

Non-operative Therapy

Unless the prolapse is small and the patient can reduce it after every bowel movement, non-operative therapy in my experience is uniformly unsuccessful and is doomed to failure. Non-operative therapy is generally directed at treating the constipation, minimizing straining and reducing the prolapse whenever it occurs.

Deciding on the Type of Surgery for Rectal Prolapse

Few conditions have generated so many operations for their correction as has rectal prolapse. Important with respect to the treatment of this condition is the fact that no matter how it is corrected surgically, there is over a 10% recurrence rate. The younger the patient, the higher the recurrence, due to the longevity of the subject. An important factor with respect to recurrence is the fact that many of these patients are chronic strainers. This and the already weakened pelvic floor are both high risk factors for recurrence.

Operative repair of rectal prolapse is divided into two broad categories of procedures: (1) perineal procedures with or without correction of the levator diastasis, and (2) abdominal procedures with fixation of the rectum with or without resection. Generally speaking, perineal procedures are reserved for older patients since they are associated with (1) loss of the rectal reservoir capacity, (2) more sphincter trauma, and (3) a higher recurrence rate. Perineal procedures can, however, be done under local anesthesia with IV sedation and are therefore suitable for even the most ill and moribund patients. Trans-abdominal procedures with or without resection are reserved for younger patients and are associated with a lower risk of recurrence.

Perineal Proctectomy

In the older debilitated patient, perineal proctectomy is the procedure of choice. Although it has a slightly higher recurrence rate, it has a low complication rate and can be performed under local anesthesia with intravenous sedation. If there is an extremely lax pelvic floor or extreme diastasis of the levator muscle, a levator plication can be performed during the same approach by plicating the levator muscle using non-absorbable suture prior to performing the colo-anal anastomosis. The entire rectum and lower sigmoid colon can be removed transanally using this approach. The downside of this procedure is that in many cases much or even the entire reservoir capacity of the rectum is removed. The symptom of fragmentation with frequent small bowel movements is common following this procedure. Although the use of the circular stapler has been reported by some, the hand sewn approach is simple, safe and cost effective. With this approach, the rectal prolapse is pulled out as far as it will come using Babcock clamps, and the rectal wall transected full thickness approximately 1 cm above the dentate line using the electrocautery (Fig. 14.2a). While the distal rectal wall is tagged using stay sutures of 2-0 polyglycolic acid, the proximal rectum is retracted distally (Fig. 14.2b). The rectal mesentery is then systematically clamped, divided, and ligated. The proximal bowel is slowly divided, as quadrant tacking sutures are placed and a one layer interrupted hand-sewn coloanal anastomosis is performed using 2-0 absorbable suture (Fig. 14.2c). Although patients have a lax anal sphincter during and at the conclusion of surgery, in approximately 50% of patients there will be a restoration of normal anal sphincter tone within 6 months of surgery. In the interim, fiber products and antidiarrheals are frequently necessary to adjust bowel function to maintain continence by providing for fewer, bulkier bowel movements. Table 14.1 shows a summary of recurrence, morbidity and mortality data for perineal proctectomy.

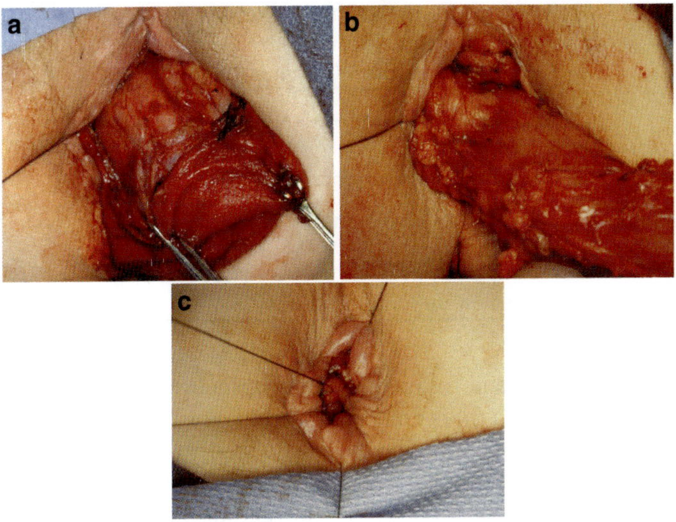

FIGURE 14.2. **a.** Perineal proctectomy is begun by inducing prolapse and grasping the prolapsed rectum with Babcock or Allis clamps. A full thickness incision is made through the rectal wall approximately 1 cm proximal to the dentate line using the electrocautery. As the bowel is divided, the distal rectum is tagged with stay sutures of absorbable suture material. I prefer 2-0 polyglycolic acid. **b.** Once the rectal wall is transected, traction is applied and the proximal rectum is pulled downward. The mesentery of the bowel is then systematically clamped, divided and ligated using absorbable suture. **c.** Once the prolapsed rectum has been resected, a single layer anastomosis is created between the proximal rectum or colon and the distal rectum using interrupted absorbable 2-0 polyglycolic acid suture. Four quadrant stay sutures are applied to the proximal colon to facilitate suturing.

Abdominal Procedures

As with low anterior resection, and ultra low anterior resection in which the majority of the reservoir capacity of the rectum is removed, patients with perineal proctectomy have

TABLE 14.1. Summary of results for perineal proctectomy for rectal prolapse (Data from Goligher, 1980).

	No. (%)
Patients reported	402
Calculated recurrence	30 (7)
Post-operative mortality	3 (1)
Complications	50 (12)
Follow-up (range in years)	1–17

fragmentation and frequent small volume bowel movements. High recurrence rates are also reported. For these reasons, in younger patients who have an expected greater longevity, transabdominal populations are more suitable. These maintain the reservoir capacity of the rectum and involve both fixation of the rectum to the sacral promontory to minimize the chance of recurrent prolapse, as well as resection of the redundant bowel to reduce the incidence of postoperative constipation. Abdominal procedures can either be done via open or laparoscopic approaches. An extensive rectal mobilization to induce fixation or scarring of the rectum to the sacral hollow is common to all of these procedures. Some fixation procedures such as the Ripstein procedure that have involved sling-type fixation of the rectum to the sacral promontory have been associated with a higher degree of postoperative constipation either due to the sling being too snug or due to sling fibrosis. In addition, in the existence of preexisting constipation, the persistence of constipation is more common following rectopexy alone than following resection and rectopexy. Other methods of fixation, such as the polyvinyl alcohol sponge that has been popular in Britain have not been used extensively in the United States. The most common abdominal procedure in the United States is abdominal rectopexy with sigmoid resection as originally described by Frickman in 1955. A summary of the recurrence rates, morbidity and mortality for Ripstein rectopexy and resection rectopexy are shown in Tables 14.2 and 14.3, respectively.

TABLE 14.2. Summary of results for Ripstein procedure for rectal prolapse (Data from Goligher, 1980).

	No. (%)
Patients reported	2,058
Calculated recurrence	60 (3)
Post-operative mortality[a]	8 (1)
Complications[b]	327 (19)
Follow-up (mean years)	5

[a]*Only reported for 947 patients.*
[b]*Only reported for 1,748 patients*

TABLE 14.3. Summary of results for sigmoid resection and rectopexy for rectal prolapse (Data from Goligher, 1980).

	No. (%)
Patients reported	243
Calculated recurrence	6 (2.5)
Post-operative mortality	2 (1)
Complications[a]	13 (6)
Follow-up (mean years)[b]	3.5

[a]*Only reported for 226 patients.*
[b]*Only reported for 215 patients.*

The Delorme procedure in which a mucosectomy is performed on the prolapsed rectum and the muscle wall plicated is not widely performed. It has been associated with a recurrence rate much higher than that reported for other procedures. The Thiersch procedure is used in children by placing absorbable suture around the distal rectum as a mechanical "vise" to keep the rectum from prolapsing, but this is not effective in adults and is essentially of historic interest.

Management of Fecal Incontinence Persisting > 6 Months Post-operatively

Nothing surgical should be done for 6 months postoperatively with respect to fecal incontinence following correction of rectal prolapse. During this time, normal restoration of sphincter tone can occur. If, however, the patient remains incontinent after this time, there are several treatment options; the first being an anterior sphincteroplasty if the patient has an obvious sphincter defect from a previous obstetrical injury that is demonstrated on endoanal ultrasound. Depending on patient age and pudendal nerve terminal motor latency, this may or may not be a viable option. In other words, if the patient is elderly, has a significant sphincter defect and significant nerve damage, functional results are likely to be poor. In this case, a better choice might be fecal diversion or implantation of an artificial anal sphincter (Acticon, American Medical Systems, Minnetonka, MN). This is an FDA-approved prosthetic device that yields functional results superior to sphincteroplasty in the presence of nerve injury, multiple sphincter defects or significant sphincter atrophy. In these cases, significant improvement from a sphincteroplasty would be unlikely. Postoperative infection is, however, a significant complication of this procedure. Other prosthetic products are available in Europe. Stimulated graciloplasty that was evaluated in clinical trials in the United States is not FDA-approved in the United States but is available in Europe.

Complications of Uncorrected Rectal Prolapse

If rectal prolapse is not corrected, incarceration of the hernia sack contents such as small bowel or even necrosis of the rectum can ensue, and in this case urgent surgery, rectal resection and colostomy are necessary (Fig. 14.3). If rectal prolapse is not corrected, it can lead to significant stretch injury to the anal sphincter and to trauma to the pudendal nerve.

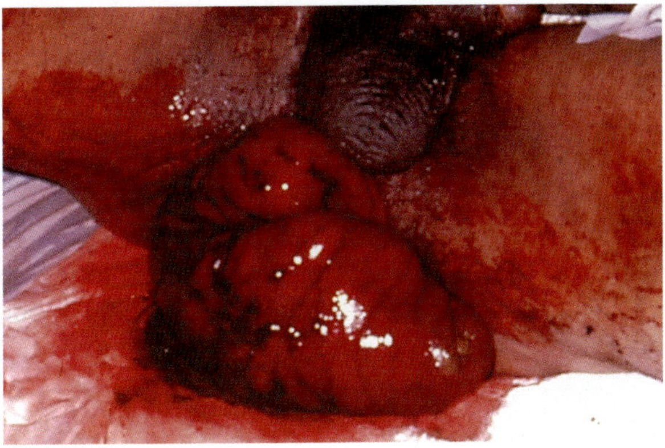

FIGURE 14.3. Incarcerated rectal prolapse containing small bowel in the cul de sac. Initially, an attempt was not made to reduce this in a timely fashion.

When the rectal prolapse is eventually corrected, severe disabling incontinence may result that does not improve over time and requires further surgical intervention.

Solitary Rectal Ulcer Syndrome

The occurrence of chronic straining can lead to the presence of solitary rectal ulcer syndrome or levator ani syndrome. The solitary rectal ulcer syndrome is an increasingly recognized nomenclature for a variety of rectal problems in which chronic constipation is common. This is also known as non-relaxing puborectalis muscle syndrome. Upon defecation, rather than relaxing in the normal fashion, the puborectalis muscle either does not relax or contracts, leading to straining and prolapse of the anterior rectal wall on the non-relaxed puborectalis muscle and chronic trauma. Rectal bleeding, mucus per rectum and tenesmus are common. The anterior rectal ulcer when seen is typically chronic and may appear polypoid rather than ulcerative. Dysfunctional defecation is a hallmark of the disease and used by many to explain the ulceration. This abnormal muscle behavior can be modified by biofeedback, it is not treated surgically. Attempts to treat this surgically without correction of the underlying abnormal muscle behavior result in prompt recurrence of the problem postoperatively. This problem may occur as early as adolescence. It is frequently characterized by bleeding and by the severe pain and tenesmus associated with the ulcer. Surgery may be necessary in cases in significant bleeding. Defecating proctography will often reveal obstructed defecation. A trial of anti-inflammatory 5-amino salicylic acid suppositories maybe helpful. If there is internal prolapse, correction of this is occasionally warranted.

Prolapse in Children

Prolapse in children is a different situation than in adults. The incidence is highest in the first 2 years of life and declines thereafter in contrast to the frequency in adults. A variety of predisposing causes have been proposed, including a failure of the rectosigmoid to follow the sacral curve; constipation, diarrhea, and excess laxative use. Boys are affected slightly more frequently than girls, and this is most frequently mucosal prolapse rather than full thickness prolapse. The mucosa may project as much as 4 cm beyond the anus, but is easily reduced. Unlike adults, rectal prolapse in children is a self limited disease and disappears with time. Treatment in the pediatric age group typically is directed at correcting constipation. Proper defecating habits and avoidance of laxatives and suppositories seem to work best. Various surgical procedures are used, including the Thiersch procedure in which an absorbable suture is placed to act like a "vise" and prevent prolapse. Resection is rarely needed.

Summary

Problems related to anatomic pelvic relaxation and functional issues with constipation and laxative use occur commonly worldwide. Rectal prolapse and its surgical treatment should take into consideration both patient age and associated pelvic floor defects. The operation must be matched to the individual patient. Irrespective of the procedure, recurrence is common.

Selected Readings

Altemeier WA, Culbertson WR, Schowengerdt CJ, Hunt J, (1971) Nineteen years' experience with the one-stage perineal repair of rectal prolapse. Ann Surg 173:993–1006

Beahrs OH, Theuerkauf FJ, Hill JR (1972) Procidentia: surgical treatment. Dis Colon Rectum 15:337–346

Frykman HM (1955) Abdominal proctopexy and primary sigmoid resection for rectal procidentia. Am J Surg 90:780–789

Goldberg SM, Gordon PH, Nivatvongs S (1985) Complications of surgery after complete rectal procidentia. In: Ferrari BT, Ray JB, Gathright JB (eds) Complications of colon and rectal surgery, prevention and management. W.B. Saunders, Philadelphia pp 251–266

Goligher JC (1980) Surgery of the anus, rectum and colon, 4th edn. Balliere Tindall, London, pp 224–258

Gordon PH (1999) Rectal procidentia. In: Gordon PH, Nivatvongs S (eds) Principles and practice of surgery for the colon, rectum, and anus, 2nd edn. Quality Medical Publishing, St. Louis, MO, pp 503–540

McMahan JD, Ripstein CB (1987) Rectal prolapse. An up-date on the rectal sling procedure. Am Surg 53:37–40

Neill NE, Parks AG, Swash M (1981) Physiological studies of the anal sphincter musculature in faecal incontinence and rectal prolapse. Br J Surg 68:531–536 take into consideration both patient age and associated pelvic floor defects. The operation must be tailored to the individual patient. Irrespective of the procedure, recurrence is common.

Selected Readings

Altemeier WA, Culbertson WR, Schowengerdt C, Hunt J (1971) [illegible] years' experience with the one stage perineal repair of rectal prolapse. Ann Surg 173:993–1006

[illegible] (19[illegible]) Procedentia: surgical treat[illegible]

15
Ischemic Colitis

Mario A. Abedrapo Moreira and Gonzalo Soto Debeuf

Pearls and Pitfalls

- The etiology of ischemic colitis is usually related to a low flow state.
- The symptoms of ischemic colitis are usually non-specific.
- One of the key points in diagnosis is a high index of suspicion by the clinician, especially in patients with risk factors.
- Currently, there are no sensitive or specific laboratory tests for detection of early ischemic colitis.
- Colonoscopy within the first 3 days of symptoms is the best diagnostic method for ischemic colitis.
- For patients without evidence of transmural ischemia, an initial trial of conservative management may be employed; conservative non-operative treatment is successful in the majority of patients with ischemic colitis (non-transmural ischemia).
- Careful observation with repeated evaluation is necessary in patients managed conservatively to assure absence of progressive disease.
- Only 15–20% of the patients require emergency operation, with mortality rates of 50–60% (transmural ischemia).
- Segmental resection of the ischemic colon with proximal diverting colostomy is recommended when emergency operation is required.
- A late sequela of ischemic colitis successfully managed conservatively is a colonic stricture.

K.I. Bland et al. (eds.), *Colorectal Surgery*,
DOI 10.1007/978-1-84996-444-9_15,

Introduction

The colon is the most common segment of the gastrointestinal tract where compromised blood flow produces clinically apparent ischemia. Ischemic colitis (IC), first described in 1963 by Boley, consists of a wide spectrum of clinical, endoscopic, and histopathologic alterations that range from a transient intramural ischemia of the colon to transmural necrosis; the latter is associated with a high mortality. This disease occurs typically in elderly patients when, as a result of inadequate tissue blood flow, the metabolic demands of the tissue supersede the delivery of oxygen, resulting in colonic ischemia. Most frequently, a non-occlusive diminution of the colonic blood flow is present, although occlusive factors can also be involved. The diagnosis of IC requires a high degree of clinical suspicion and confirmed by colonoscopy, the diagnostic method of choice. Most patients have intramural ischemia and a good prognosis, requiring only conservative management, whereas when transmural ischemia is evident, aggressive operative resection is indicated.

Epidemiology and Etiology

Approximately 1 in 2,000 acute hospital admissions are attributed to IC. The incidence of IC has been reported between 4.5 and 44 cases per 100,000 person-years. This incidence, however, may be underestimated due to the difficult diagnosis, especially in mild cases. In fact, after aortic surgery, in only 50% of patients with endoscopic and histologic confirmation of IC was the diagnosis suspected initially. IC is the most frequent form of ischemic changes of the gastrointestinal tract, representing approximately 50–60% of such cases. Generally, IC affects elderly people in the seventh and eight decades, with 90% of patients being older than 60 years of age. Irrespective of age, risk factors include cocaine use, hypercoagulable states, vasculitis, trauma, and marathon runners. There is a slight predilection for women (55–64%) in most reported series. In many cases, the exact etiology of IC is difficult to find. The most common etiology of IC is a hypoperfusion state secondary to shock or cardiac failure. Additional etiologies include mesenteric arterial thrombosis or embolism producing an occlusive type of ischemia. IC may also develop after procedures where technical factors may contribute, such as vascular surgery (especially those after repair of an abdominal aortic aneurism) and left colectomy (Table 15.1).

Pathophysiology

Perfusion of the colon and rectum depends on inflow from the mesenteric arteries (superior and inferior) and on the internal iliac vessels. In the region of the splenic flexure, the arc of Riolan and the marginal artery of Drummond join the superior and inferior mesenteric systems, producing a zone potentially vulnerable to ischemia (also called the watershed area) where the blood supply between both arterial territories is suboptimal. Up to 30% of the patients do not have a sufficient communication between both systems, predisposing this area of the splenic flexure to ischemia. Despite this, IC is usually not confined to the splenic flexure, and any segment of the colon can be affected, leading some to question whether IC is really an ischemic phenomenon at all. IC occurs most commonly in the descending and sigmoid colon (40%), followed by the transverse colon and splenic flexure (17%), the splenic flexure alone (11%), the right colon (12%), and the rectum (6%). The ischemia is secondary to alterations of the systemic circulation or of the mesenteric circulation itself. The colon is particularly sensitive to decreased mesenteric blood flow, because the colonic circulation does not have an adequate self-regulation and because there is poor microcirculation in the muscular walls. The histologic alterations consist initially of edema and hemorrhage of the mucosa and submucosa, with the potential for progression to ulceration, transmural ischemia, necrosis, and eventual perforation. In cases of non-transmural colonic ischemia, parietal fibrosis with secondary colonic stricture may develop in the long term.

TABLE 15.1. Etiology of ischemic colitis.

I. Non-occlusive factors
1. Idiopathic
2. Shock
(a) Septic
(b) Hemorragia
(c) Cardiogenic
(d) Hypovolemic
3. Drugs
(a) Catecholamines
(b) Diuretics
(c) Digitalis
(d) Estrogens, oral contraceptives
(e) NSAIDs
(f) Cocaine
4. Colon obstruction
(a) Colon cancer
(b) Fecal impaction
II. Occlusive factors
1. Arterial
(a) Embolus
(b) Thrombosis
(c) Post aortic reconstructive surgery
(d) Trauma
(e) Vasculitis
2. Venous
(a) Hypercoagulable status
(b) Pancreatitis

Clinical Presentation

The central point in the clinical presentation and diagnostic evaluation of the patient with IC is clinical suspicion. The clinician must consider the diagnosis of IC in elderly patients with abdominal symptoms and risk factors such as recent aortic surgery (ligated inferior mesenteric artery), patients in shock and under the effect of vasoconstrictor drugs (diminution of the mesenteric and specially colonic blood flow), and patients with predisposing factors to mesenteric insufficiency (atherosclerotic vascular disease, ischemic heart disease, congestive heart failure). Although this is the classic history of a patient with IC, this diagnosis must also be considered in young patients (especially women) using cocaine or oral contraceptives, patients with known vasculitis or hypercoagulable states, and in long distance runners. The clinical presentation is dependent frequently on the degree of colonic ischemia. IC should be suspected in patients with risk factors who present with slight to moderate abdominal pain (2/3 of the patients), bloody diarrhea (2/3 of the patients), nausea/vomiting (1/3 of the patients), or abdominal distention. The pain is generally sudden in onset, crampy, located in the left side of the abdomen, and associated with urge to defecate. Rectal bleeding, red or darker, according to the location of the ischemia, is generally self-limiting, and transfusion is required only rarely. Initially, the patient with IC is generally stable, without hemodynamic compromise and without signs of peritonitis, reflecting the fact that most of the patients do not have transmural ischemia; however, when transmural ischemia is present, the patients will develop peritoneal signs, and the risk of perforation is imminent.

Diagnosis

Patients with suspected IC must undergo appropriate evaluation to confirm the diagnosis. The biochemical markers are generally non-specific; however, leukocytosis may be present.

Serum lactate determination deserves special mention due to its frequent use when intestinal ischemia is suspected. Although it is true that serum lactate increases in some patients with advanced IC, the serum lactate level is non-specific and lacks adequate sensitivity. Second, in intestinal ischemia, lactate is removed from the portal circulation by the liver; therefore, its utility is extremely low, especially in the initial phase of IC.

In the evaluation of patients with abdominal pain, abdominal and chest radiographs may be useful to exclude other diagnoses, such as visceral perforation or intestinal obstruction. The radiographic findings in IC are also generally non-specific. Air/barium contrast enemas have the risk of further decreasing the effective colonic blood flow by increasing the parietal pressure, may interfere with subsequent study by computed tomography (CT), and are not recommended when IC is suspected. CT of the abdomen and pelvis allows for screening of other abdominal pathologies and, in the case of IC, can demonstrate a non-specific segmental thickening of the colonic wall, air within the colon wall, or free air. Angiography is generally not useful because of its low sensitivity. Colonoscopy is the preferred diagnostic modality in patients with suspicion of IC.

In emergency cases, in which the colon cannot be prepared (e.g., patients in the intensive care unit), careful endoscopic examination requires gentle water flush to clean the colonic mucosa for inspection. Minimal insufflation of the colon during colonoscopy is necessary to avoid perforation when transmural ischemia is present. In more clinically stable patients where time allows, it may be possible to give an oral bowel preparation prior to endoscopy. The endoscopic study must be made as early as possible to determine presence of ischemia and allow appropriate intervention to avoid progressive ischemia or perforation. The endoscopic view is fundamental for the diagnosis, evaluation of the magnitude of the ischemia, management, and follow-up of the patient. In mild cases, the mucosa and submucosa appears edematous and erythematous with hemorrhagic nodules or with disrupted zones of mucosa, submucosa, and abundant fibrin. In advanced cases, the colonic mucosa is edematous with a greenish, grayish, or even black appearance corresponding to transmural ischemia or frank necrosis. Patients treated conservatively must be followed endoscopically based on the initial degree of ischemia and the patient's clinical evolution.

Patient Management

Most patients have a slight, reversible ischemia that never progresses to transmural disease. When the definitive diagnosis is made, all potentially contributing factors contributing to the ischemia must be corrected. Treatment includes intestinal rest, rehydration, optimization of cardiac function, and discontinuation of vasoconstrictor drugs. Although there is no evidence-based proof of the benefit of antibiotic use in IC, their use is recommended typically because of the theoretic protection against bacterial translocation and because of the possible progression toward gangrene. The patient requires regular and frequent (every 6–8 h) clinical, endoscopic, and laboratory reevaluation in order to detect signs of ischemic progression. In the case of ischemic progression despite aggressive conservative management, operative intervention is recommended. Other indications for urgent operative intervention are patients who present with peritoneal signs, patients diagnosed with transmural necrosis during colonoscopy, fulminate colitis, and, rarely, massive lower GI bleeding. Typically, a segmental colectomy is adequate, resecting the ischemic colon with a margin of normal, non-ischemic bowel and performing a proximal diverting colostomy. The distal end may be matured as a mucous fistula or can be left in the abdomen as a Hartmann's pouch. Only in cases of ischemia of the right colon and in hemodynamically stable patients should a ileocolic primary anastomosis be considered. Indications for semi-elective operative intervention are for those patients with persistent symptoms and signs of colitis for more than 2 weeks, patients who develop a protein-losing colopathy, or patients with recurrent septic

TABLE 15.2. Operative indications in ischemic colitis..

1. Acute
(a) Peritonitis
(b) Massive lower GI bleeding
(c) Fulminant colitis
2. Subacute
(a) Segmental colitis with persistent symptoms
(b) Protein-losing colopathy
(c) Recurrent sepsis attributable to IC
3. Chronic
(a) Symptomatic stricture
(b) Symptomatic segmental IC

episodes attributable to the IC. In these patients, a segmental colectomy with a primary anastomosis may be performed according to the clinical condition of the patient. Finally, there are also indications for elective colectomy, such as chronic IC with development of colonic stricture or the unusual patient with chronic segmental colitis. When symptomatic, segmental resection with primary anastomosis is warranted (Table 15.2).

Prognosis and Results

Of all patients with IC, approximately 80–85% have a non-transmural ischemia. Of them, 70% recover completely with conservative therapy and are asymptomatic after 1–2 weeks. Nearly 10% eventually will go on to develop a symptomatic ischemic stricture that requires operative resolution, and up to 20% will develop a chronic ischemic colitis that also will need a partial colectomy (Fig. 15.1). Patients who require emergency operation because of transmural disease (15–20%) have a mortality rate near to 50–60% because of sepsis or related complications. The

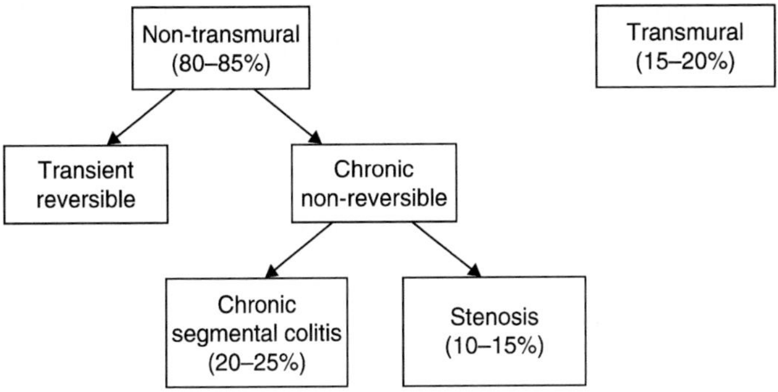

FIGURE 15.1. Classification of ischemic colitis.

factors associated with a poor prognosis after operative treatment of IC are early hemodynamic instability, IC secondary to aortic surgery (mortality approaching 80%), IC after operations employing extracorporeal circulation (mortality of 75%), and total colonic ischemia (mortality of 70%).

Conclusion

A high clinical suspicion and early endoscopic diagnosis are the most important determining factors in evaluation and management of the patients with IC. Most patients with IC will require only conservative management. Nevertheless, those patients who have a rapid progression of transmural disease require prompt and aggressive surgical treatment. This group of patients has a high mortality associated generally with their frequent and complex co-morbidities, sepsis, and multiple organ failure.

Selected Readings

Brandt LJ (2000) AGA technical review on intestinal ischemia. Gastroenterology 118:954–968

Church J (1995) Ischemic colitis. In: Church J (ed) Endoscopy of the colon, rectum and anus. Igaku-Shoin, New York/Tokyo, 328–331

Higgins PDR, Davis KJ, Laine L (2004) Systematic review: the epidemiology of ischemic colitis. Aliment Pharmacol Ther 19:729–738
MacDonald PH (2002) Ischemic colitis. Best Pract Res Clin Gastroenterol 16:51–61
Medina C, Vilaseca J, Videla S, et al. (2004) Outcome of patients with ischemic colitis: review of fifty-three cases. Dis Colon Rectum 47:180–184
Sreenarasimhaiah J (2005) Diagnosis and management of ischemic colitis. Current Gastroenterology Reports 7:421–426

16 Hemorrhoids

Francis Seow-Choen and Kok-Yang Tan

Pearls and Pitfalls

- Hemorrhoidal tissue is a normal anatomical structure that is only of concern when symptomatic.
- Factors predisposing to hemorrhoids include: hereditary factors, straining during defecation, squatting during defecation, and pregnancy.
- Use of a high fiber diet is controversial and may aggravate symptoms.
- Other sinister colorectal conditions may mimic hemorrhoid symptoms.
- Only symptomatic hemorrhoids require treatment.
- Hemorrhoids are traditionally divided into 4 degrees. Each degree should, however, be subdivided into large and small piles.
- Some small fourth-degree hemorrhoids may be treated conservatively, however, large first-degree piles may require operative intervention.
- Single pedicle rubber band ligation is efficacious and superior to injection sclerotherapy.
- Stapled hemorrhoidopexy is efficacious in most patients that require operative intervention.
- Patients with filiform skin tags or singular hemorrhoid prolapse should be treated with conventional operative excision.

K.I. Bland et al. (eds.), *Colorectal Surgery*,
DOI 10.1007/978-1-84996-444-9_16,

Pathophysiology

Hemorrhoidal tissues are derived from the anal vascular cushions. Hemorrhoids are present as normal structures in every individual beginning in fetal life. These vascular cushions consist of mucosa, submucosal fibro-elastic connective tissues, smooth muscle, and arterio-venous channels. These arterio-venous channels, which control the size of the anal cushions, are involved in the fine control of continence to liquids and gases, and function normally when they are in their proper position in the anal canal. Fixation is by submucosal smooth muscle and elastic fibers, which act as suspensory ligaments anchoring the anal cushions to the anal sphincters.

Even totally asymptomatic people can engorge their anal cushions massively by bearing down. Performing a Valsalva maneuver during proctoscopy will confirm this fact. Vascular engorgement of anal cushions is also made more obvious by straining in the squatting position. We believe that the propensity of the Asian population to have larger hemorrhoids (piles) is in part related to many Asian toilets being of the squatting type. Prolonged and repeated straining on a sitting toilet also results in engorgement of these cushions. As such, reading in the toilet and prolonged and repeated straining with chronic constipation or frequent diarrhea also predispose to symptomatic hemorrhoids. Pregnancy and delivery exert tremendous pressure or bearing down and are also common causes of large, congested, and prolapsed piles.

Once prolapse occurs, further engorgement of these arteriovenous channels occurs. This leads to pain and inflammation. Anal spasm then prevents reduction of the prolapsed tissue and edema, and inflammation and thrombosis ensue. As long as thrombosis has not occurred, these engorged cushions will shrink rapidly once they are reduced into the anal canal.

Chronic prolapse occurs when there is repeated prolapse and congestion of the hemorrhoids and the hemorrhoidal suspensory ligaments are sheared and fragmented. (Fig. 16.1)

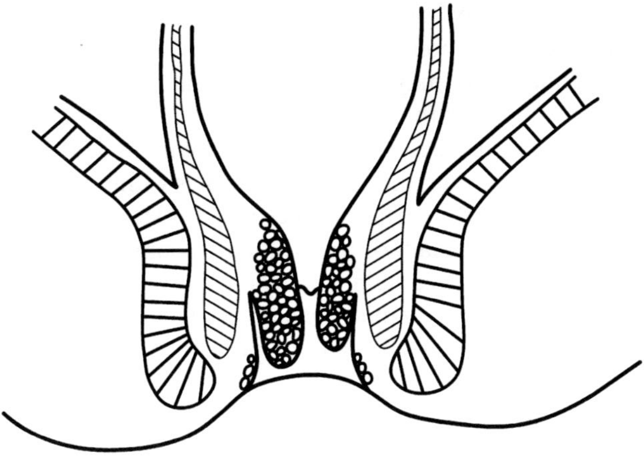

FIGURE 16.1. Prolapse of hemorrhoids results from partial or complete rupture of suspensory ligaments which anchors the hemorrhoidal tissues above the anorectal junction.

The vascular cushions can then prolapse easily, and when anal sphincters contract, there is further aggravation of edema and congestion. In genetically predisposed individuals, symptomatic prolapse may occur at a much younger age without conscious straining of stool.

Clinical Presentation

Many patients remain asymptomatic despite having prolapsed hemorrhoids. Hemorrhoids should not be treated unless they are symptomatic.

The most common symptoms of hemorrhoids are bleeding, prolapse, pain, and perianal pruritus.

While most patients suffering from piles are aware of bleeding symptoms, it is often remarkable that many are unaware as to whether their hemorrhoids are prolapsed or not. This may not be entirely surprising, considering that not everyone is aware of the normal anatomy of the anal region. Many patients with large prolapsed hemorrhoids will answer in the negative when asked if they had any prolapsed hemorrhoids. Prolapse may be reducible spontaneously after defecation, may require digital reduction, or may be irreducible. Pain may be caused by acute thrombosis of the prolapsed tissue, edema, or strangulation. Pain may also be secondary to concomitant anal fissures. Bleeding occurs when the vascular channels within the hemorrhoidal tissues rupture. This may occur at any stage of prolapse. Patients often complain of fresh blood dripping after defecation; others experience staining only on wiping. Perianal pruritus is commonly due to mild fecal or mucus discharge around the perianal area, which leads to perianal inflammation or dermatitis.

It is important to note that hemorrhoids are very common and may coexist with other more sinister colorectal conditions. Rectal cancer may present with symptoms similar to those of hemorrhoids. Indeed, there have been patients who were treated for bleeding hemorrhoids and were later found on colonoscopy to harbor rectal cancers.

Any patient who has blood or mucus mixed with stools, change in bowel habits, abdominal symptoms, or a family history of colorectal cancer should undergo endoscopic evaluation. We recommend colonoscopy in patients above 40 years of age. Younger patients should at least have a sigmoidoscopy, as one encounters young patients, even those without a family history, with silent colorectal cancer or inflammatory bowel disease.

Diagnosis and Staging of Hemorrhoids

The diagnosis of hemorrhoids is clinical. A proper anorectal examination is essential to assess fully the severity of the hemorrhoids and exclude concomitant anorectal pathology. We examine our patients in the left lateral position with good lighting. Careful inspection of the perianal region and anus is performed to exclude anal fissures, fistulae, and tumors. This examination is followed by proctoscopy with a wide and beveled Graeme-Anderson proctoscope.

TABLE 16.1. Classification of internal hemorrhoids.

Degree	Description
1	Hemorrhoids protrude into anal canal and often bleed, but do not prolapse
2	Hemorrhoids may protrude beyond anal verge with straining or defecation, but reduce spontaneously when straining ceases
3	Hemorrhoids protrude spontaneously or with straining, and require manual reduction
4	Hemorrhoids chronically prolapse and cannot be reduced. They usually contain both internal and external component and may present with acute thrombosis or strangulation

Prolapsed piles are conveniently graded into the various degrees of prolapse for purposes of treatment (Table 16.1). First-degree hemorrhoids are due to circulatory disturbances within the anal cushions leading to engorgement and swelling of the hemorrhoidal tissues. These hemorrhoidal tissues are located anatomically at the anorectal junction in the submucosal plane and are fixed in place by perihemorrhoidal condensed fibers of the longitudinal layer of the internal anal sphincter. These fibers are especially thick at the dentate line, where they are known as the suspensory ligaments of Parks. Partial rupture of these ligaments allows the hemorrhoidal tissues to slide downward during defecation; however, because there is sufficient residual contractile activity in intact fibers, hemorrhoids are withdrawn spontaneously after defecation. These are considered to be second-degree hemorrhoids.

In third-degree hemorrhoids, these ligaments are ruptured almost completely. Once prolapsed, spontaneous reduction is not possible, and manual reduction is required. The perianal skin is stretched in fourth-degree hemorrhoids, and thus, complete reduction is not possible or prolapse recurs immediately after reduction.

Patients often have mixed degrees of prolapse, with one portion at a different severity from the others. Surgeons normally assign the degree of prolapse as that of the most severely affected hemorrhoid.

Physicians should be aware that at every level of prolapse, the hemorrhoidal tissues can be large or small. Hence, there are large first-degree hemorrhoids which may demand therapy because of incessant bleeding and small fourth-degree hemorrhoids that are asymptomatic and do not require treatment.

Treatment

Two important issues are worthy of re-emphasis. First, in the assessment of hemorrhoidal symptoms, it is very important to ensure that symptoms are not attributed to hemorrhoids prior to screening the rectum. Second, hemorrhoids are treated on the basis of symptoms and not just on the degree of prolapse. The degree of prolapse and the size of the hemorrhoids help to determine the appropriate therapy.

Nonoperative Treatment

Because hemorrhoids have an important function in fine-tuning continence, one should first use non-operative methods of treatment if hemorrhoids are prolapsing minimally. The first thing to do is to correct toilet habits. Sitting toilets are preferred to squatting toilets. Reading and other habits that emphasize straining or prolong the time required for defecation should be discouraged.

Although many health authorities recommend a high fiber diet as a treatment for constipation, our experience has been that in up to 60% of patients, high fiber diet often aggravates constipation by producing bigger, harder, and more compact stools. Many constipated patients actually require a decrease or stoppage of dietary fiber to ease the act of defecation. Adequate fluid intake is essential and must be encouraged. Many patients with prolapsed hemorrhoids drink inadequate fluids secondary to various lifestyle reasons.

Micronized diosmin and hesperidin (Daflon 500) have pharmacologic properties that include venous contraction, reduction in blood extravasation from capillaries, and inhibition of the inflammatory response. These properties have proven to reduce hemorrhoidal symptoms. Thus, these agents can be useful as primary treatment and also as an adjunct to other forms of treatment.

Rubber band ligation is useful for first-and second-degree hemorrhoids that are not too large but sufficiently symptomatic for patients to seek treatment. One or two small rubber bands are applied to the pedicle of the hemorrhoid tissue *above* the dentate line. This results in a pulling inwards of the bulk of the hemorrhoid tissue (Fig. 16.2). Four to 5 days later, the ligated tissue necroses and sloughs off. The wound then

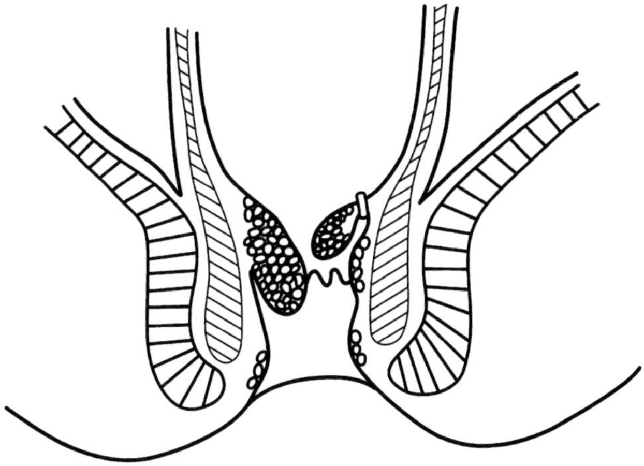

FIGURE 16.2. Rubber band ligation of hemorrhoids. A small rubber band is applied to the pedical of the hemorrhoidal tissue above the dentate line.

undergoes fibrosis with resultant fixation of the mucosa and prevention of engorgement and prolapse. Banding is 60–80% effective, but there is a 2–5% risk of secondary hemorrhage occurring 4–7 days postoperatively.

Sclerosant agents used include phenol (5%) in almond oil or sodium tetradecate. These solutions are injected into the submucosa of the pedicle. We do not favor this method, because we find that the results are inferior to those of rubber band ligation. The injection needle causes bleeding, which on occasion may be dramatically brisk. There is also the risk of intra-vaginal or prostatic injection. We do not recommend infrared photocoagulation unless patients are in coagulopathy. Similarly, cryotherapy is not recommended by us, as it is associated with an unpleasant and odorous discharge. Hemorrhoidal artery ligation using a Doppler-guided anoscope shows promise with regard to technical ease and effectiveness. Further studies are needed on these novel surgical approaches.

Operative Treatment

When the hemorrhoids are large and are at the third-or fourth-degree stage, operative management gives the most durable results. Traditionally, conventional operative excision of these hemorrhoids is recommended. There are numerous techniques that have been described pertaining to whether the wound after excision should be left open to granulate or closed primarily with sutures. There are also different techniques described with regard to the equipment used to perform the excision. The aim, however, is to excise the prolapsing hemorrhoidal tissue by dissecting it off the internal sphincter, while preserving adequate mucocutaneous bridges between the excision margins.

We believe that this form of treatment is not ideal for the following reasons. First, conventional operative excision focuses only on the symptoms without addressing the pathophysiology of hemorrhoids. The primary aim of restoring normal physiology is to restore the fixation of congested anal cushions rather than to excise them completely. Second, conventional excision is associated with substantial pain and discomfort from the time of operation and up to 3 months postoperatively. There are also frequent cases of anal incontinence, especially in the first few months after operative resection. Finally, operative excision in patients with massive circumferential hemorrhoids often results in residual or recurrent symptoms even after the performance of a Whitehead hemorrhoidectomy.

Nonetheless, excision is still performed widely. In this regard, we have found open hemorrhoidectomy using diathermy to give the best results. A trial using lateral sphincterotomy with hemorrhoidectomy to reduce sphincter spasm after excision demonstrated increased rates of incontinence and this is no longer performed. Another recent randomized, controlled, double-blind trial from Singapore using glyceryl trinitrate ointment on the postoperative wound showed that the wound healing rate was faster in the glyceryl trinitrate ointment group compared with placebo, although there was no significant difference in the pain and analgesic use. Excision using the Harmonic Scalpel and the Ligasure has been shown in recent trials to have marginal benefits in terms of operative blood loss, but larger studies and cost analysis are not available to justify their widespread use.

Compared with operative excision, however, stapled hemorrhoidopexy corrects the primary pathology, resulting in resolution of hemorrhoidal symptoms; this approach is now our preferred technique for patients with advanced piles. This technique excises redundant lower rectal mucosa, impressively reduces the prolapsed hemorrhoidal tissue, and fixes the prolapse back into its proper place on the wall of the anal canal (Fig. 16.3). Fixation onto the muscle wall of the anal canal may be important to prevent subsequent dislodgement and recurrence. Once reduced, the engorged hemorrhoidal tissues decongest and shrink rapidly. We have found a modification of this technique suitable for acute thrombosed

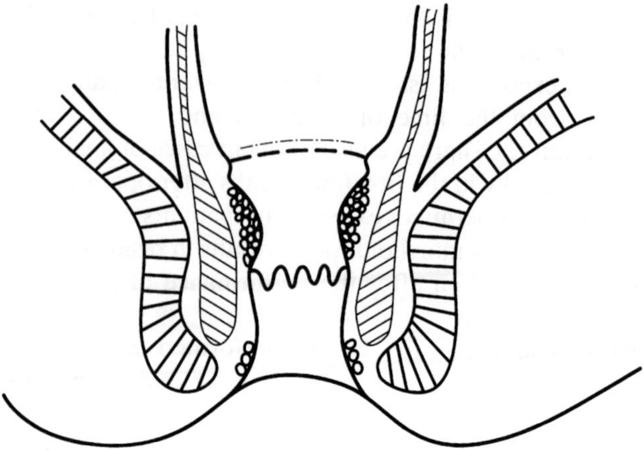

FIGURE 16.3. Stapled hemorrhoidopexy excises redundant lower rectal mucosa, reduces the prolapsed hemorrhoidal tissues, and fixes them back into their proper place.

hemorrhoids as well. The preservation of the anal cushions within the anal canal may contribute to the low rate of incontinence after this operation.

Even stapled hemorrhoidopexy on its own may not deal with massive circumferential hemorrhoidal prolapse. Prolapse more that 3–4 cm beyond the anal verge may not be housed adequately in the staple gun, and much residual hemorrhoidal tissue will remain prolapsed. Residual skin tags or external components may also result in less than ideal outcome. Various novel techniques to deal with these difficult issues have been described, ranging from elliptical mucosal excision after stapling to mucosal excision before insertion of the purse-string. Minor complications of acute urinary retention and bleeding occur in about 5% of patients undergoing operative excision or stapling. Postoperative pain requiring readmission and anorectal stricture occurs in 1–2% of patients. The recurrence rate after a median follow-up of 16 months was 0.3%. These results confirm the safety and efficacy of stapled hemorrhoidopexy.

Conclusion

In the treatment of hemorrhoids, an understanding of the pathophysiology is essential and efforts should be directed at restoring the weakened support for anal cushions in order to produce the best results.

Treatment should be instituted only if symptomatic, and efforts to exclude concomitant sinister colorectal disease should not be spared. Rubber band ligation remains the best non-operative option, while stapled hemorrhoidopexy is efficacious for most patients who require operative intervention.

Selected Readings

Ho YH, Tan M, Seow-Choen F, Goh HS (2000) Micronized purified flavonidic fraction compared favorably with rubber band ligation and fiber alone in the management of bleeding hemorrhoids. Randomized controlled trial. Dis Colon Rectum 43:66–68

Lloyd D, Ho KS, Seow-Choen F (2002) Modified Longo's hemorrhoidectomy. Dis Colon Rectum 45:416–417

Ng KH, Ho KS, Ooi BS, et al. (2006) Experience of 3711 stapled hemorrhoidectomy operations. Br J Surg 93:226–230

Seow-Choen F (2002) Surgery for hemorrhoids: ablation or correction. Asian J Surg 25:265–266

Tan KY, Sng KK, Tay KH, et al. (2006) Randomized double blind clinical trial 0.2 percent glyceryl trinitrate ointment on wound healing and pain reduction after open diathermy hemorrhoidectomy. Br J Surg 93:1464–1468

Thomson WHG (1975) The nature of hemorrhoids. Br J Surg 62:542–552

Part II
Malignant

17 Premalignant Polyps of the Colon and Rectum

David J. Maron and Robert D. Fry

Pearls and Pitfalls

- Most colorectal cancers arise from benign polyps that transform histologically into neoplasms.
- The "adenoma-carcinoma sequence" describes the process by which a benign polyp develops into an invasive cancer.
- The removal of benign polyps detected during colonoscopy has been shown to decrease the incidence of colorectal cancer.
- The possibility of a polyp containing carcinoma increases with size and with villous architecture.
- A tubular adenoma smaller than 1 cm has a less than 5% chance of containing cancer.
- A villous adenoma larger than 2 cm has a greater than 50% chance of containing cancer.
- Familial adenomatous polyposis (FAP) is a hereditary syndrome caused by a mutation in the APC gene and characterized by over 100 polyps arising in the colon and rectum; the incidence of colorectal cancer approaches 100%.
- Attenuated familial adenomatous polyposis is characterized by a significant risk for cancer, but with colorectal polyps (average of 30).
- Patients suspected of having attenuated familial polyposis, but in whom genetic testing fails to reveal an APC mutation, should be investigated for an MYH genetic mutation.

K.I. Bland et al. (eds.), *Colorectal Surgery*,
DOI 10.1007/978-1-84996-444-9_17,

- Hereditary nonpolyposis colorectal cancer syndrome (HNPCC) is caused by a mutation in DNA repair genes and is associated with an increased cancer risk of not only colorectal cancer, but other organ sites including: endometrium, stomach, gall bladder, kidney and small intestine.
- Cancer incidence in patients with HNPCC can be decreased by surveillance colonoscopy, performed every 2 years after age 20 and annually after age 35.
- Colon cancer in the patient with HNPCC should be treated by abdominal colectomy and ileorectal anastomosis.
- The risk of metastases from cancer arising in a colorectal polyp can be assessed by determining the depth of invasion into the polyp (Haggit's level).

Introduction

A colorectal polyp may be defined as a mass that arises from the surface of the intestinal epithelium and projects into the intestinal lumen. These lesions may be characterized by their gross appearance as sessile (relatively flat) or pedunculated (with a stalk). The histological pattern of the epithelium of a polyp may also be used to further describe the lesion. The epithelium of a colorectal polyp is generally characterized by pathologists as being of one of three common varieties: tubular (with branched, tubular appearing glands), villous (with long frond-like projections of surface epithelium), or tubulovillous (containing both tubular and frond-like epithelium). Tubular adenomas are the most common polyps of the large bowel (comprising about three fourths of all polyps), and are typically pedunculated. About 15% of polyps are tubulovillous, and a slightly lesser number are villous adenomas, which are most often sessile.

The basic definition of a polyp given above is usually used to initiate a discussion of benign, or at least minimally invasive, early neoplasms. However, a "mass of surface epithelium that projects into the lumen of the intestine" also describes the majority of cancers of the large bowel. Although polyps may bleed and can (rarely) cause obstructive symptoms by serving as a lead point for an intussusception, their importance lies in the close relationship between benign growths and invasive cancer of the large bowel. The purpose of this chapter is to examine that relationship in the light of evidence that has been gathered by surgeons, gastroenterologists, pathologists, epidemiologists, and molecular geneticists, with emphasis on relatively recent observations and discoveries that have enhanced our understanding of that relationship.

The Adenoma-Carcinoma Sequence

Although a quarter of a century ago there was considerable controversy over the concept that a benign polyp is a precursor to cancer, the evidence from many fronts provides such strong support for the adenoma-carcinoma sequence that this concept is generally unquestioned today. It is naïve to assume that all colorectal polyps are predestined to become cancerous, and there have been documented cases (especially in the Japanese literature) that occasionally large bowel cancers can arise directly from the mucosa without being associated with a benign precursor. Nevertheless, our understanding of the process of colorectal carcinogenesis assumes the fact that most cancers arise from benign polypoid precursors.

Evidence that supports the notion that benign polyps may be premalignant include the observation that microscopic examination of a colonic cancer will often reveal elements of a benign tubular or villous adenoma adjacent to, and often inseparable from, the cancer. In fact, the pathologist may often describe the cancer as "arising from a villous adenoma."

The incidence of both benign polyps and colon cancers increases with patients' age, with the polyps' rising incidence preceding that of the cancers' by about 7–10 years. This suggests a 7–10-year "dwell time" for a benign polyp to acquire malignant characteristics.

Colonic polyps occur more frequently in patients who have colorectal cancer. At least one third of patients with a colorectal cancer will have a polyp elsewhere in the large bowel. Removal of benign polyps by screening colonoscopy reduces the expected incidence of colorectal cancer in the population undergoing screening.

Large polyps are found to contain cancer much more often than small polyps, and the larger the polyp, the higher the chance that it is cancerous. The histological pattern of the polyp is also important; a tubular adenoma smaller than 1 cm in size has less than a 5% chance of containing invasive cancer, while the risk of cancer in a tubular adenoma larger than2 cm is at least 35%. A villous adenoma larger than 2 cm has an approximately 50% chance of containing cancer.

Patients with familial polyposis, in which there are literally hundreds of adenomatous polyps throughout the colon, will invariably develop colorectal cancer if not treated. The adenomatous polyps in these patients are indistinguishable from the colorectal polyps that occur in the general population, both histologically and by genetic markers.

Perhaps most convincing of all these observations in the support of the adenoma-carcinoma sequence is the discovery of the molecular model of carcinogenesis by Fearon and Vogelstein, which describes the step-by-step progression from normal epithelium through benign adenoma to invasive cancer at the molecular level(Fig. 17.1).

Polyps and Hereditary Colorectal Cancer Syndromes

APC-Associated Polyposis Syndromes

There are several recognized inherited syndromes which predispose a carrier to colorectal cancer. APC-associated polyposis syndromes include *familial adenomatous polyposis (FAP), attenuated FAP, Gardner's syndrome,* and *Turcot syndrome*. These syndromes are all caused by mutations in the APC gene, located on chromosome 5q. FAP is characterized by hundreds to thousands of adenomatous polyps arising in the large bowel, usually appearing after puberty and increasing

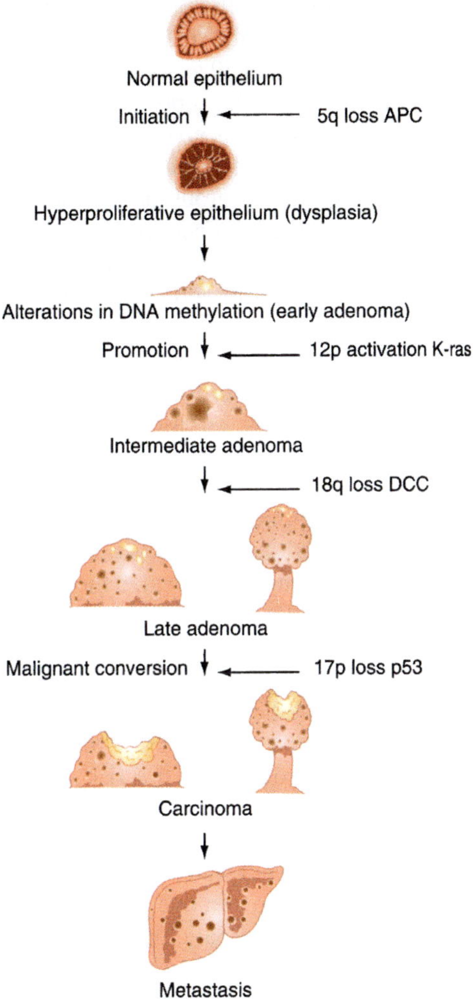

FIGURE 17.1. Model of colorectal carcinogenesis (Modified from Corman, 1998. With permission; after Fearon and Vogelstein, 1990. Copyright 1990. With permission from Elsevier).

in number with age. Patients with this syndrome will invariably develop colorectal cancer if not treated, with a mean age of cancer in untreated patients of 39 years. The appropriate surgical treatment depends somewhat upon the number of polyps involving the rectum, but there is no controversy involving the importance of removing the colon that is harboring the numerous benign appearing adenomatous polyps, one or more of which will certainly progress to cancer. The rectum may be preserved in some instances (by abdominal colectomy with anastomosis between the ileum and rectum) with the understanding that surveillance (proctoscopy) is required every 6 months to detect and eradicate any polyps that subsequently arise. If the rectum should harbor too many polyps to consider this approach (which is usually the case), the appropriate treatment is restorative proctocolectomy with ileal pouch anal anastomosis.

Attenuated FAP is characterized by a significant risk for colorectal cancer, but with fewer polyps (average of 30) than classic FAP. The polyps tend to be located more proximally in the colon than in classic FAP, and the average age of cancer diagnoses in individuals with attenuated FAP is 50–55years (10–15years later than in patients with classic FAP, but earlier than in patients with sporadic colorectal cancer). Management is significantly different than that of FAP, but the importance of recognizing the syndrome and the risk associated with numerous premalignant polyps is obvious. Abdominal colectomy with ileorectal anastomosis is the preferred treatment for individuals with this syndrome, but segmental colectomy with annual colonoscopy to remove any new polyps is an acceptable approach for some patients.

Gardner's syndrome is FAP associated with osteomas and soft tissue tumors (epidermoid cysts, fibromas, desmoid tumors). Usually these tumors are innocuous, but retroperitoneal or mesenteric desmoid tumors arising after colectomy may be very problematic. The treatment of desmoids arising in patients with FAP includes surgical excision, radiation, nonsteroidal anti-inflammatory drugs (NSAIDS), anti-estrogens, and cytotoxic chemotherapy.

Gardner's syndrome was once thought to be a distinct clinical entity, but it is now recognized that mutations in the APC gene are responsible for both classic FAP and Gardner's syndrome. Some correlation exists between extraintestinal growths and the mutation location in APC.

Turcot syndrome is the association of CNS tumors, usually medulloblastomas, with colorectal polyposis. The numbers of polyps that occur, as well as the phenotypic features of Gardner's syndrome and Turcot syndrome, relate to the location of the APC mutation. (Two thirds of Turcot syndromes are associated with APC mutations, but one third are associated with HNPCC mutations, described below. The CNS tumors in individuals with HNPCC are usually glioblastoma multiforme.)

APC-associated polyposis syndromes are inherited in an autosomal dominant fashion. Approximately 75–80% of patients with APC-associated polyposis will have an affected parent, with the remaining individuals representing a new mutation. Molecular genetic testing of APC detects disease causing mutations in up to 95% of probands with typical FAP.

Chemoprevention with FAP

Several studies have demonstrated temporary regression of adenomas in patients with FAP treated with nonsteroidal anti-inflammatory drugs (NSAIDs). Celecoxib received accelerated Food and Drug Administration approval based on data showing a reduction of polyp burden in individuals with FAP, although the clinical benefit of this COX-2 inhibitor was not proven. Unfortunately, these somewhat optimistic results were tempered with data showing that rofecoxib, a COX-2 inhibitor, increases the risk of cardiovascular events.

COX-2 inhibitors are unlikely to play a role in colorectal cancer prevention in the general population, but they currently are recommended by some for FAP patients with a low polyp burden in the rectum who have been treated with abdominal colectomy and ileorectal anastomosis in the hopes of delaying or preventing the need for proctectomy.

MYH-Associated Polyposis

MYH is a DNA repair gene that corrects DNA base pair mismatch errors in the genetic code prior to replication. Mutations in the MYH gene are associated with a high risk of colorectal cancer and a syndrome of premalignant polyps is similar to that seen with attenuated FAP. However, the disorder is inherited in an autosomal recessive manner, so two copies of the gene must carry a mutation. If an APC mutation is not identified in a patient suspected of having FAP or attenuated FAP, molecular genetic testing of MYH should be considered.

Hereditary Non-polyposis Colorectal Cancer

HNPCC is an autosomal dominant colorectal cancer syndrome with polyps that appear grossly similar to APC-associated polyps that arise with somewhat greater frequency in the proximal colon. The "dwell time" during which cancer arises in these polyps appears to be relatively short, and apparently benign polyps have progressed to cancer within the time span of a year ("accelerated carcinogenesis"). There are far fewer colorectal polyps appearing in this syndrome than in patients with FAP, but there is an increased incidence of other malignancies, including cancer of the endometrium, ovary, stomach, small intestine, pancreas, ureter and renal pelvis. HNPCC is caused by mutations in DNA mismatch repair genes, primarily MLH1, MSH2, and to a lesser frequency MSH6 and PMS2. Microscopically the tumors appear aggressive (poorly differentiated, Signet cells) and the tumors are characterized by microsatellite instability (MSI) that can be demonstrated on testing a tumor block from the cancer.

A family history is critical to detect patients with HNPCC. Before the genetic mutations responsible for the syndrome were recognized, the diagnosis was made based upon three elements known as the Amsterdam criteria: (1) colorectal cancer in three family members (first-degree relatives), (2) involvement of at least two generations, and (3) at least one affected individual being younger than the age of 50 at the time of diagnosis. The initial Amsterdam criteria has since been modified, recognizing the risk of other cancers found in the syndrome. The modified Amsterdam criteria considers not only colorectal cancer, but also endometrial, ovarian, gastric small intestinal, pancreatic and upper urinary tract cancers.

Patients with known or suspected HNPCC should have surveillance colonoscopy every 2 years beginning at age 20, and annually after age 35. In women, periodic vacuum curettage is begun at age 25, as well as pelvic ultrasound and determination of *CA-125 levels*. Annual tests for occult hematuria should also be obtained, because of the risk of upper urinary tract cancer.

Annual colonoscopy with removal of benign polyps has been shown to decrease the cancer incidence in patients with HNPCC. If colon cancer is detected, abdominal colectomy with ileorectal anastomosis should be considered. Women with known HNPCC who develop colon cancer should consider hysterectomy and bilateral oophorectomy at the time of colectomy.

The hereditary colorectal cancer syndromes account for only a small portion of all colorectal cancer. However, the identification of the genetic causes of these particular cancers, and the observations of the progression from normal mucosa to benign polyp to invasive cancer that occurs, has provided insight into the development of nonhereditary colorectal carcinogenesis. The genetic abnormalities that cause APC, MYH and HNPCC syndromes are known to arise spontaneously and play a major role in the pathogenesis of noninherited colorectal cancer.

Genomic Instability

Colorectal cancer arises as a multistep progression sequence at both the molecular and morphologic levels. This observation is not incompatible with the view that many (even most) benign polyps remain forever benign and do not progress to cancer. It does not exclude the fact that cancer can arise directly from the epithelium, without a benign polypoid precursor, although this form of pathogenesis is relatively uncommon. However, most colorectal cancers arise from a polyp that acquires certain alterations transforming it from a benign growth to a lesion capable of invasion and metastasis.

It is also generally accepted that genetic and epigenetic alterations promote colorectal cancer formation because they provide a clonal growth advantage to the cells that acquire these alterations. A key molecular step that occurs early in the pathogenesis of colorectal cancer is the loss of genomic stability. Three significant forms of *genomic instability* have been identified in colon cancer: (1) microsatellite instability (MSI), (2) chromosome instability (CIN), and (3) chromosomal translocations. In addition to genomic instability, a form of epigenomic instability has been identified that results in the aberrant methylation of tumor suppressor genes. Much research is ongoing regarding the exact role of genomic and epigenomic instability in the process of tumorigenesis. It is not clear whether genomic instability commonly initiates the adenoma-carcinoma sequence or whether it arises during this process and facilitates the development of cancer. However, both CIN and MSI can be observed in adenomas, so it would appear that at least in some cases chromosomal instability appears during adenoma initiation but before progression to frank cancer.

CIN is the most common type of genomic instability observed in colorectal cancer, occurring in approximately 85% of tumors. However, despite the high incidence of CIN in colorectal cancer and the fact that aneuploidy is a well-known characteristic of cancer, our understanding of the significance of chromosomal disarray is still incomplete. It is not clear if aneuploidy is a nonspecific occurrence arising during carcinogenesis which is tolerated by the tumor, or if the chromosomal disarray reflects an active process of CIN that is an important factor in tumorigenesis.

Colorectal Polyps: Assessment of Virulence

The treatment of an adenomatous or villous colorectal polyp is removal, usually by colonoscopy; distal polyps may be removed through a transanal approach. Pedunculated polyps are usually removed by severing the stalk with a snare passed through the colonoscope. Sessile polyps may not be amenable to excision using endoscopic techniques, although in some circumstances it is possible to elevate the polyp from the underlying muscularis with saline injection, thus permitting transluminal excision without perforation of the bowel wall. However, large sessile polyps often require segmental colectomy for complete removal, even if the presence of cancer is not confirmed prior to resection.

In view of the preceding discussion, polyps should be considered premalignant, and consideration given to assessment of the presence of cancer, and to its virulence, or metastatic potential of a cancer found in the polyp. Careful histological assessment of the polyp may reveal the presence of malignant cells. If these cells are confined to the muscularis mucosae (whether the polyp is pedunculated or sessile), the potential for metastases is negligible, such a finding is usually termed "atypia", and polypectomy is sufficient treatment. However, malignant cells penetrating the muscularis mucosae possess the ability to metastasize, and such polyps contain "invasive cancer". Appropriate treatment of such polyps requires consideration of the risk of lymph node metastasis and local recurrence. Haggitt proposed a classification for polyps containing cancer based upon the depth of invasion. Haggitt's criteria is as follows (Fig. 17.2):

Level 0: Cancer cells do not invade the muscularis mucosae (carcinoma-in-situ or intramucosal carcinoma)
Level 1: Cancer penetrates the muscularis mucosae (into submucosa), but is confined to the head of the polyp
Level 2: Cancer invades the level of the neck of the polyp (junction between the head and stalk)
Level 3: Cancer invades the stalk
Level 4: Cancer invades the submucosa below the stalk but above the muscularis propria

By this classification, all sessile polyps with invasive carcinoma are classified as Haggitt's Level 4.

Other factors to be considered when assessing the risk of metastases from a polyp containing cancer include the cellular

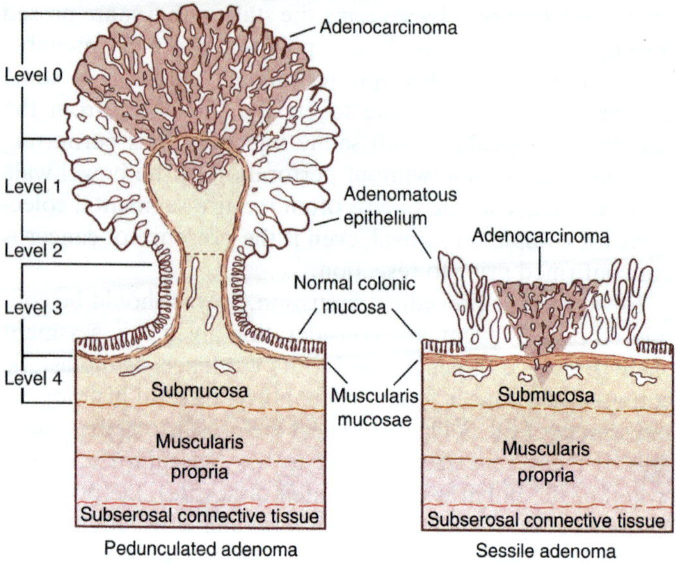

FIGURE 17.2. Anatomic landmarks of pedunculated and sessile polyps (Reprinted from Haggitt et al., 1985. Copyright 1985. With permission from the American Gastroenterological Association).

differentiation of the tumor (poorly differentiated cancer is more virulent than well differentiated, with moderately differentiated cancer assuming carrying an intermediate risk). Invasion of the lymphovascular spaces by cancer cells is also a poor prognostic factor, with at least a 10% chance of metastases to lymph nodes even if the cancer appears confined to the submucosa.

A pedunculated polyp with invasion to Haggitt's Levels 1, 2, and 3 has a low risk of lymph node metastasis or local recurrence, and complete excision of the polyp is adequate if the cancer is not poorly differentiated and there is no invasion of the lymphovascular channels in the specimen. Sessile cancers containing invasive cancer have at least a 10% chance of lymphatic metastasis, and generally require resection of the involved segment of intestine.

Selected Readings

Burt RW, Leppert MF, Slattery ML, et al. (2004) Genetic testing and phenotype in a large kindred with attenuated familial adenomatous polyposis. Gastroenterology 127:444–451

Corman ML (ed) (1998) Colon and rectal surgery, 4th edn. Lippincott-Raven, Philadelphia, p 593

Fearon ER, Vogelstein BL (1990) A genetic model of colorectal cancer tumorigenesis. Cell 61:759–767

Grady WM (2006) Genomic instability and colorectal cancer. Current Colorectal Cancer Reports 2:66–71

Haggitt RC, Glotzbach RE, Soffer EE, et al. (1985) Prognostic factors in colorectal carcinomas arising in adenomas: Implications for lesions removed by endoscopic polypectomy. Gastroenterology 89:328–336

Haggitt RC, et al. (1985) Prognostic factors in colorectal carcinomas arising in adenomas: implications for lesions removed by endoscopic polypectomy. Gastroenterology 89:328–336

Vogelstein B, Fearon ER, Hamilton SR, et al. (1988) Genetic alterations during colorectal tumor development. N Engl J Med 319:525–532

Wang L, Baudhuin LM, Boardman LA, et al. (2004) MYH mutations in patients with attenuated and classic polyposis and with young-onset colorectal cancer without polyps. Gastroenterology 127:9–16

18
Management of Colon Cancer

Robin S. McLeod and Robert Gryfe

Pearls and Pitfalls

- There is strong evidence that colorectal cancer screening with fecal occult blood testing reduces cancer related mortality and decreases the incidence of colon cancer in average risk individuals.
- Taking a family history is essential in individuals with colorectal cancer since 15–20% will have a family history of colon cancer. This information may change the management of the individual with cancer and change screening recommendations in family members.
- Familial adenomatous polyposis accounts for approximately 1% of colorectal cancers while HNPCC accounts for between 3% and 5% of colorectal cancers.
- Deaths due to colorectal cancer have decreased in the past 20 years in western countries.
- Laparoscopic colon resections can be performed safely with less pain and a modest decrease in time to the return of gastrointestinal function and length of stay and similar long-term outcomes.
- There is Level I evidence that mechanical bowel preparation is unnecessary in patients having colon resections.
- Patients with cancers that have microsatellite instability (MSI) have a better prognosis although these same individuals do not appear to derive benefit from 5-fluorouracil-based adjuvant chemotherapy.

K.I. Bland et al. (eds.), *Colorectal Surgery*,
DOI 10.1007/978-1-84996-444-9_18,

- Colectomy and ileorectal anastomosis may be the procedure of choice in individuals who have obstructing or perforating cancers and those who have synchronous cancers, HNPCC or attenuated familial adenomatous polyposis.
- Outcome is similar irrespective of the anastomotic configuration and whether it is stapled or handsewn.

Epidemiology, Incidence, Genetics

Colon cancer is among the most common cancers in the Western World. In the USA, it is estimated that more than 145,000 individuals were diagnosed with colorectal cancer in 2005 and more than 55,000 deaths were attributed to the disease; thus, making colorectal cancer the third most common cancer among males and females. Cancer is fundamentally a genetic disease in which a number of genetic alterations present in a cancer cell allow for its uncontrolled growth, evasion of cell death, local invasiveness and metastatic potential. Approximately 20% of individuals with colorectal neoplasia will have an affected first degree family member but only 5% of all patients with colorectal cancer will have an identifiable inherited genetic disorder. Inherited syndromes that predispose to colorectal cancer are generally categorized based on the presence of large numbers of adenomatous polyps, few (if any) adenomatous polyps or the presence of hamartomatous polyps (Table 18.1). Rational treatment recommendations for patients with inherited colorectal cancer syndromes are tailored to these variable disease phenotypes.

Although genetic abnormalities are fundamental to cancer development, various behavioral risk factors have been identified which are associated with colorectal cancer. Physical activity has been shown to be protective against the development of polyps. Smoking, alcohol consumption and dietary factors have all been causally linked with colon cancer. Controversy exists as to whether fiber or animal fat content is the important factor in diet since diets high in fiber tend to

TABLE 18.1. Inherited colorectal cancer syndromes and their associated genes.

Syndrome	Associated gene
Adenomatous polyposis syndromes	
Familial adenomatous polyposis (FAP)	APC
MYH-associated polyposis (MAP)	MYH
Nonpolyposis syndrome	
Hereditary nonpolyposis colorectal cancer (HNPCC)	MSH2, MLH1, MSH6, PMS2
Hamartomatous polyp syndromes	
Peutz-Jeghers syndrome (PJS)	LKB1
Juvenile polyposis syndrome (JPS)	SMAD4, BMPR1A
Cowden disease, including Bannayan-Ruvalcaba-Riley syndrome	PTEN

be low in animal fat and vice versa. It is therefore difficult to disassociate these two factors.

Staging of Colon Cancer

Several staging systems have been described but the most widely used system is the TNM Staging System developed by the American Joint Commission on Cancer (AJCC). To be considered invasive, cancers must extend into the muscularis mucosae. Malignant cells superficial to this layer lack malignant potential and such lesions are considered to be carcinoma in situ or to be dysplastic. Four stages are recognized (Table 18.2) and the prognosis worsens as the stage increases. Although a number of variables have been shown to have prognostic significance, the depth of invasion and the status of the nodes are the greatest independent predictors of outcome in colon cancer. The degree of differentiation (moderate or poorly differentiated) and the presence or absence of lymphovascular invasion are also

TABLE 18.2. AJCC staging classification.

	Depth	Nodal status	Distant metastasis
Stage 1	T1, 2	N0	M0
Stage 2	T3, 4	N0	M0
Stage 3	Any T	Any N (except N0)	M0
Stage 4	Any T	Any N	M1

TX, primary tumor cannot be assessed; T0, no evidence of primary tumor; Tis, carcinoma in situ; T1, tumor invades into submucosa; T2, tumor invades into muscularis propria; T3, tumor invades through muscularis propria; T4a tumor perforates visceral peritoneum; T4b tumor directly invades other structures; NX, regional lymph nodes cannot be assessed; N0, no regional lymph nodes; N1, 1–3 regional lymph nodes; N2, more than 4 regional lymph nodes; N3, regional lymph nodes along a named vascular trunk; MX, presence of distant metastasis cannot be assessed; M0, no distant metastases; M1, distant metastases.

considered to be predictors of outcome. While no genetic marker has yet to gain widespread acceptance in terms of prognosis, high frequency-microsatellite instability (MSI-H), observed in approximately 15% of sporadic colorectal cancers and most cases of HNPCC, has been consistently observed to be prognostic of improved survival independent of clinical factors such as tumor stage and grade. Additionally, while it appears that patients with microsatellite stable (MSS) cancers derive a survival benefit from adjuvant 5-fluorouracil-based chemotherapy, patients with MSI-H cancers do not appear to benefit similarly.

Prevention of Colorectal Cancer

Primary Prevention

Despite strong epidemiological evidence that populations consuming diets high in animal fat and low in fiber have an increased risk of colorectal cancer, to date, modifications to diet and administration of supplements with fiber, vitamins and minerals have not been shown to decrease the risk of polyps or cancer. This apparent discrepancy may be because there is a complex association between dietary factors, and trials have tended to include only adults; modify or supplement only one or a few factors; and tend to be relatively short in duration such that a therapeutic effect may be missed.

There are several non experimental studies and randomized controlled trials assessing the effectiveness of aspirin and other non steroidal anti-inflammatory agents. NSAIDS are potent inhibitors of cyclooxygenase (COX) enzymes and animal studies suggest that they produce their antineoplastic effect through both COX dependent and independent pathways. Most studies have included individuals who had a previous cancer or polyp. There appears to be some benefit in this group, although there is no evidence to date that the frequency of colonoscopic surveillance can be decreased. Furthermore, the side effects of these drugs, including gastrointestinal bleeding and cardiovascular complications, mean that further studies are required to ensure that the benefits outweigh the risks. There is also evidence from one trial that calcium may decrease the risk of adenomas (but not cancer) but this trial has inadequate power to determine whether the risk of cancer is reduced and, furthermore, does not address the issue of whether colonoscopic surveillance recommendations can be modified.

Secondary Prevention

There are several screening options available including fecal occult blood testing (FOBT), flexible sigmoidoscopy, barium enema and colonoscopy. Other tests such as fecal DNA studies and virtual colonoscopy are promising but have not been adopted for general use. Screening recommendations vary depending on the personal and family history of the individual.

In average risk individuals (i.e., those without a personal or family history of colon cancer), it is usually recommended that screening be started at age 50 years. Fecal occult blood testing lacks sensitivity and specificity but it is the easiest test to perform. There is Level I evidence that annual or biennial screening with FOBT decreases cancer specific mortality as well as the incidence of colon cancer. However, approximately 1,000 individuals must be screened for 10 years to prevent one death. The evidence is less strong for the other modalities but they have been recommended as follows: (1) flexible sigmoidoscopy every 5 years, (2) combined FOBT and flexible sigmoidoscopy every 5 years, (3) colonoscopy every 10 years, and (4) double contrast barium enema every 5 years.

For individuals with a first degree relative with colon cancer, it is generally recommended that screening colonoscopy be performed starting at age 40 years or 10 years younger than the earliest stage of diagnosis in the family. Individuals at risk for HNPCC should have colonoscopy every 1–2 years beginning at age 20–25years. However, the evidence supporting this recommendation is weak. Finally, individuals who are at risk for familial adenomatous polyposis should have genetic testing if the mutation has been identified in the proband. If so, then genetic testing in the at-risk relative can be performed with 100% accuracy. Those individuals who are known to carry the APC gene or are at-risk but cannot have genetic testing require annual flexible sigmoidoscopy beginning in puberty.

Preoperative Evaluation

Patients presenting with a colon cancer require evaluation of their entire colon since polyps and synchronous cancers maybe present in up to 30% of individuals and might alter management decision making. Endoscopic examination is preferred since it may also be therapeutic if another lesion is found. In some instances, it may not be possible to evaluate the proximal colon because the cancer has narrowed the lumen. If so, a careful inspection should be performed intraoperatively and colonoscopy performed post operatively. Since many colon cancer procedures are now performed laparoscopically, the tumor should also be tattooed with India ink so that it is readily identifiable at the time of surgery.

To assess the patient for metastatic disease, a CT scan should be performed. This may provide valuable information regarding the presence of metastatic disease as well as the extent of local lesion invasion. If CT scanning is not available, an ultrasound maybe performed. A chest x-ray or CT scan of the chest should be performed to assess the lungs for metastatic disease.

Perioperative Care

There is Level I evidence supporting many of the perioperative measures prescribed in patients undergoing colorectal cancer surgery. Recent evidence suggests that a mechanical bowel preparation may not only be unnecessary but harmful to patients. Guenga and colleagues performed a Cochrane review that included nine trials and 1,592 patients. Following colonic surgery, both leak (2.9% vs. 1.6%; OR 1.80, 95% CI 0.68–3.26) and wound infection rates (7.4% vs. 0.4%, OR 1.46, 95% CI 0.97–2.18) were insignificantly higher in the cohort having bowel preparation.

The need for prophylactic antibiotics is well accepted. Various routines have been studied including different combinations and different routes of administration (oral or intra-venous). What is well established is that antibiotics should be administered prior to the skin incision being made so there are adequate tissue levels. Secondly, post-operative antibiotics do not appear to be required. Intraoperative doses may be required only when the case is greatly extended. There is also level I evidence that intra-operative warming reduces the risk of wound infections by approximately 50% as well as decreasing the risk of cardiac complications. Supplemental oxygenation given both pre and intraoperatively also appears to be effective in reducing the risk of surgical site infections by 50%. In addition, clipping rather than shaving may be preferable. Similarly, prophylaxis against the development of thromboembolic complications is required. Kehlet and colleagues have been proponents of

TABLE 18.3. Care program in patients undergoing resection with fast-track care.

Preoperatively	Information of surgical procedure, expected length of stay and daily milestones for recovery
Day of surgery	Mobilized at 2 h
	Drink at 1 l h
	Two protein-enriched drinks
	Solid food
Postoperative day 1	Mobilized > 8 h
	Drink > 2 l
	Four protein-enriched drinks
	Solid food
	Remove bladder catheter
	Plan discharge
Post operative day 2	Normal activity
	Remove epidural catheter
	Discharge after lunch

"fast track" surgery (Table 18.3). They have been able to show that functional capabilities return earlier and length of hospital stay can be reduced with a fast track approach.

Surgical Therapy

Surgical resection remains the mainstay of treatment of cancers of the colon. Since cancers spread locally, through the lymphatics and hematogenously, the oncological principles of colon cancer surgery include resection of the tumor with adequate resection margins plus removal of all lymph node bearing tissue. Depending on the site of the cancer, the segment of colon resected may vary. For most cancers, a segmental resection and primary anastomosis can be performed. However, if the patient has more than one cancer, has a family history of HNPCC or attenuated FAP, or has no family history of colon cancer but is young (i.e., less than 40 years), a colectomy and ileorectal anastomosis is often recommended depending on the site of the cancer. This is based on the rationale that the risk of a second primary cancer is high and also, surveillance of the rectum can be performed more easily. If colectomy and ileorectal anastomosis are performed the anastomosis should be carried out at the sacral promontory. Removing more of the rectum might result in a poor functional result. For patients with familial adenomatous polyposis, colectomy with ileal pouch anal anastomosis is the preferred option by most experts. However, colectomy and ileorectal anastomosis may be an acceptable option in patients who have few or no polyps in their rectum and whose family history is negative for more numerous polyposis or desmoid tumors.

For cancers of the right colon, a right hemicolectomy is performed with ligation of the ileocolic vessels. In most instances, it is necessary to mobilize the hepatic flexure in order to complete the anastomosis. Cancers of the hepatic flexure and proximal transverse colon are treated usually with an extended right hemicolectomy with ligation of both the ileocolic and middle colic vessels. For technical reasons, it is easier to perform an anastomosis between the terminal ileum and distal transverse or descending colon for transverse colon cancers rather than attempting to mobilize the hepatic flexure and perform a colo-colonic anastomosis. Left sided lesions require ligation of the inferior mesenteric vessels or their branches. There is no strong evidence to suggest that a high ligation of the inferior mesenteric vessels improves outcome but in many situations it is technically easier to divide the vessels at the origin of the inferior mesenteric artery rather than more distally. Splenic flexure cancers and cancers high in the left colon are often difficult to mobilize, particularly if they are large. The left branch of the inferior mesenteric artery must be divided to remove the lymph nodes. While theoretically, an anastomosis can be performed between the proximal transverse colon and proximal sigmoid colon, in reality this may be difficult and an ileosigmoid anastomosis may be necessary.

The type of anastomosis can be done at the discretion of the surgeon. There is level I evidence that sutured and stapled anastomoses can be performed with similar complication rates with the exception of stricture which is somewhat more common in stapled anastomoses. However, strictures usually are not significant and do not cause symptoms. Similarly, the configuration of the anastomosis may be based on the surgeon's preference: side to side, end to end or end to side. For sigmoid cancers, the patient should be placed in stirrups in the lithotomy position so one has the option of performing an end to end anastomosis by passing a circular stapler per anum. Otherwise the patient can be placed in the supine position unless one expects invasion of other organs.

The complication rate following elective surgery for colon cancer tends to be low. The leak rate in most series is less than 5%. Thus, it is unusual in the elective situation that a defunctioning ileostomy is required except in situations where there is a perforation, an abscess or contamination of the abdomen, if a multivisceral resection is performed or other unusual findings are encountered.

Laparoscopic Versus open Resection

Laparoscopic colon resection was first described in 1991. It has been adopted much slower than other laparoscopic abdominal procedures such as cholecystectomy and anti reflux procedures likely because it can be a technically challenging procedure. Early reports, however, suggested that laparoscopic assisted colectomy is associated with less pain, lower analgesic requirements, and a more rapid recovery. However, there was hesitancy in adopting the approach because of early reports of recurrences occurring at the site of port sites. In 1995, Ortega and colleagues reported a port site recurrence rate of 1.2% in 504 patients registered in The American Society of Colon and Rectal Surgeons database. Further concerns were raised about whether an adequate oncological resection could be performed laparoscopically since the oncological outcomes far outweigh the early functional outcomes in importance.

Multiple randomized controlled trials have been performed in Europe, South America, Asia, Australia and North America over the past decade. At present, mainly short term results are available. These results suggest that laparoscopic resection takes longer to perform, but time to pass flatus, time until solid diet is tolerated, and time to hospital discharge are decreased by approximately 30%. In absolute terms these differences are approximately 30–60 min longer for surgery but approximately 1 day shorter in the other outcomes in the laparoscopic group. Pain and narcotic requirements are similarly reduced. Interestingly though, both the CLASICC and the COST studies were not able to demonstrate differences in quality of life using several validated instruments between the two groups of patients.

Early data suggest that laparoscopic procedures can be performed equally as well and safely as open procedures with several studies showing similar numbers of nodes harvested as well as post-operative complication rates being similar or even lower. To date, four trials have reported long term data with follow-up of 1,528 patients for between 3.5 and 5 years. Reza and colleagues combined the data from these trials and reported no difference in overall mortality (OR 0.81, 95% CI 0.58–1.11); cancer related mortality (OR 0.70, 0.28–1.72) or recurrence (OR 0.88, 0.61–1.27).

The COST trial is the largest trial to report long-term outcome data. Overall, survival was 86% in the laparoscopic group and 85% in the open-colectomy group with no significant differences between groups in the time to recurrence or survival for patients with any stage of cancer. On the other hand, Lacy and colleagues reported a significantly higher cancer-related survival in patients in the laparoscopic group with the improvement being mainly due to improved outcome in the Stage III group of patients.

The evidence to date suggests that laparoscopic colectomy is an acceptable alternative to open surgery for colon cancer. Short term outcomes are modestly better; patient satisfaction appears to be high with a laparoscopic approach and oncological results appear to be similar. Laparoscopic colectomy is being quickly adopted by surgeons yet it is a difficult procedure to master and there is a definite learning curve. Some guidelines suggest that a surgeon should perform at least 20 laparoscopic colectomies in patients with benign disease before undertaking a laparoscopic colectomy for malignant disease. Even that number may be inadequate and certainly patients should be chosen carefully during the early phase of adoption.

Most procedures are actually laparoscopic assisted procedures. For malignant disease, the colon should be mobilized and vessels taken intracorporeally before exteriorizing the bowel to do the anastomosis. Most authors recommend making an adequate incision and using a wound protector to exteriorize the bowel to minimize the chance of a local recurrence.

Special Situations

Obstructing Cancers

Cancers are the most common cause of large bowel obstruction. Left sided cancers are more likely to cause obstruction, but obstruction may be caused by cancers at virtually any location. Obstructing cancers tend to be large and are usually associated with a poorer prognosis with many already having distant metastases.

Treatment will depend to some extent on whether the patient is partially obstructed or completely obstructed. If possible, it is always worthwhile to delay surgery to allow the obstruction to resolve. However, if the patient is completely obstructed, emergency surgery may be necessary. For patients with right sided obstructing lesions, a right hemicolectomy with a primary anastomosis can usually be performed unless there are extenuating circumstances. A defunctioning stoma is not necessary. Treatment options for obstructing lesions of the left colon include the following: Hartmann procedure, subtotal colectomy and ileorectal or ileosigmoid anastomosis or a washout procedure followed by resection and anastomosis. In rare circumstances, a defunctioning colostomy alone may be the preferred option but it should probably be reserved for patients with significant comorbidities or who are systemically unstable or as a palliative procedure. Each of the other procedures has both advantages and disadvantages. The Hartmann procedure is the standard operation and is probably the most straight forward procedure. Mobilization of the splenic flexure, which might be difficult if the bowel is greatly distended, is not required. It is the preferred option for unstable patients or those in whom it might not be safe to perform an anastomosis. The disadvantage of a Hartmann procedure is that a second operation is required. In fact, reconstruction is never performed in a large proportion of patients who are elderly or have comorbidities. Colectomy and ileorectal or ileosigmoid anastomosis eliminates the need for a second operation. Furthermore, it eliminates stoma problems and deals with a synchronous cancer if present and unsuspected. It, however, should not be performed if the resection line is below the sacral promontory or in elderly patients as functional results might be suboptimal. In younger patients, it is probably the procedure of choice. It may also be required if there are ischemic changes or tearing of the caecal serosa due to the obstruction.

Theoretically, colonic washout followed by segmental resection and anastomosis is the best option. However, surgery for obstructing cancers is usually performed in the middle of the night and the washout tends to be tedious and fraught with mishaps so this technique has not gained popularity with many surgeons. If undertaken, the resection is performed in the usual way. Intravenous tubing is then threaded into the appendix and anesthetic tubing is inserted into the bowel at the proximal resection margin. An umbilical tape is used to fasten securely the tubing. The distal end of the anesthetic tubing is placed in a bucket. The splenic flexure needs to be mobilized so one can assist with the passage of the fluid and stool. Several liters of saline are required to wash out the colon but once completed, an anastomosis is performed.

The operative morbidity and mortality following emergency or urgent surgery for obstructing cancers is higher than following elective surgery and vary widely depending on the site of the tumor and the type of procedure performed as well as the status of the patient. Furthermore, obstructing cancers tend to be more advanced than non obstructing cancers and therefore a curative operation may be possible in only half of them. Long term survival is also significantly lower, even when adjusted for stage. Some authors have reported the survival is approximately half of that of non obstructing cancers.

Perforation

Perforation is an uncommon complication but portends a poor prognosis. The perforation may be at the site of the tumor or may occur secondarily at a proximal site, usually the caecum, in obstructing cancers. There may be invasion of other structures and organs. Primary resection is the preferred treatment and if there is a contained perforation, it may be possible to undertake a primary anastomosis. Otherwise, a colostomy or an anastomosis with a defunctioning stoma may be necessary. If the perforation is in the right colon due to an obstructing left sided lesion, a subtotal colectomy is required.

Resection in the Setting of Metastatic Disease

Approximately 25% of patients with colon cancer present with Stage IV disease. Of those, it is estimated that approximately 20% have potentially resectable primary lesions. In the vast majority of these patients, their metastatic disease is not resectable and therefore surgery, if it were performed, would be for palliative purposes only. If the patient is symptomatic (bleeding, anemia or obstruction) from the primary lesion, surgery is indicated. In the asymptomatic patient, there is controversy as to whether surgery is worthwhile. With modern chemotherapeutic regimens, median survival in this group is approximately 20 months and during this time the patient may become symptomatic from the lesion. Theoretically, surgical removal of the primary might improve survival, improve quality of life, obviate the need for surgery and likely a stoma in the future when patients may have more advanced disease and are less well systemically. On the other hand, only 10% of patients who are not resected seem to require surgery in the future. Operative mortality tends to be low but not insignificant. Results of treatment (surgery and chemotherapy vs. chemotherapy alone) are available from only a few retrospective studies which may be biased by patient selection. These results suggest that there may be a small improvement in survival in the surgery group but there are no data pertaining to quality of life. Thus, at the present time, decision making must be individualized based on the burden of metastatic disease present, the site and symptomatology of the primary tumor, the ease with which it could be resected and the age and comorbidities of the patient.

Follow-Up

Patients having curative resections for colon cancer are at risk of recurrence. There is some evidence from a small number of trials that more intensive post-operative follow-up leads to a small survival benefit. The benefit is likely due to the early diagnosis and resection of recurrent, limited disease, particularly in the lungs, liver and locally. However, it is not clear what tests or group of tests are optimal nor what the optimal timing of tests is due to the heterogeneity of the trials. There is further uncertainty since the risk of recurrence varies depending on the stage of the disease, and therefore, the follow-up regimen should perhaps be altered depending on the stage of the disease.

The rationale for surveillance is first, to detect recurrence of the cancer, and secondly, to detect polyps or other cancers at an early stage since metachronous cancers may occur in up to 5% of patients. The evidence supporting surveillance of the colon is stronger than for other sites. Based on the National Polyp Study, it is recommended that a colonoscopy be performed 1 year following surgery (unless the colon was not fully evaluated preoperatively and then colonoscopy should be performed earlier) and if that is normal, then at 3 and 5 year intervals.

Otherwise, recommendations for surveillance are somewhat arbitrary. Cancer Care Ontario, in Canada, recommends follow-up in patients with Stage IIb or III cancers when they are symptomatic and at 6 monthly intervals provided they can tolerate the diagnostic tests and surgery if recurrent disease is detected. Patients with earlier disease likely require less intense follow-up. Furthermore, if patients are deemed too old or unfit for surgery, then follow-up examinations are unnecessary.

Prognosis

Based on SEER data from the USA, the overall survival of colon cancer is approximately 65%. However, survival varies according to the stage of the disease. Thus, the mean 5-year survival of patients with Stage I disease is over 90%, with Stage II disease is approximately 75–80%, Stage III disease is 50–60% and Stage IV disease is less than 5%.

References

Figueredo A, Rumble RB, Maroun J, et al., and members of the Gastrointestinal Cancer Disease Site Group (2004) Follow-up of patients with curatively resected colorectal cancer. Practice Guideline Report #2–9, www.Cancer care Ontario/program in evidence-based care

Selected Readings

Geerts WH, Pineo GF, Heit JA, et al. (2004) Prevention of venous thromboembolism: the Seventh ACCP Conference on Antithrombotic and Thrombolytic Therapy, http://www.chestjournal.org/cgi/content/full/126/3_suppl/338S

The Clinical Outcomes of Surgical Therapy Study Group (2004) A comparison of laparoscopically assisted and open colectomy for colon cancer. N Engl J Med 350:2051–2059

Gryfe R (2006) Clinical implications of our advancing knowledge of colorectal cancer genetics: inherited syndromes, prognosis, prevention, screening and therapeutics. Surg Clin N Am 86:787–817

Guenaga K, Atallah AN, Castro AA, et al. (2006) Mechanical bowel preparation for elective colorectal surgery. The Cochrane Database of Systematic Reviews, vol3

Jacobsen DH, Soone E, Andreasen J, Kehlet H (2006) Convalescence after colonic surgery with Fast-Track vs. Convention Care. Colorectal Dis 8:683–589

Reza MM, Blaxco JA, Andradas E, et al. (2006) Systematic review of laparoscopic versus open surgery for colorectal cancer. Br J Surg 93:921–928

Sanga S, Yao M, Wolfe MM (2005) Non-steroidal anti-inflammatory drugs and colorectal cancer prevention. Postgrad Med J 81:223–227

Schwent W, Haase O, Neudecker J, Muller JM (2006) Short term benefits for laparoscopic colorectal resection. The Cochrane Database of Systematic Reviews, vol3

Song F, Glenny AM (2006) Antimicrobial prophylaxis for colorectal surgery. The Cochrane Database of Systematic Reviews, vol 3

Winawer S, Fletcher R, Rex D, et al. (2003) for the US Multisociety Task Force on Colorectal Cancer. Colorectal cancer screening and surveillance: clinical guidelines and rationale-update based on new evidence. Gastroenterology 124:544–560

19 Appendiceal Epithelial Neoplasms and Pseudomyxoma Peritonei, a Distinct Clinical Entity with Distinct Treatments

Paul H. Sugarbaker

Pearls and Pitfalls

- Appendiceal epithelial malignancies present as either a malignant mucocele of the appendix or as a perforated appendiceal malignancy.
- If the disease presents as a contained process, then surgical removal of the mucocele with negative margins and negative appendiceal lymph nodes offers a curative approach to the disease process.
- In a majority of patients, the mucocele has perforated and epithelial cells in mucoid ascites have distributed themselves throughout the abdomen and pelvis (pseudomyxoma peritonei syndrome). Patients with pseudomyxoma peritonei syndrome should be treated with cytoreductive surgery which includes peritonectomy procedures and intraperitoneal chemotherapy washing usually with hyperthermic mitomycin C.
- The pseudomyxoma peritonei syndrome may present with large volume disease requiring knowledgeable selection of patients for this combined approach.
- Use of systemic chemotherapy in patients with mucinous appendiceal carcinomatosis remains controversial in the absence of a definitive clinical trial.
- In the absence of further evidence, these patients with aggressive carcinomatosis from appendix cancer are treated with systemic chemotherapy after cytoreduction and perioperative intraperitoneal chemotherapy.

K.I. Bland et al. (eds.), *Colorectal Surgery*,
DOI 10.1007/978-1-84996-444-9_19,

Background Clinical Science

In the 9th International Classification of Disease (ICD-9) revised in 2004, primary epithelial neoplasms of the appendix are grouped together with colorectal malignancy. In future revisions, appendiceal neoplasms may be reclassified as a distinct clinical entity, because of profound differences in natural history and pathology of colorectal cancer compared with appendiceal neoplasms. Consequently, there are profound differences in the treatment of these two disease processes. Table 19.1 contrasts the clinical and pathologic features of colorectal cancer and appendiceal neoplasms. The clinical presentation, histology, extent of tumor invasion, and difference in tumor differentiation separate colorectal cancer and appendiceal neoplasms as distinct pathologic and clinical diseases.

The age of onset of appendiceal epithelial neoplasms is lower than colorectal cancer with a mean age for initial presentation of 48 years. Although the proportion of patients

TABLE 19.1. Contrast of the clinical and pathologic features of colorectal cancer and appendiceal neoplasms.

Feature	Colon	Appendix
Mean age of onset (years)	68	48
Peritoneal dissemination at onset	10%	85%
Adenocarcinoma histology	85%	10%
Mucinous histologic type	10–15%	90%
Minimally invasive	1%	75%
Signet ring adenocarcinoma	1/1000	1/10
Adenocarcinoid	0%	2.5%
Differentiation of adenocarcinoma		
Well-differentiated	10%	80%
Moderately differentiated	80%	10%
Poorly differentiated	10%	10%

with an unruptured mucocele is not known, many of these patients have peritoneal dissemination at the time of their initial presentation. The great majority of the tumors are of a mucinous histopathologic type. Also, about 75% of appendiceal neoplasms are minimally invasive, such that they layer out on the peritoneal surfaces rather than invade into parietal peritoneum or visceral structures. There is, however, a wide spectrum of aggressiveness, and some patients show signet ring morphology or poorly differentiated cancer with dissecting mucus penetrating deeply through the peritoneal layer of structures in the abdomen and pelvis. Because they usually present with peritoneal dissemination, even the most minimally aggressive of these malignancies should be regarded as a uniformly fatal condition, sometimes over several decades, unless unique, specialized treatments are initiated.

Management of a Mucocele

The clinical presentation of a mucocele is usually nonspecific. Up to 50% are found incidentally at the time of operation, and about half of patients will be asymptomatic. In those with symptoms, 30% will have abdominal pain, 15% an abdominal mass, 15% weight loss, 10% nausea, vomiting, or both, and the remainder acute appendicitis. Presence of symptoms suggests a higher incidence of cystadenocarcinoma.

Diagnostic Studies

Diagnosis of a mucocele, often made by computed tomography of the abdomen, is characterized by a well-encapsulated cystic mass 2–20 cm in diameter that occurs usually in the right lower quadrant. Curvilinear mural calcification is present about 50% of the time. Enhancing nodules in the mucocele wall suggest cystadenocarcinoma. In women, these findings are accompanied by enlargement of the ovaries from mucinous, tumor cell entrapment within the ovarian tissues (pseudomyxoma ovarii). Mucoceles of benign origin are rarely larger than 2 cm. A mucocele caused by cystadenoma or cystadenocarcinoma is usually larger and associated with a 20% incidence of perforation. Mucinous ascites in the pelvis and in right upper quadrant between liver and right hemidiaphragm indicates rupture of the mucocele and pseudomyxoma peritonei syndrome.

Diagnosis of a mucocele is sometimes made by an ultrasonography based on a sausage-shaped cystic structure in the appendiceal region but may include images suggesting mucous ascites. The target lesion imaged by ultrasonography is secondary to a thickened appendiceal wall. In some patients, multiple echogenic layers along the dilated appendix may be pathognomonic for mucocele.

An Intact Mucocele is a Benign Process

One of the cardinal principles of surgical management of an appendiceal mucocele is that an intact mucocele presents no future risk for the patient. In contrast, just the opposite is true if the mucocele has ruptured and epithelial cells escape into the peritoneal cavity. In the review by Misdraji and colleagues, none of 39 patients with intact mucoceles had progression of disease; however, patients with epithelial cells in the mucus within the peritoneal cavity developed mucinous neoplasms on peritoneal surfaces. Thus, it is crucial to maintain the mucocele intact during operations. When a mucocele is visualized at the time of laparoscopic examination, although it may be possible to remove it intact without rupture, the safer approach is to convert the laparoscopic examination to an open laparotomy for safe mucocele excision to prevent rupture of the mucocele and seeding of trocar sites.

Conversion of a laparoscopy to a laparotomy for excision of a mucocele aids in managing this disease process in two ways. First, this approach ensures that a benign process will not be changed to a malignant one by rupture of the mucocele. Second, it allows the surgeon to explore more thoroughly the remainder of the abdomen to exclude the presence of mucoid fluid accumulations. These accumulations are most commonly found in the right retrohepatic space or deep in the pelvis. Also, mucinous tumor nodules within the omentum are very common. Another site where mucoid neoplasms can accumulate is the in cul-de-sac created in the left paracolic space just above the junction of the sigmoid and descending colon. Thorough exploration of all these anatomic sites may be difficult by laparoscopic examination. An open laparotomy enables palpation and direct inspection of all sites that are of high risk for progression of the mucinous carcinomatosis.

At the time of laparoscopy or laparotomy for mucocele, all mucinous fluid within the abdomen should be harvested carefully for a cytospin of the fluid collected. If epithelial cells are found outside the appendix within the mucoid fluid, the diagnosis of pseudomyxoma peritonei syndrome or mucinous peritoneal carcinomatosis of appendiceal origin is established.

Right Colectomy is not Required in the Management of Mucinous Appendiceal Malignancies

In the past, all patients with epithelial malignancy of the appendix have been recommended for right colectomy. This practice was suggested on the basis of retrospective data; right colectomy appeared to produce a survival advantage. But recent prospective data by Gonzalez-Moreno and associates3 showed that in treating appendiceal mucinous carcinomatosis and the pseudomyxoma peritonei syndrome, there is no survival benefit with a right colectomy. The standard of practice of right colectomy with appendiceal mucinous neoplasms has changed such that open operation for removal of mucoceles associated with mucinous carcinomatosis should not be extended for a right colectomy.

Although appendiceal epithelial malignancies can metastasize to regional lymph nodes, this pattern for mucinous appendiceal neoplasms is unusual. Nevertheless, a second important part of the open laparotomy for an appendiceal mucocele is the generous resection of the appendiceal lymph nodes. The entire mesoappendix should be resected with the appendiceal mucocele to provide additional information about the natural history of the disease. The indications for a right colectomy in these patients would be the gross appearance or frozen sections showing malignancy in the appendiceal or the ileocolic lymph nodes.

Similarly, the base of the appendix should be evaluated carefully when removing the mucocele. If there is any doubt about extension of the tumor mass longitudinally through the appendix, frozen sections of the surgical margin is indicated. Another indication for a right colectomy or, preferably, a cecectomy, is a positive margin at the appendectomy site.

Mucocele Progression and the Pseudomyxoma Peritonei Syndrome

Perforated mucoceles may be associated with mucoid material in the peritoneal cavity. This mucoid material may be acellular or can contain cells with either low-or high-grade dysplasia. Patients with appendiceal mucinous neoplasms with peritoneal dissemination have a lethal condition without treatment. Gough and colleagues established that there is no disease-free survival in the absence of either intraperitoneal 5-fluorouracil or intraperitoneal 32-phosphorus. More recently, Misradji and associates showed a median survival of 5–8 years; at 10 years, only a few patients were available for study.

Combined Treatment for the Pseudomyxoma Peritonei Syndrome

About half of patients with mucinous neoplasms of the appendix have perforation at the time of exploration with mucinous peritoneal carcinomatosis or pseudomyxoma peritonei found at the time of appendectomy. In the past, this was a lethal condition without exception. More recently, peritonectomy combined with hyperthermic intraperitoneal chemotherapy has been employed to treat pseudomyxoma peritonei and peritoneal carcinomatosis. The essential features of this approach are diagrammed in Fig. 19.1. The surgeon is responsible for removing as much neoplasm on peritoneal

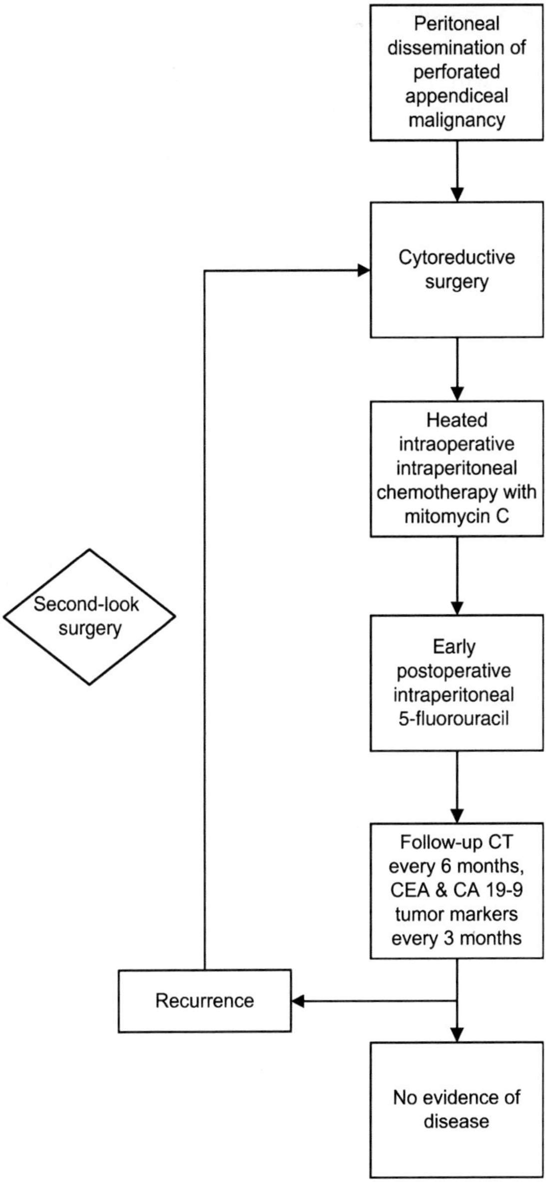

FIGURE 19.1. Approach to the treatment of peritoneal carcinomatosis from appendix cancer.

surfaces as possible. This approach of cytoreductive therapy involves a greater and lesser omentectomy and splenectomy combined with peritonectomy procedures to strip neoplasm from the abdominal gutters, pelvis, right subhepatic space, and right and left subphrenic spaces.

Perioperative Intraperitoneal Chemotherapy

After the operative cytoreduction and with the abdomen open, the peritoneal space is washed extensively by the surgeon's hand using gauze debridement of all surfaces. This is done in the presence of a warm mitomycin C chemotherapy solution (Fig. 19.2). Also, a window of time exists in which all intraperitoneal surfaces are available for intraperitoneal chemotherapy utilizing 5-fluorouracil in the early postoperative period. Uniformity of treatment with intraperitoneal chemotherapy to all peritoneal surfaces, including those surfaces dissected by the surgeon, can be achieved if the intraperitoneal chemotherapy is used during the first postoperative week. As the 5-fluorouracil chemotherapy solution is indwelling in the early postoperative period, intraperitoneal distribution is maximized by turning the patient alternately onto his or her right and left side as well as into the prone position.

This perioperative intraperitoneal chemotherapy (combination of heated, intraoperative mitomycin C and early postoperative 5-fluorouracil) has been utilized in over 850 patients and has not been associated with an increased incidence of anastomotic disruptions. In patients with prior operative procedures who require many hours of lysis of adhesions, there is an increased incidence of postoperative bowel perforation, presumably a result of the combined effects of damage to small bowel from electrosurgical dissection of adhesions (seromuscular damage) and effects of intraperitoneal chemotherapy on the intestine (mucosa and submucosa damage). In patients with high-grade, appendiceal mucinous peritoneal carcinomatosis, intravenous chemotherapy is also recommended after combined treatment is completed. Usually capecitabine and oxaliplatin for 6 months are appropriate. In selected patients,

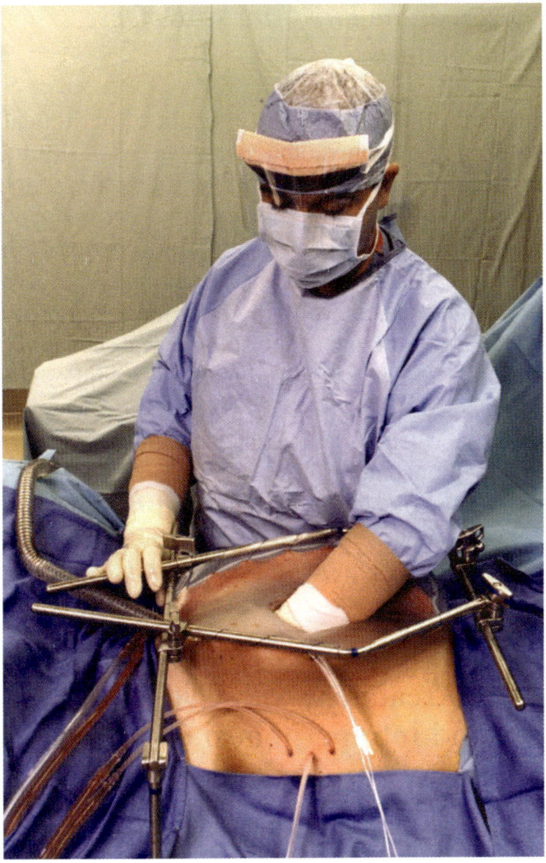

FIGURE 19.2. Intraoperative hyperthermic intraperitoneal chemotherapy. The skin edges are suspended on a self-retaining retractor. Warm (41–42°C) chemotherapy solution is circulated while distributed manually throughout abdomen and pelvis.

usually those who require ostomy closure, a second-look operation is recommended at 6 months after the cytoreduction with perioperative chemotherapy. If at staging celiotomy small tumor foci are found on peritoneal surfaces of the abdomen or pelvis, the nodules are resected, and a final intraperitoneal chemotherapy treatment is performed.

Peritoneum as the First Line of Defense in Carcinomatosis

It is important that definitive treatment of peritoneal carcinomatosis or pseudomyxoma peritonei be instituted in a timely fashion. Each non-definitive (debulking) operative intervention makes potentially curative cytoreductive surgery more difficult. Respect for the peritoneum as the first line of defense of the host against carcinomatosis is a requirement of optimal results using the peritonectomy procedures. Also, the relative sparing of the small bowel seen early in the natural history of peritoneal carcinomatosis and pseudomyxoma peritonei disappears after several surgical procedures have been performed. The fibrous adhesions that result inevitably will become infiltrated by neoplastic cells, leading to extensive involvement of the small bowel. Eventually, effective cytoreductive therapy is impossible, and the effects of intraperitoneal chemotherapy are not adequate to keep the patient disease-free.

Results of Treatment with Cytoreductive Surgery and Intraperitoneal Chemotherapy

The results of this aggressive combined treatment for peritoneal surface dissemination of appendiceal malignancies are unexpectedly good. The mean follow-up of our 385 patients with appendiceal malignancy was 38 months; all appendiceal malignancy patients including adenomucinosis and mucinous adenocarcinoma subtypes were included. All had documented peritoneal surface disease, and a majority had large volume disease. After completion of cytoreductive surgery, the abdomen was inspected for the presence of residual disease. A completeness of cytoreduction score (CC) was obtained based on the size of individual tumor nodules remaining. A CC-0 score indicated no visible tumor remaining; CC-1 indicated tumor nodules less than 2.5 mm; CC-2 indicated tumor nodules between 2.5 mm and 2.5 cm;

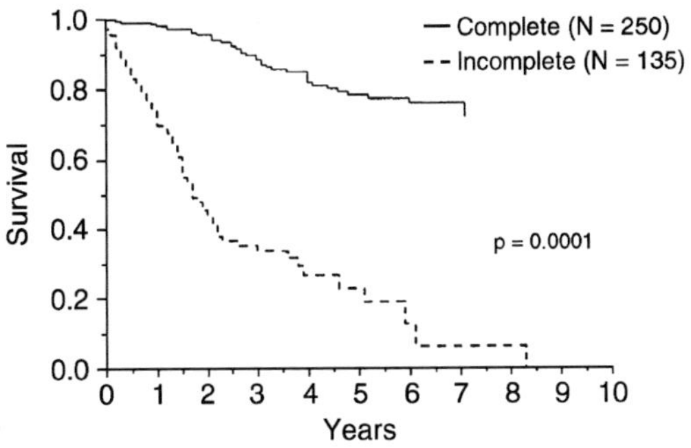

FIGURE 19.3. Survival by cytoreduction of appendiceal malignancy with peritoneal dissemination (Reprinted from Sugarbaker and Chang (1999). With kind permission of Springer Science and Business Media).

and CC-3 indicated tumor nodules larger than 2.5 cm or a confluence of implants at any site. In Fig. 19.3, the survival of patients with CC-0 and CC-1 is compared with those with an incomplete cytoreduction (CC-2 and CC-3). Survival differences were statistically significant; patients with tumor nodules smaller than 2.5 mm in diameter were more likely to survive in the long term than were those with an incomplete cytoreduction. There were no differences in survival between patients with CC-2 and CC-3.

Survival by Histology

From specimens removed at the time of cytoreductive surgery and whenever possible from review of the primary appendiceal malignancy, a histologic assessment was made. Histologic subtypes of adenomucinosis, hybrid, and mucinous adenocarcinoma have been described. Adenomucinosis includes minimally aggressive peritoneal neoplasms that produce large volumes of mucous ascites usually with a primary appendiceal neoplasm described as a cystadenoma. Hybrid malignancies showed adenomucinosis combined with isolated

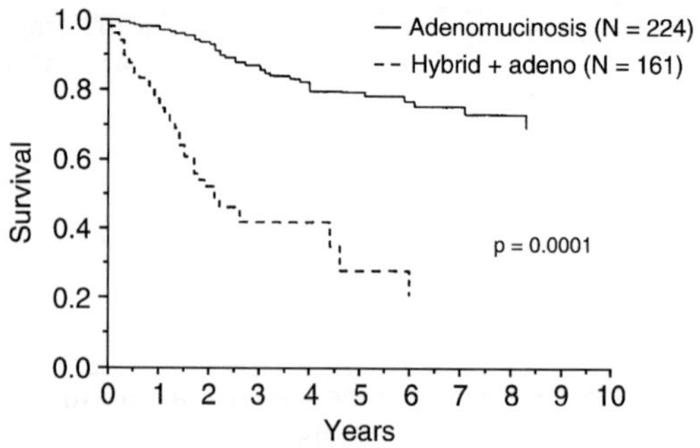

FIGURE 19.4. Survival by histology of appendiceal malignancy with peritoneal dissemination. (Reprinted from Sugarbaker and Chang (1999). With kind permission of Springer Science and Business Media).

foci of mucinous adenocarcinomas (less than 5%). Mucinous adenocarcinoma involves a truly invasive process, often of the signet ring morphology with poor differentiation.

Figure 19.4 shows the survival distribution of these appendix malignancy patients by histology. Survival differences were evident between patients with adenomucinosis and those with hybrid or mucinous adenocarcinoma. No differences were noted between patients with hybrid and mucinous adenocarcinoma histology. A noninvasive histopathology is extremely important in selecting patients most likely to benefit from the treatment strategy of aggressive combined therapy.

Survival by Prior Surgical Score

When the previous operative notes on these patients were reviewed, a judgment was made regarding the anatomic sites of previous surgical dissections. The summation of these dissections from all prior surgical interventions was recorded on a diagram of the abdominopelvic regions which allowed an assessment of the anatomic locations in which previous surgery had been performed. In patients with a prior surgical score (PSS) of 0, diagnosis of peritoneal carcinomatosis was obtained through biopsy only or by laparoscopy plus biopsy. PSS 1 indicated only a previous exploratory laparotomy, while PSS 2 indicated exploratory laparotomy with some resections, usually greater omentectomy with or without right colectomy. With a PSS of 3, patients had an attempt at a complete cytoreduction, usually involving a greater omentectomy, right colectomy, hysterectomy, and bilateral salpingo-oophorectomy with the possibility of other resections from both abdominal organs or parietal peritoneal regions. Patients with PSS scores of 0 through 2 had an improved survival compared with those with a PSS of 3. When analyzed by a multivariate type analysis, complete versus incomplete cytoreduction proved the most important variable with a relative risk of 9.98.

Morbidity and Mortality

Extensive cytoreductive surgery combined with early postoperative intraperitoneal chemotherapy presents a major physiologic insult. Nevertheless, operative mortality remains at 2% in this group of patients. Pancreatitis and fistula formation represent the major complications. Anastomotic leaks were no more common in this group of patients than in a routine general surgical setting (2.4%). Substantial morbidity was 20%. There was no morbidity or mortality associated directly with the intraperitoneal chemotherapy. Rather, the incidence of complications depended on the extent of the operation, number of peritonectomy procedures, and time required to complete the cytoreduction.

Selected Readings

Gonzalez-Moreno S, Sugarbaker PH (2004) Right hemicolectomy does not confer a survival advantage in patients with mucinous carcinoma of the appendix and peritoneal seeding. Br J Surg 91:304–311

Gough DB, Donohue JH, Schutt AJ, et al. (1994) Pseudomyxoma peritonei: long-term patient survival with an aggressive regional approach. Ann Surg 219:112–119

Misdraji J, Yantiss RK, Graeme-Cook FM, et al. (2003) Appendiceal mucinous neoplasms: a clinicopathologic analysis of 107 cases. Am J Surg Pathol 27:1089–1103

Sugarbaker PH (2003) Peritonectomy procedures. Surg Oncol Clin N Am 12:605–621

Sugarbaker PH, Chang D (1999) Results of treatment of 385 patients with peritoneal surface spread of appendiceal malignancy. Ann Surg Oncol 6:727–731

Sugarbaker PH, Alderman R, Edwards G, et al. (2006) Prospective morbidity and mortality assessment of cytoreductive surgery plus perioperative intraperitoneal chemotherapy to treat peritoneal dissemination of appendiceal mucinous malignancy. Ann Surg Oncol 13:635–644

Sugarbaker PH, Ronnett BM, Archer A, et al. (1997) Pseudomyxoma peritonei syndrome. Adv Surg 30:233–280

20
Anal Cancer

Graham Branagan and Brendan Moran

Pearls and Pitfalls

- Eighty-five percent of anal cancers arise in the anal canal with 15% in the anal margin.
- Eight-five percent of anal canal cancers are squamous cell carcinomas (SCC).
- Anal intraepithelial neoplasia (AIN), thought to be a precursor of SCC, is associated with human papillomavirus infection of the perianal skin and anal canal, and iatrogenic immunosuppression in patients who receive an organ allograft.
- Delay and misdiagnosis are common as the signs and symptoms of SCC of the anal canal are similar to those of common, benign perianal conditions, such as hemorrhoids or fissures.
- Histological diagnosis often requires examination and biopsy under anesthesia.
- A record should be made of: (1) position and size of the tumor, including the extent of the tumor within the rectum, perineum, and ischiorectal fossa; and (2) fixity of the tumor to surrounding structures.
- Optimal staging of patients with anal cancer includes a pelvic magnetic resonance imaging (local invasion and pelvic/inguinal lymphadenopathy) and abdominal/thoracic computed tomography for distant spread. This could be complemented by sentinel node biopsy where local expertise exists.

K.I. Bland et al. (eds.), *Colorectal Surgery*,
DOI 10.1007/978-1-84996-444-9_20,

- Compared with surgery, primary chemoradiotherapy offers superior local control and survival with the added benefit of avoiding a permanent stoma in many patients.
- Patients with severe anal symptoms may require fecal diversion, best performed laparoscopically.
- Studies have confirmed the benefits of both combined chemoradiotherapy over radiotherapy alone and that of mitomycin.
- Debate continues regarding the most appropriate radiotherapy dose and overall treatment time.
- Radical salvage surgery by abdominoperineal resection (APR) is the only option offering the possibility of long-term survival for patients with persistent or recurrent disease.
- The major morbidity after salvage APR is perineal wound problems.
- A vertical rectus abdominis flap to primarily close the defect has excellent primary healing rates and acceptable morbidity.

Introduction

The anus is composed of the anal margin and the anal canal. The anal margin extends from the anal verge outwards to include 5 cm of perianal skin. The anal canal extends from the anorectal ring to the anal verge and is usually 3.5–4 cm in length. At the proximal end of the anal canal is a transition zone known as the dentate line, where the squamous lining of the anus meets the glandular mucosa of the rectum. The fundamental distinction between the anal canal and anal margin is important as early squamous tumors of the anal margin can be treated by a similar approach to that of skin lesions by wide local excision with an 80% 5-year survival.

Anal cancer is a rare disease accounting for less than 4% of all anorectal neoplasms, with an annual incidence of 1 per 100,000 population. Historically, anal cancer is more common in women and the elderly. However, the incidence is rising dramatically in the young, especially among the male homosexual population. Incidence rates among this population are 25–30 times that of the general population. Infection with the human immunodeficiency virus (HIV) significantly increases the risk of developing anal cancer, whilst HIV-positive homosexual males have a relative risk 84 times that of the general population.

The etiology of anal cancer seems to be more closely related to genital malignancies than other malignancies of the gastrointestinal tract. Data suggest associations between incidence of anal cancer and infection with human papillomavirus (HPV), lifetime number of sexual partners, cigarette smoking, genital warts, receptive anal intercourse, and infection with HIV.

Anal intraepithelial neoplasia (AIN) is thought to be a precursor of squamous cell carcinoma (SCC) of the anus, similar in many respects to cervical intraepithelial neoplasia. AIN is associated with HPV infection of the perianal skin and anal canal, including the anal transition zone. As infection with these oncogenic viruses persists, the anal tissues may progress through low-grade to high-grade dysplasia and eventually cancer. Long-term follow up suggests that approximately 5% of advanced AIN undergoes malignant change. AIN is also associated with iatrogenic immunosuppression in patients who receive an organ allograft with an estimated increased risk for developing anal cancer of between 10 and 100 times that of the general population. Treatment aims to eradicate AIN and prevent development of anal cancer. Available treatment options include HPV-based vaccines, immunomodulation, local ablation and surgery. However, reported success rates are variable and larger randomized trials are needed. Surgery is associated with significant recurrence rates, especially in HIV positive patients.

Eighty-five percent of anal cancers arise in the anal canal with the remainder arising in the anal margin. Eight-five percent of anal canal cancers are SCC. Approximately, 10% are adenocarcinomas of the anal ducts or glands, behave similarly to low rectal adenocarcinomas and are treated in the same fashion. Other rare anal tumors include melanomas, sarcomas and neuroendocrine tumors.

Anal melanoma is a particularly aggressive tumor that does not respond to chemotherapy or radiotherapy and prognosis is poor. There appears to be no advantage in abdomino-perineal resection (APR) over simple wide local excision of these tumors with median survival rates of 17 and 21 months, respectively.

Clinical Presentation and Diagnosis

Misdiagnosis and delays in diagnosis are common as the signs and symptoms of SCC of the anal canal are similar to those of common, perianal conditions, such as hemorrhoids or fissures. Physicians should be alerted by persistent symptoms that do not respond to treatment.

The majority of patients present with either bright red rectal bleeding (60%) and/or perianal pain (60%). Other common presenting symptoms are the presence of a mass (25–30%) and pruritus or anal discharge (25%). Anal cancers are often locally aggressive with spread to adjacent organs. At first presentation 30–50% of patients will have locally advanced disease. Symptoms of tenesmus or fecal incontinence suggest involvement of the anal sphincter. The passage of feces or offensive discharge per vagina in females is suggestive of a recto-vaginal fistula. Other organs at risk of invasion are the urethra and the prostate gland in men.

A careful inspection of the perianal region, digital rectal examination and proctosigmoidoscopy are of paramount importance. A record should be made of the position and size of the tumor either at the anal margin or within the anal canal, including the extent of the tumor within the rectum, perineum and ischiorectal fossa. Other important details are the fixity of the tumor to surrounding structures, such as the vagina, prostate and pelvis. In some patients it may be possible to palpate enlarged mesorectal lymph nodes. Both groins should be carefully palpated to check for inguinal lymphadenopathy. Recording these details is important as they act as a reference for further examination after chemoradiotherapy.

A histological diagnosis is mandatory and may be best performed during an examination under anesthesia (EUA), which may also facilitate the careful examination described above. Evaluation of the remaining colon has been demonstrated as not to be necessary.

Systemic spread of anal cancer is usually via the lymphatics and less commonly via the bloodstream. Distal anal canal cancers (below the dentate line) spread to the inguinal and femoral node basins whereas proximal cancers drain to mesorectal, internal iliac and para-aortic nodes. About one third of patients with anal cancer will have palpable inguinal nodes but only half of these will have metastases.

Clinically palpable nodes should be evaluated histologically which has been done historically by fine-needle aspiration cytology. Recently some clinicians have advocated the use of sentinel node biopsy techniques to stage these patients more accurately.

Staging and Imaging

Staging of anal cancer patients is based on information gained from pre-treatment clinical, endoscopic and radiological assessments. It is performed using the Union Internationale Contre le Cancer/ American Joint Committee on Cancer (UICC/AJCC) TNM classification (2002) (Table 20.1).

Tumor stages T1–T3 are defined on the basis of size, and imaging has little role to play in the staging of these lesions. However, imaging is of paramount importance in determining the presence and extent of invasion into surrounding structures (T4). Magnetic resonance imaging (MRI) and endoanal ultrasound (EUS) are useful in this respect as they are both able to distinguish the different layers of the bowel wall and identify the interface between the outer layer of the bowel and surrounding structures.

EUS is a relatively inexpensive investigation but the availability of the necessary expertise is limited and the procedure is operator dependent. There is a learning curve with experience of over 50 patients recommended to achieve good results.

TABLE 20.1. Union Internationale Contre le Cancer/American Joint Committee on Cancer (UICC/AJCC) TNM classification (2002).

Primary tumor (T)

TX: Primary tumor cannot be assessed

T0: No evidence of primary tumor

Tis: Carcinoma in situ

T1: Tumor < 2 cm in greatest dimension

T2: Tumor between 2 and 5 cm in greatest dimension

T3: Tumor > 5 cm in greatest dimension

T4: Tumor of any size that invades adjacent organs, e.g., vagina, urethra, bladder (involvement of the sphincter muscle alone is not classified as T4)

Regional lymph nodes (N)

NX: Regional nodes cannot be assessed

N0: No regional lymph node metastases

N1: Metastasis in mesorectal lymph node or nodes

N2: Metastasis in unilateral internal iliac and/or inguinal node or nodes

N3: Metastasis in mesorectal and inguinal nodes and/or bilateral internal iliac and/or inguinal nodes

Distant metastases

MX: Distant metastases cannot be assessed

M0: No distant metastases

M1: Distant metastasis

Stage grouping

Stage 0: Tis N0 M0

Stage 1: T1 N0 M0

Stage 2: T2/3 N0 M0

Stage 3: T4 N0 M0, any T N1 M0

Stage 4: T4 N1 M0, any T N2 M0, any T N3 M0

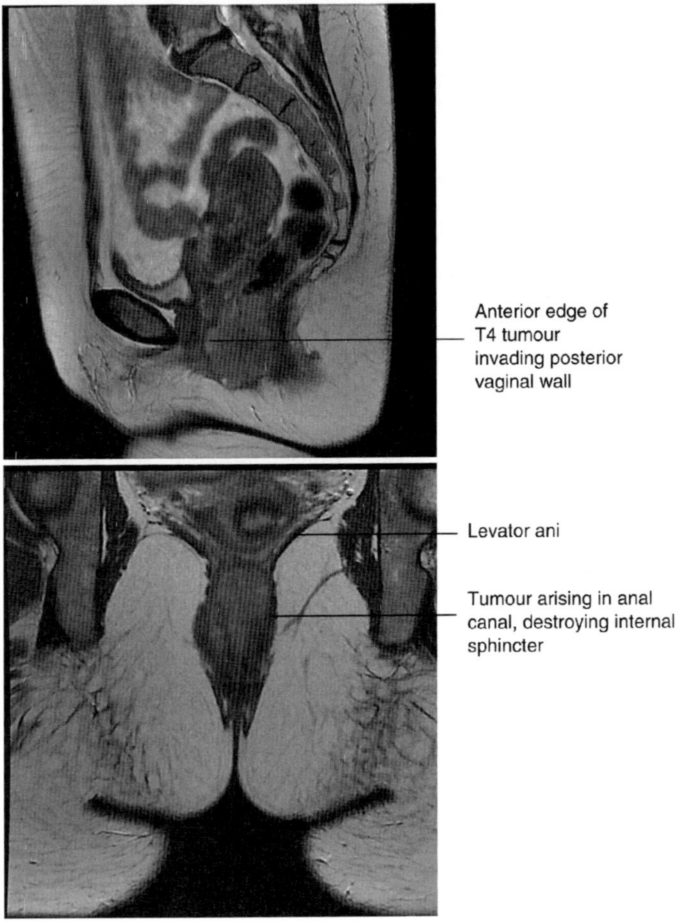

FIGURE 20.1. Coronal and sagittal MRI images of a patient with a T4 cancer invading vagina.

MRI is now used extensively in the staging of rectal cancer, particularly in Europe. However, the experience of MRI staging of anal cancer is limited. Although more expensive than EUS, MRI has two distinct advantages. Firstly, MRI has multiplanar capability allowing sagittal and coronal imaging (Fig. 20.1). Secondly, tumor visualization can be enhanced by intravenous/intraluminal contrast and fat suppression imaging techniques. There are no published data comparing EUS with MRI in staging anal cancer but data from studies in rectal cancer have shown benefits in local staging of advanced disease by MRI.

Local response to therapy is based usually on clinical assessment but can be augmented by EUS. Magnetic resonance imaging (MRI) has been shown to be accurate in assessing the extent of recurrent local disease. Abdominal and pelvic computed tomography (CT) or MRI scanning have high sensitivity for identifying pelvic, inguinal and retroperitoneal lymphadenopathy. However, neither modality is accurate at characterizing lymphadenopathy as benign or malignant.

Current treatment of primary anal cancer does not involve surgical resection and thus the histological status of the lymph nodes is not known. The status of the pelvic nodes is clinically less important than the status of inguinal nodes as the former are included routinely as part of the primary pelvic radiotherapy fields. The approach to management of inguinal nodes remains open to debate. Prophylactic groin irradiation has been shown to decrease the incidence of metachronous inguinal metastases but the majority of patients will probably be overtreated with this regime, receiving larger doses of radiation and an increased risk of toxicity, especially when combined with chemotherapy.

Several authors advocate the use of lymphatic mapping by sentinel node biopsy (SNB) to identify the status of inguinal nodes. This technique is based on the premise that the sentinel node is the first to receive drainage from a primary tumor and is the node most likely to contain metastatic disease. Hence the presence of a negative sentinel node suggests that the remainder of the draining nodal basin is at minimal risk of containing metastases.

Published data for the use of SNB in anal cancer are limited but 5 small series have been reported including a total of 84 patients. In the largest series the sentinel node was identified in all 33 patients and was histologically positive in 7 (21%). None of the patients with histologically negative sentinel nodes received groin irradiation and at 18 months follow up none had developed inguinal metastases. Advocates of SNB suggest that the technique allows a more selective approach to treatment of the inguinal nodes in anal cancer.

Distant metastases are present in 10% of patients at diagnosis with the most common sites being liver and lung. The liver can be assessed by either CT or MRI and the chest by CT.

An optimal approach to staging of patients with anal cancer is to undertake a pelvic MRI to assess local invasion and both pelvic and inguinal lymphadenopathy with an abdominal and thoracic CT to assess for distant spread. This could be complemented by sentinel node biopsy where local expertise exists.

Treatment and Outcomes

Historically, treatment of most patients with anal cancer was by abdominoperineal resection (APR) of the rectum and anal canal, with local excision reserved for patients with well-differentiated tumors smaller than 2 cm or tumors confined to the mucosa and submucosa. APR was a radical surgical option with significant morbidity and formation of a permanent end colostomy. It resulted in local treatment failure in 30–50% of patients and 5-year survival of 50–70%. Local excision was suitable for less than 10% of patients with anal cancer and reported results were variable. Results for local excision of advanced lesions were extremely poor with local recurrence rates greater than 60% and few 5-year survivors.

Pioneering work by Nigro et al. in the 1980s has led to the adoption of combined chemoradiotherapy as the recommended first-line treatment for SCC of the anal canal. In this study patients with locally advanced anal cancers were treated with neoadjuvant external beam radiotherapy and concurrent chemotherapy with fluorouracil (5-FU) and mitomycin C. Complete pathological responses were observed in 81% patients.

Subsequent studies have confirmed the benefits of combined chemoradiotherapy over radiotherapy alone (Table 20.2). Both the European Organisation for Research and Treatment

TABLE 20.2. Results of randomized clinical trials of chemoradiation in anal cancer.

Trial	N	DXT (phase 1)	Boost	Chemotherapy	Outcome
UKCCCR ACT I	585	45 Gy in 20-25 fractions	15 Gy after 6 weeks	5-FU days 1-4 and 29-32; mitomycin day 1	Significant improvement in local control in chemoradiotherapy group ($p < 0.0001$)
EORTC	110	45 Gy in 25 fractions	15-20 Gy after 6 weeks	5-FU days 1-5 and 29-33; mitomycin day 1	Significant improvement in local control in chemoradiotherapy group ($p < 0.02$)
RTOG	291	45-50.4 Gy in 25-28 fractions	None	5-FU days 1-4 and 29-32 (both groups); mitomycin days 1 and 29 (1 group only)	Significant improvement in local control with mitomycin ($p < 0.001$)

UKCCCR ACT I: UK Coordinating Committee on Cancer Research Anal Cancer Trial; EORTC: European Organisation for Research and Treatment of Cancer; RTOG: Radiation Therapy Oncology Group; 5-FU: fluorouracil.

of Cancer (EORTC) trial and the UK Coordinating Committee on Cancer Research (UKCCCR) Anal Cancer Trial (ACT)1 demonstrated that chemoradiotherapy is more effective than radiotherapy alone in terms of local control, with a clear improvement in colostomy free survival. However, neither trial demonstrated any difference in overall survival between the two groups.

Currently, debate continues regarding the most appropriate radiotherapy dose and overall treatment time. Recent data suggest that the shortening of radiotherapy treatment times by eliminating the gap between the initial phase of radiotherapy and subsequent boost dose results in improved local control.

The use of mitomycin C is associated with significant toxicity including prolonged thrombocytopenia. However, the Radiation Therapy Oncology Group (RTOG 87-04) trial reported a higher complete response rate (92% vs. 85%), better local control (72% vs. 51%), improved disease-free survival (73% vs. 51%) and a lower colostomy rate (9% vs. 22%) in the group that received mitomycin C and 5-FU in combination with radiotherapy compared with the group that received radiotherapy and 5-FU alone (Table 20.2). Overall 4-year survival was similar (75% vs. 70%) but toxicity (Grade 4 + 23% vs. 7%) was significantly greater in the mitomycin arm.

Cisplatin is superior to mitomycin C as a radiosensitizer with greater activity against squamous cell solid tumors. It also has a more favorable side-effect profile with less myelosuppression. There are some data to suggest that cisplatin based regimes may be superior to those containing mitomycin C with similar local control and survival rates, but reduced toxicity. However, the numbers are small and most of the trials involving cisplatin use higher radiation doses than mitomycin based trials. Several trials investigating the role of cisplatin in the treatment of anal cancer are currently under way. In particular, two large phase III randomized trials, RTOG 98-11 and the UKCCCR-ACT II trials are comparing mitomycin C-based with cisplatin-based chemoradiotherapy.

The maximum clinical and pathological response to chemoradiotherapy may not be reached until 6–9 months after completion of treatment. Hence, patients that have residual tumor clinically on completion of treatment require intense follow-up examination every 6 weeks. Tumors that persist or progress require biopsy. For patients with a complete clinical response, any new growth requires a biopsy to exclude recurrence.

Persistent disease is defined as tumor that remains after maximum treatment response or tumor that recurs within 6 months of a complete response. Recurrent disease is defined as tumor that reappears more than 6 months after a complete response.

Although surgery is no longer the primary treatment for anal cancer it still has an important role in the management of these patients. As already described, EUA and biopsy of the primary tumor is required for most primary tumors, and SNB is increasingly accepted as optimal staging of the inguinal lymph nodes. Formation of a temporary colostomy may be necessary in patients who have incontinence of feces due to invasion of the sphincter by advanced tumor or those who are at risk of continence problems secondary to the acute side, effects of pelvic radiotherapy. Currently, laparoscopy with laparoscopic stoma formation is the best method for peritoneal and liver surface imaging, with rapid recovery compared to open surgery.

Finally, for patients with persistent or recurrent disease that cannot have or do not respond to further chemotherapy and/or radiotherapy, radical salvage surgery in the form of APR with wide skin margins is the only option offering the possibility of long-term survival. Patients being considered for salvage surgery require careful assessment. Where clear resection margins cannot be achieved, radical excisional surgery should not be considered as there is no survival benefit and significant risk of morbidity. In these cases, diversion of the faecal stream by a defunctioning stoma may be necessary for palliation.

Overall survival after salvage surgery ranges from 24% to 53% with most of the reported series having small numbers. The largest reported series of 57 patients demonstrated a 5-year survival of 33% with median survival of nearly 3 years. Patients with curative resection (negative margins and no new intraoperative metastases) had a 5-year survival of 40% with a median survival of over 4 years.

Factors which predicted poor outcome after salvage surgery included positive resection margins (0% 5-year survival, median survival 10 months), nodal disease at surgery (11% 5-year survival, 8 months median survival) and tumors which were large (> 5 cm) or invaded adjacent organs (0% 5 year survival, median survival 19 months). Most reported series demonstrate worse outcomes for patients with persistent disease (5-year survival 56–82%) compared with patients with recurrent disease (5-year survival 23–33%).

The major morbidity after salvage APR is perineal wound complications almost certainly related to the radiotherapy component of the initial treatment. Perineal breakdown occurs in 30–60% of patients resulting in persistent non-healing wounds for 6–9 months or longer. The large perineal wounds resulting from radical salvage APR present problems due to a combination of the difficult anatomical position, the propensity for infection and the potential need for further management of the underlying pathology. This has led to the introduction of plastic surgical techniques which aim to reduce this considerable complication rate. Local flaps, such as the posterior thigh flap, tensor fascia lata flap and vastus lateralis flap have been used. However, there is a complication rate of 20–50% for these flaps and they do not always have sufficient bulk to close the defect.

Currently, the most commonly used technique is the use of a trans-pelvic vertical rectus abdominis myocutaneous (VRAM) flap based on the inferior epigastric vessels, providing a long pedicled flap with a large bulk of muscle. There are a number of small series reporting excellent primary healing with acceptable morbidity with VRAM flaps.

The treatment of the inguinal node basins may differ with the advent of SNB. Currently, some centers irradiate the groins as part of the pelvic radiotherapy regime. Others pursue a "watch and wait" policy after careful clinical assessment of the groins and fine needle aspiration cytology of any suspicious nodes. SNB allows more accurate staging of these nodes and a selective policy for groin irradiation.

For patients with synchronous groin node disease, chemoradiotherapy results in disease control in 65–90% patients. For persistent inguinal disease, block dissection of the groin can be offered, although in an irradiated field this procedure has high morbidity. In patients who have not received groin irradiation, metachronous or recurrent groin disease can be treated with radiotherapy and additional chemotherapy or with inguinal node dissection.

Currently, treatment of distant metastatic disease is palliative with a uniformly poor prognosis. Complete response to treatment is rare and duration of response usually short. Palliative radiotherapy and chemotherapy have a role to play in the management of symptomatic metastases.

Conclusion

Whilst no longer the primary modality of treating patients, surgery still has an important role to play in the management of patients with anal cancer and the surgeon remains a key member of the multidisciplinary team. The majority of patients present to surgeons with local anal symptoms and confirmatory histological diagnosis may require biopsy under anesthesia. Chemoradiotherapy offers good disease control and 5-year survival and avoids a permanent stoma in the majority of patients. Individual patients with severe anal symptoms may require fecal diversion prior to chemoradiotherapy. In selected patients with persistent or recurrent disease, radical salvage surgery may be necessary and in specialized units is associated with reasonable 5-year survival and good palliation in incurable cases.

Selected Readings

Abbasakoor F, Boulos PB (2005) Anal intraepithelial neoplasia. Br J Surg 92:277–290

Bell SW, Dehni N, Chaouat M, Lifante JC, et al. (2005) Primary rectus abdominis myocutaneous flap for repair of perineal and vaginal defects after extended abdominoperineal resection. Br J Surg 92:482–486

Damin DC, Rosito MA, Schwartsmann G (2006) Sentinel lymph node in carcinoma of the anal canal: a review. Eur J Surg Oncol 32:247–252
Mackay SG, Pager CK, Joseph D, et al. (2003) Assessment of the accuracy of transrectal ultrasonography in anorectal neoplasia. Br J Surg 90:346–350
Nilsson PJ, Svensson C, Goldman S, Glimelius B (2002) Salvage abdominoperineal resection in anal epidermoid cancer. Br J Surg 89:1425–1429
Roach SC, Hulse PA, Moulding FJ, et al. (2005) Magnetic resonance imaging of anal cancer. Clin Radiol 60:1111–1119
Welton ML, Sharkey FE, Kahlenberg MS (2004) The etiology and epidemiology of anal cancer. Surg Oncol Clin N Am 13:263–275
Yue-Kui B, Wen-Lan C, Ji-Dong G, et al. (2004) Surgical salvage therapy of anal canal cancer. World J Gastroenterol 10:424–426

21 Rectal Cancer: Issues for the 21st Century, a Practical Update for the Surgeon

Richard J. Heald

Pearls and Pitfalls

- Mobility of the tumor (on pubo-rectal sidewall) remains the key physical sign.
- Think embryology: What is removed is an intact envelope of the midline hindgut with its surrounding lymphovascular "mesentery."
- Circumferential surgery is the key – move from one quadrant to another.
- As Goethe said, "Man recognizes only what he knows." Learn the "holy plane" by careful visualization and three-directional traction to open its avascular areolar "cobweb."
- Learn the hypogastric plexuses and preserve them.
- The plane leads to the visceral muscle tube of the internal sphincter. Triple stapling is expensive but safe and a wash-out below to seal the specimen wise.
- Never forget to do both rectal and vaginal examinations before neo-adjuvant treatment and always on the table at the start of surgery. Mobility is the key.
- If you lose the "holy plane" or make something bleed go across the pelvis 180° and develop the plane elsewhere, whilst maintaining pressure on the bleed.
- Avoid tearing from excessive traction.

K.I. Bland et al. (eds.), *Colorectal Surgery*,
DOI 10.1007/978-1-84996-444-9_21,

- During the circular stapling never catch any external sphincters. Be sure you can see the edge of the anvil through the single layer of anorectal smooth muscle.
- It is usually wiser to defunction the very low anastomosis.

Introduction

There can be few areas of surgical practice around which change seems so frenetic but yet in which cynics might feel that hard evidence of survival benefit so slow to appear. Rectal cancer offers more opportunity for improvement in outcome, both in terms of cure and in the reduction of "collateral damage," than any of the other common malignancies. Nevertheless, competing pressures from the various disciplines that are now involved have created more unanswered questions and less truly convincing hard evidence of real benefit than we need for the many decisions we must help our patients to make. Examples of outstanding and pressing areas of confusion include:

- Radiotherapy (RT)
- Should it be short course or long?
- Conformal anal preserving or conventional?
- Should it be combined with chemotherapy?
- Which combinations of drugs and how should the two modalities be scheduled?
- The criteria for selection and the use of modern imaging modalities
- Should a rectal cancer operation in 2006 ever be undertaken without a fine slice magnetic resonance imaging (MRI)?
- The emergence of the "complete response" phenomenon (cCR)
- Should we be following Habr-Gama's lead and observing selected cases with the now widespread use of chemoradiotherapy (CRT) combinations?

All of these add to the already rich tapestry of surgical challenges and potential improvements to which this chapter seeks to provide an update. In the background is the understanding in the minds of many experienced surgeons that details of their operative technique probably matter more to most patients than the decisions that may be made at a distance on their behalf by distinguished members of the multidisciplinary team(MDT). Perhaps the most worrying aspect of advances into the 21st century is the staggering escalations in cost that the involvement of other disciplines has brought with it. Many European cancer centers now regard preoperative chemoradiotherapy as the "new European standard" so that the first 5 years of the new century have seen the cost of these therapies surpass the total cost of hospitalization, surgery and all other aspects of the patient's management added together. The second 5 years of the new century are likely to see this situation become even more out of proportion with even more potentially devastating financial implications for the funding of cancer care especially in poorer countries. A further serious consequence of multiple therapies with changes and modifications that appear almost monthly is that the practice of "evidence-based medicine" becomes impossible because so many aspects of care are changing simultaneously. Fortunately there is much that can be achieved by the affordable application of MRI staging, refinements in surgical technique, and the introduction of histopathological audit.

Preoperative Assessment and Work Up

It is self-evident that each patient must be assessed clinically with particular regard to comorbidity that may influence operative decisions. By government edict most patients are now discussed by a MDT covering the whole range of relevant specialists although specialist advice on comorbidity is often not available at such meetings. Key elements of this presurgery conference about each patient are a full computed tomography (CT) scan of the chest and abdomen with particular reference to the detection of metastatic disease. In the UK the Pelican Centre has been working for a number of years on the MERCURY project which has demonstrated close correlation between specialist preoperative fine slice phased array coil MRI examinations and the subsequent histology. For tidy comparison the whole specimen is not cut right open by the surgeon but preserved intact, fixed, and subsequently sliced axially to conform with the preoperative axial images. Where the necessary radiological and histological skills have been developed in the same hospital the focal point of most MDT discussions is now these special MRI scans, which show very accurately the relationship of the cancer and its extramural extensions to the enveloping mesorectal fascia which will subsequently guide the surgeon's "holy plane" dissection around the total mesorectal excision(TME) specimen. The operator's grasp of the anatomy and the levels in the pelvis is much enhanced by reference to these scans if they are skillfully presented. It should not be forgotten, however, that these fine slice examinations do not generally extend up to the root of the inferior mesenteric artery, so that some lymph nodes, which might be removed in a good TME may not be assessed by this method. Similar limitations apply to all the routine RT pelvic fields, so that high nodes escape irradiation and the dissection around the aortic root of the inferior artery becomes more important. The MERCURY study reports the practice of a network of hospitals in three countries (England, Germany, and Wales) and centered on the Pelican Centre in Basingstoke in using a minimum of 1mm mesorectal clearance within the mesorectal fascia on MRI as the principal indication for avoiding preoperative RT (predicted clear margins). Exception is made when there is extensive intra-mesorectal disease, either N2 lymphatic spread or extensive extramural venous invasion, all factors known to increase the risk of local failure. Somewhat arbitrarily also the involvement of internal iliac nodes visualized on MRI is taken as an indication for preoperative chemoradiotherapy, since the management of such nodes surgically is generally avoided except in Japan.

Choice of Operation – Clinical and Radiological Assessment

Local excision. This is probably most safely restricted to T1 cancers in the anorectal area or possibly more advanced tumors in people in whom the risk of a major operation or of major adjuvant therapy tips the balance towards a relatively minor procedure. We consider that the combination of local excision with chemo-radiotherapy is currently suspect in relation to the hazard of converting an entirely curable early lesion into a preventable late disaster.

Transanal endoscopic microsurgery(TEM) has been extensively practiced in some centers and claims for its suitability for some T2 tumors have been made by certain specialists. The excision of a disk of rectal wall in the upper anal canal and distal rectum is considered by our unit to be intrinsically dangerous in that it may compromise the peri-mesorectal "holy" plane if a subsequent anterior resection and TME were to become necessary.

Anterior resection (AR) and abdominoperineal excision (APE). Advances in imaging have in no way diminished the need for the surgeon to establish the following by digital examination:

1. The size and the mobility of the primary tumor in relation to the pubo-rectal sling in the conscious patient and therefore tone in the pubo-rectal sling (i.e., not simply examination under anesthetic when the pelvic floor may be relaxed).
2. The position and the size of the cancer and its relationship to left or right pelvic sidewalls, prostate, vesicles or vagina in front, and the coccyx and sacrum behind. Mobility on the vaginal wall is particularly important to establish since we do not consider its excision necessary unless it is threatened or invaded by the cancer.
3. The discrete nature and palpability of the precise distal margin of the cancer together with an assessment of the amount of healthy normal mucosa below the tumor and above where the surgeon judges the dentate line to be.

The palpable lower edge of a rectal cancer is almost invariably its microscopic lower edge.

Selection for sphincter preservation. It is the author's opinion that most cancers with (a) a discrete distal margin, which is mobile on the pubo-rectal sling with the patient awake and (b) in whom there is 1–2 cm of clear smooth anorectal mucosa between an anorectal discrete edge and the dentate line, will be best treated, in expert hands, by the TME operation. After the full mesorectal mobilization achieved by this operation, provided the patient has a healthy functioning anal sphincter, an ultralow stapled reconstruction with a colon pouch or side to end anastomosis will provide good or acceptable anorectal function. This, however, may not be true in the new century if the patient has undergone, or later undergoes, radiation therapy—as is now very common in European practice. Data from Sweden suggest that incontinence and frequency of bowel function is rather common after anterior resection procedures in patients who have undergone RT. Frank discussion of these risks with the patient is now essential.

Technical Advances in Total Mesorectal Excision

The basic steps of TME have been fully described elsewhere. The surgeon who is likely to achieve the best results is the one who is prepared to take infinite pains to perfect the creation of a perfect cancer specimen according to the embryological principles which underlie the concept of TME. The "holy plane" around the mesorectum was created in utero when the midline hindgut, distinct from the essentially paired embryonic parities, returned into the abdominal cavity during intrauterine life. All the surgical planes around gut derivatives—pancreas, duodenum, retromesocolic on right or left, the holy plane itself within the pelvis, etc.—are recognizable as dissection planes and provide the key to optimal curative colorectal cancer surgery. This is most particularly true in rectal carcinoma where the main field of spread is usually locoregional, metastases are so often late, and intra-peritoneal spread somewhat uncommon.

If the concept is so simple, how can there be continuing "advances" in the 21st century? Quintessentially these are those improvements that surgeons are making in every field of surgery but applied here to *das koncept der TME totalen mesorectalen excisionen*. Firstly there can be few procedures where it is so true that two really experienced specialist surgeons achieve better results and more perfect specimens than one senior with an inexperienced assistant. This was one of the secondary observations on the data collected for the MERCURY project. Most of the relevant technical advances relate to newer methods of visualizing accurately what we are actually doing. Thus in open surgery improvements in the shaping and illumination of retractors, based on the St. Mark's pattern and the reversed mesorectal retractor with built-in fiber-optic illumination designed by Bolton Surgical, are significant. The use of a pair of retractors, both illuminated but one concave and the other convex, combines the provision of excellent illumination with traction and counter-traction in the difficult depths of the human pelvis. The addition of a third direction of retraction further helps to put areolar tissue continuously on stretch so that it may be divided in an avascular manner by modern diathermy dissection. All these methods combined with the effective aspiration of smoke and the creation of a dry operation field facilitate better and more anatomically correct surgery for this technically challenging malignancy. In addition to this there have been major advances in the use of electro-coagulation and ultrasonic hemostatic devices such as Ligasure. The application of these same principles in laparoscopic surgery is little short of revolutionary in its impact on the potential of the laparoscope in the whole of colorectal surgery. It is interesting in this regard that open surgery and laparoscopic surgery are both making progress but it is the retraction which remains the greatest problem in laparoscopy and the hemostasis which still represents the greatest problem in open surgery. Probably each discipline can learn from the other so that the next few years will see better and better mesorectal specimens with more consistently clear surgical margins. At the present time, however, it is probably sensible to warn laparoscopic surgeons against attempting to excise large cancers in the true pelvis, most particularly in large male patients or patients with a narrow small pelvis. It is literally true that the planar anatomy of the lower pelvis is only now being fully understood because the planes are difficult to demonstrate in the cadaver and difficult to develop during live surgery due to access and bleeding. It is interesting that in laparoscopic surgery the lessons of open surgery are being applied by many of the leading exponents, i.e., sharp monopolar diathermy dissection and more sophisticated methods of opening up tissue planes by ingenious traction and counter-traction devices.

Abdominoperineal Excision

Whilst this has been frequently described elsewhere there are developing ideas which are appropriate for this "update." It has been observed by Quirke and others that the frequently published poor results that are often achieved in APE correlate with a much higher incidence of margin involvement by cancer on the histological specimens than is observed in anterior resection TME specimens. Interestingly these apply both to the perineal and the TME component of the APE – an operation which should encompass the whole mesorectum and the enveloping levators and sphincters. This has led to widespread calls for a more cylindrical operation specimen and the careful avoidance of the development of a "waist" on the APE specimen. This waist comes about because the peri-mesorectal holy plane tapers into the top of the two-layered sphincter mechanism and it is around this area between the dentate line and about 5 cms above it that perforation of the bowel or involvement of the specimen margin most commonly occurs. The author's view is that modern MRI can demonstrate reasonably clearly whether the outside of the sphincter complex is threatened at any point by the carcinoma and it is in these cases that preoperative CRT should be considered—rather than after all ultralow cancers undergoing APE as is practiced in many centers. The specific disadvantage of giving RT to patients undergoing APE is that delayed perineal wound healing becomes extremely common.

It is the author's personal opinion that the widespread advocacy of "cylindrical APE" has perhaps pushed us towards removing more ischiorectal fat than is really necessary. It appears logical, provided the outside of the sphincter complex is not penetrated by cancer, as visualized on MRI, to preserve most of the ischiorectal fat and dissect in the recognizable plane just outside the anal sphincters and to follow the levator ani muscles up to their point of origin on the inner aspect of the obturator internus muscles. Many surgeons believe that this can be best done and the best "waist-free" specimens achieved with the patient in the prone jackknife position for the perineal dissection. Removal of the coccyx may also be a wise precaution, particularly in the more advanced cancers, as the larger "hole" thus created makes it safe to deliver the upper part of the specimen first without risking rupture of the cancer which is an operative error to be avoided at all costs. Laparoscopy for the abdominal dissection has obvious advantages in APE, which are not so clear when the method is used for anterior resection, because this perineal delivery of the specimen makes an abdominal incision completely unnecessary. Furthermore, it is desirable to discontinue dissection from the abdominal aspect in APE at the point of origin of the levator muscles around to the coccyx at the back, i.e., the most difficult and challenging part of peri-mesorectal dissection. As in anterior resection, however, the anterior plane remains a major dissection challenge, and anterior tumors have a higher incidence of local failure than posterior or posterolateral tumors.

High Anterior Resection and Mesorectal Transection (Partial Mesorectal Excision)

Partial mesorectal excision (PME) applies to rectal cancers with their lower margin above between 10 and 14 cm from the anal verge according to the size and build of the patient. The degree of extra mobilization that can be achieved by avascular dissection is the final determinant. The decision as to whether a TME or a PME is to be undertaken is made after every avascular component of the dissection has been completed down to the point which used to be described as the "lateral ligament." At this point, where the inferior hypogastric plexus is on the pelvic sidewall, surgeons in the past have used big clamps to divide what are often called the "lateral stalks." Provided peri-mesorectal dissection is pursued in a TME operation very precisely only small vessels are generally found here and no middle rectal artery of any significant size actually exists except in a small minority of patients (Sato & Sato). After dissection has proceeded to this level, if there is a 5 cm mesorectum available distal to the lower edge of the tumor, the mesorectum may be divided at this point using ligasure or ligation. This is only a worthwhile exercise if it enables a significantly higher anastomosis to be effected, as this will obviate the need for a temporary loop stoma. Indeed the whole procedure becomes a less "major" operation with clear advantages for the patient.

The Colon Pouch and the Coloplasty

Each of these methods has been widely described elsewhere and each provides satisfactory improvement in the functional outcome of the very low anastomosis. If a pouch is to be used, however, we would counsel against it being larger than around 2° 6 cm for fear of obstructed defecation developing over time. This is the only risk of pouch surgery which may get worse rather than better over time.

Anastomotic Leakage and the Temporary Stoma

The author's extensive traveling and performance of TME in different countries has given him an insight into the variations that exist in attitudes to this problem. It has been made very clear throughout the world that the principal risk factor for anastomotic leakage is the lowness of the anastomosis, i.e., its proximity to the anal sphincters themselves. Rullier put the difference at eight times increase in risk for anastomoses below6 cm. This places most true TME operations, as opposed to PMEs for higher tumors, in the high-risk category. Multiple discussions in China reveal the fact that there and probably in many parts of the world the defunctioning stoma is not routine but the use of a wide bore soft tube drain for 7 days or more is standard practice against the risk of fecal fistula. In Europe, however, the defunctioning stoma for the ultralow anastomosis has become very widespread indeed whilst drainage is generally restricted to low tension suction drainage for only 2 days to evacuate potential hematoma in the pelvic space. Many factors are relevant to these differences. RT is rarely used in China where anal stretch is considered a convenient and cost-effective method of protecting the anastomosis. The latter is, however, considered inappropriate in Europe by most colorectal authorities who consider that it may lead to long-term anal incontinence. Reconstitution of the pelvic peritoneum in some parts of the world has been common and may be relevant in helping to confine the leakage within the pelvis but this does become virtually impossible if a full TME is undertaken along the lines that have been described by us. Our own view is that significant leakage should be avoided if possible and its consequences minimized since clinically detectable leakage in our own series not only increases mortality but also diminishes the chance of good ano-rectal function. We therefore advocate either ileostomy or colostomy with closure at 6 weeks—before adjuvants if these are planned.

As in so many aspects a multitude of factors contributing to anastomotic leakage make reliable hard data unobtainable. One long-standing misconception has, however, been recently corrected by workers from Orebro in Sweden. They have confirmed that defunctioning does not only minimize or abolish the consequences of a low leak, but it also reduces the risk of this actually occurring. Risk factors which should be borne in mind and which probably make defunctioning in

Western practice imperative include smoking, widespread vascular disease, and diabetes. Operative factors that are certainly relevant include pulsatile blood supply on the colonic side of the anastomosis, lack of tension and adequate length to fill the pelvis with redundant colon, optimal hemostasis within the pelvic cavity, and possibly the use of effective suction drainage to remove any blood, which does so readily collect. Good stapling technique and the use of either a colon pouch or a side to end anastomosis are probably important.

The Complete Pathological Response

A "new dilemma" is posed by the apparent complete disappearance of the cancer. This is compounded by the progressive but variable timescale of the down-staging process which continues over many months after the CRT has finished. Somewhat arbitrarily only 6–10 weeks delay is usual before operating—a time perceived as a "window of opportunity." Radical surgery is considered mandatory because regrowth within the irradiated area is believed inevitable. This has been challenged by Habr-Gama and her coworkers in Sao Paolo, Brazil. Her series lacks MRI staging and includes some early tumors, whereas CRT here is usually reserved for advanced cancers threatening the mesorectal margin on MRI, or with other adverse MRI features. The Brazil data, however, show that cancers which seem to have disappeared may indeed have done just that (complete clinical response, CR or cCR), i.e., the patient may be cured. As many as 99/360 patients treated between 1991 and 2005 were clinical cCRs and a further 24 patients who had resections had no identifiable cancer in the specimen (ypT0N0). Only 2% of the 99 cCR patients observed without surgery have died of cancer in a follow-up extending for up to 10 years. Five percent regrowths detected during follow-up were all amenable to "delayed resection."

British surgeons have generally regarded the Habr-Gama series as interesting but without immediate relevance. Widespread CRT and mandatory involvement in MDTs does, in our opinion, make this viewpoint no longer tenable – at least for patients about to undergo APE with permanent colostomy. This operation is viewed with dread by many patients who might well prefer a surveillance option. Furthermore, the mandatory positive biopsy before APE is somewhat illogically scrapped if the tumor has "disappeared." Positive biopsy is unlikely in cCR cases because cancer often cannot be found in whole specimens when surgery is undertaken.

It is important that enthusiasm for the exciting possibilities that cCR opens up should be kept in proportion. Specialized primary surgery will continue to be the cornerstone of management, backed by specialized MRI selection for CRT plus histopathological audit to maintain standards. It is probable that 50–70% of patients are best treated by optimal surgery alone, and that most of the downstaged CRT cases will need surgery but will achieve clear margins when these appear threatened. In the short and medium term it is unlikely that more than around 10% of all rectal cancers will be in line for the nonsurgical option. Nevertheless, our fundamental understanding of modern cancer treatment for all solid tumors demands that this special group be properly investigated. Furthermore, if Habr-Gama's experience is confirmed, a significant minority each year may one day be spared the necessity for major surgery.

Summary

Rectal cancer is no longer a disease for the generalist. Rather it has become the paradigm and test bed for the future multidisciplinary specialist management of all solid tumors. The relative importance of surgical technique, modern RT, and the arrival of the new drugs represent one of the most fascinating and complex scenarios in modern medicine. Advances in surgery are individually small but together create one of the most spectacular improvements in actual cancer "cure" of the modern era. The challenge is to organize our cancer services so that all may benefit and so the other (so expensive) modalities may be tested against a standard (high quality) "product" standardized and audited oncological surgery.

Selected Readings

Adam IJ, Mohamdee MO, Martin IG, et al. (1994) Role of circumferential margin involvement in the local recurrence of rectal cancer. Lancet 344:707–711

Heald RJ, Moran BJ, Ryall RDH, et al. (1998) The Basing-stoke experience of total mesorectal excision 1978–1997. Arch Surg 133:894–899

Hermanek P, Wiebelt H, Staimmer D, Riedl S (1995) The German Study Group Colorectal Carcinoma (SGCRC). Prognostic factors of rectal carcinoma -experience of the German Multicentre Study. Tumori 81:60–64

MacFarlane JK, Ryall RD, Heald RJ (1993) Mesorectal excision for rectal cancer. Lancet 341:457–460

Martling AL, Holm T, Rutqvist L, et al. (2000) Effect of a surgical training programme on outcome of rectal cancer in the County of Stockholm. Stockholm Colorectal Cancer Study Group, Basingstoke Bowel Cancer Research Project. Lancet 356:93–96

MERCURY Study Group (2006) Diagnostic accuracy of preoperative magnetic resonance imaging in predicting curative resection of rectal cancer: prospective observational study. BMJ 333:779

Quirke P, Scott N. (1992) The pathologist's role in the assessment of local recurrence in rectal carcinoma. Surg Oncol Clin North Am 1:1–17

Stelzner F (1996) Das echte und das falsche Lokalrezidiv nach der Kontinenzresektion des rektumkarzinoms. Chirurg 67:611

Wibe A, Moller B, Norstein J, et al. (2002) A national strategic change in treatment policy for rectal cancer— implementation of total mesorectal excision as routine treatment in Norway. A national audit. Dis Colon Rectum 45:857–866

22
Adjuvant and Neoadjuvant Therapy for Colorectal Carcinoma

Anne Y. Lin, Deborah Schrag, and W. Douglas Wong

Pearls and Pitfalls

Colon Cancer

- Adjuvant chemotherapy with 5-FU-based chemotherapy is used for the treatment of patients with Stage III colon cancer to minimize local recurrence and metastatic spread of disease.
- Combination regimens with oxaliplatin/5-FU/leucovorin (FOLFOX) have improved disease-free survival rates for patients with Stage III disease. The main side effect of oxaliplatin therapy is peripheral neuropathy.
- Novel targeted therapies with the monoclonal antibodies bevacizumab (anti-VEGFR) and cetuximab (anti-EGFR) are being investigated for use in the adjuvant setting.
- The risk of recurrence is approximately 20–25% for patients with Stage II colon cancer. There is an increasing trend towards treating Stage II colon cancer patients with adjuvant chemotherapy, particularly those with poor prognostic clinicopathologic features.

K.I. Bland et al. (eds.), *Colorectal Surgery*,
DOI 10.1007/978-1-84996-444-9_22,

Rectal Cancer

- An adequate total mesorectal excision (TME) including circumferential margin is important for decreasing local recurrence rates.
- Adjuvant chemotherapy and radiation are recommended for Stages II and III disease.

Introduction

The risk of recurrence in colorectal cancer has decreased with optimal surgery and the addition of adjuvant and neoadjuvant therapy. However, even with an adequate resection for colorectal carcinoma, the risk of recurrence remains present. Adjuvant therapy is thus aimed at the subset of patients who may potentially harbor occult microscopic disease or who have deeper transmural extension of the neoplasm, in an attempt to minimize local recurrence and metastatic spread of disease. Adjuvant chemotherapy is the standard of care for Stage III colon cancer patients. Although controversial, there is an increasing trend toward treating Stage II colon cancer patients with adjuvant chemotherapy. For rectal cancer, adjuvant chemotherapy and radiation are recommended for Stages II and III disease.

Stage III Colon Cancer

5-Fluorouracil-based chemotherapy is currently the standard of treatment for patients with advanced stage colon cancer. Historically, the added benefit of adjuvant chemotherapy for Stage III colon cancer was established in a series of trials by the National Cancer Institute Intergroup and the National Surgical Adjuvant Breast and Bowel Project in the 1980s. Since then, a 5-year follow-up has shown that levamisole-modulated 5-FU chemotherapy for Stage III colon cancers reduced recurrence and mortality (40% and 33%, respectively). An important finding from the Intergroup-0089 study showed that a 6-month regimen of leucovorin (LV)-modulated 5-FU is comparable to longer-duration therapy and to a levamisole-modulated 5-FU combination. 5-FU can be administered in a bolus or via an infusional fashion. Infusional therapy achieves a higher concentration of the drug with less toxicity. Intergroup 0153 showed that infusional 5-FU therapy was as effective as, but less toxic than, bolus 5-FU in patients with Stage III and high-risk Stage II disease. A preliminary report from a multi-center randomized trial showed a trend toward improved 5-year recurrence-free survival (RFS) and overall survival with less toxicity. Neutropenia and diarrhea were less frequent with infusional therapy; hand-foot syndrome, however, was seen more frequently.

An alternative means of administering 5-FU is via the orally active fluoropyrimidines, specifically capecitabine (Xeloda) and UFT. Capecitabine is activated by the enzyme thymidine phosphorylase within malignant cells. The X-ACT trial was a non-inferiority study that compared capecitabine to the 5-FU/LV Mayo Clinic bolus regimen. This study showed that oral capecitabine is equivalent to the intravenous regimen, with disease-free survival (DFS) as the primary endpoint. Although the incidence of hand-foot syndrome was greater in the capecitabine subgroup, and half of the group required a dose reduction, the overall incidence of adverse effects was less than with bolus 5-FU/LV administration. The NSABP C-06 study assigned 1,608 patients with resected Stage II or III colon cancer to oral UFT plus LV versus the Mayo Clinic 5-FU/LV bolus regimen and found comparable efficacy and toxicity.

As for combination adjuvant therapies, recent trials have examined the effect of adding oxaliplatin to 5FU/LV regimens, with 5FU/LV administered via an infusional (de Gramont) versus bolus (Roswell Park) method. The MOSAIC trial, for example, compares infusional 5-FU/LV versus infusional 5-FU/ LV/oxaliplatin (FOLFOX4). Although there was no difference in overall survival, patients with Stage III disease in the infusional-FU/LV/oxaliplatin treatment arm had a significantly improved 4-year DFS (70% vs. 61%); this difference was not significant in patients with Stage II disease (85% vs. 81%). The NSABP C-07 study comparing bolus 5-FU/LV(Roswell Park) versus bolus 5-FU/LV/oxaliplatin(FLOX) showed an improvement in 3-year DFS in the bolus 5-FU/LV/oxaliplatin group (77% vs. 72%) for the overall group of patients with both Stage II and III disease. The National Comprehensive Cancer Network (NCCN) guidelines now include FOLFOX as an alternative to 5-FU/LV or capecitabine for Stage III colon cancer.

The primary side effect of oxaliplatin therapy is peripheral neuropathy. Ninety-two percent of patients who received FOLFOX in the MOSAIC trial experienced peripheral neuropathy; 12% had severe (grade3) neuropathy. Although generally reversible, 4% had persistent grades 2 or 3 neuropathy at 18 months post-treatment. Other side effects of FOLFOX therapy include febrile neutropenia and severe diarrhea (2% and 11%, respectively). Bolus 5-FU/LV/oxaliplatin therapy is associated with more grade 3–4 diarrhea than infusional 5-FU/LV/oxaliplatin.

Another chemotherapeutic agent that has been the focus of many trials is irinotecan. The CALGB trial comparing bolus 5-FU/LV versus bolus 5-FU/LV/irinotecan (IFL) for adjuvant therapy in resected Stage III disease showed greater toxicity and no clinical benefit for the irinotecan subgroup. The preliminary results for infusional 5FU/Folinic acid (FA) and irinotecan (FOLFIRI) versus 5FU/FA alone in the adjuvant setting for Stage III colon cancer showed no difference in DFS between the two groups. The NCCN guidelines advise against the use of bolus irinotecan in the adjuvant setting; final recommendations for infusional irinotecan are pending.

Novel targeted therapies such as bevacizumab, an antibody against the vascular endothelial growth factor receptor, and cetuximab, an antibody against the epidermal growth factor receptor, have been used successfully in metastatic colorectal cancer and are currently being investigated for use in the adjuvant setting. Current adjuvant trials underway include the following: NSABPC-08, which compares FOLFOX with and without the addition of bevacizumab in Stages II and III disease; Intergroup 0147 (ECOG/ NCCTG), which compares FOLFOX versus FOLFOX, and cetuximab in patients with Stage III disease. As for side effects associated with these targeted therapeutic agents, bevacizumab has been associated with hemorrhage, thromboembolism, proteinuria, hypertension, and gastrointestinal perforation. Toxicities associated with cetuximab include an acneiform rash, malaise, and magnesium wasting.

Stage II Colon Cancer

While adjuvant therapy for Stage III colon cancer is clearly beneficial, the role of adjuvant therapy for Stage II colon cancer, with a 20–25% risk of recurrence, is less clear. A pooled analysis of Stage II colon cancer patients randomized to receive either adjuvant treatment with 5-FU/LV or observation showed no significant improvement in overall or event-free survival. The MOSAIC trial, which compared infusional 5-FU/LV versus infusional 5-FU/LV/oxaliplatin (FOLFOX4), showed no difference in overall survival or DFS in patients with Stage II disease. Based on a systematic meta-analysis of 12 randomized trials of 5-FU-based therapy, the American Society of Clinical Oncology (ASCO) reported no statistically significant improvement in overall or event-free survival. Because of the favorable prognosis of Stage II disease, i.e. 75–80% of patients never develop recurrent disease, larger trials are necessary in order to have adequate power to detect a less than 5% (2–4%) benefit. Preliminary results from the QUASAR trial, consisting of 3,239 subjects with colorectal cancer (91% with Stage II disease), showed a small but significant survival benefit in the adjuvant treatment group. This additional benefit, although small, may justify its use in selected high-risk Stage II patients. Individually customized treatment decisions that take into account risk factors and preferences are recommended in this circumstance. For example, consideration of adjuvant therapy may be warranted in patients with poor prognostic features, including inadequately sampled nodes (fewer than 12 nodes), poorly-differentiated histology, T4 lesions, obstructing or perforating neoplasms, venous invasion, and close, indeterminate, or positive margins. The importance of adequate lymph node sampling was demonstrated further in a recent study of patients with Stage II disease; the subset of patients with a greater number of nodes evaluated showed an improvement in overall 5-year survival. Identification of molecular characteristics, such as 18q loss of heterozygosity and microsatellite instability, may help stratify patients with Stage II disease into low-risk and high-risk subgroups. An ongoing trial ECOG E5202, incorporates not only patient stage (IIA versus IIB), but also tumor microsatellite instability and loss of heterozygosity at 18q into the stratification process for treatment with FOLFOX versus FOLFOX with bevacizumab. Assigning therapy based on molecular characteristics is a novel concept that will likely be the aim of additional future trials.

The MOSAIC trial, as previously mentioned, showed a slight improvement in 4-year DFS for patients with Stage II disease receiving infusional 5-FU/LV/oxaliplatin versus 5-FU/LV alone (85% vs. 81%). One may argue that this 4% benefit, in addition to the small benefit (2–4%) gained from adjuvant 5-FU/LV therapy compared with operation alone, provides an additional incremental benefit (up to 7%) with adjuvant treatment. The potential benefits, particularly in average-risk individuals lacking any adverse features, are limited, but for those with high-risk features (obstruction, perforation, and poorly differentiated histology), treatment may be worth considering. Our current recommendation is that the decision regarding adjuvant treatment of Stage II disease should be individualized after forthright patient-physician discussion of the potential benefits (up to 7%) versus risks of treatment-related mortality (<1%) and morbidity.

Rectal Cancer

Heald and colleagues introduced the concept of total mesorectal excision (TME) in rectal resection for improved local control and emphasized the importance of adequate circumferential, proximal, and distal margins. The introduction of adjuvant therapy for Stages II and III rectal cancer resulted in improvements in both locoregional control and overall survival. There are many trials historically evaluating postoperative and preoperative radiotherapy. At the time of introduction of TME, trials aimed at evaluating postoperative radiotherapy showed decreased local recurrence rates without survival benefit. The Swedish Rectal Cancer trial and the Dutch study were designed to examine the benefit of preoperative therapy, given the theoretical advantages of preoperative radiation, which include more tissue oxygenation, potential downsizing of the tumor, and decreased small bowel toxicity. The Swedish Rectal Cancer trial showed a significant decrease in local recurrence and improvement in overall survival with preoperative, short-course radiotherapy of 25 Gy in five fractions. Not all patients in this trial, however, had a standard TME resection. Thus, the Dutch study randomized patients to TME versus short-course radiotherapy followed by TME to assess the potential value of radiotherapy. Prior to initiation of the study, surgeons were trained to perform TME. Short-course radiotherapy, followed by TME, reduced 2-year local recurrence rates from 8% to 2%, but there was no difference in overall survival.

Similar attention was given to adjuvant chemoradiation during this time period. For example, trials by the GITSG and NCCTG showed improved overall survival for the subgroup treated with postoperative CMT. Thus, based on these trials, the NIH consensus statement in 1990 recommended treatment of patients with Stages II and III rectal cancer with 5-FU-based chemotherapy with radiation.

Multiple single-institution studies have demonstrated the potential benefits of neoadjuvant CMT, which provides complete or partial responders with improved resectability, as well as improved overall survival and recurrence rates. Recently, the German Rectal Cancer Trial, a randomized controlled trial, compared preoperative versus postoperative CMT. Patients in the preoperative group received 50.4Gy in 28 fractions with continuous infusion 5-FU, followed by operative resection in 6 weeks' time. The postoperative group received an extra 5.4 Gy boost to the pelvis. Subsequent to surgery or radiotherapy, each group received an additional four cycles of bolus 5-FU. The preoperative CMT group showed several advantages compared with the postoperative subgroup, including a lesser rate of local recurrence (6% vs. 13%), less grades 3 and 4 toxicity including diarrhea (12% vs. 18%), a higher sphincter-preservation rate (39% vs. 19%), and a lower rate of anastomotic strictures (4% vs. 12%).

Although there are many benefits to preoperative therapy, there are potential limitations, which are related mostly to inaccurate preoperative clinical staging. A few examples are provided by data from the postoperative treatment subgroup: 18% were found to have pathologic Stage I disease; thus, they were overstaged and would have been overtreated with neoadjuvant therapy. Furthermore, another 10% were found to have metastatic disease at the time of the resection or thereafter, and therefore may not have benefited from neoadjuvant therapy. Despite these limitations, at the present time, neoadjuvant CMT has been embraced for the reasons listed above, which include increased sphincter-preservation rates, decreased bowel toxicity, and potential tumor down-sizing for improved operative control. One must be mindful, however, of the potential side effects of adjuvant therapy, including increased rates of bowel incontinence, as well as dissatisfaction with bowel function compared with the TME alone subgroup. Patients at potential risk of overtreatment include those with superficial T3N0 disease and adequate TME with at least 12 sampled nodes negative for metastasis, and those with disease in the proximal rectum. A subset of patients with favorable prognostic features, including pathologic as well as superficial radial extension on imaging by endorectal ultrasonography (<2 mm into perirectal fat), were found to have improved local control and RFS. A final recommendation for this subgroup will require randomized controlled trials, but subject recruitment may be difficult. More adequate staging techniques are needed before subjects will decide to have more limited treatment.

As for postoperative chemotherapy for rectal cancer, the optimal regimen still remains to be determined. Using data extrapolated from colon cancer trials such as the MOSAIC study, our standard is to give patients with clinical Stage III disease eight cycles of postoperative infusional 5-FU/LV/oxaliplatin following neoadjuvant CMT and resection. For patients with clinical Stage II disease, our preference is for either 5-FU/LV versus 5-FU/LV/oxaliplatin or no treatment, based on absence or presence of favorable-risk characteristics. As in adjuvant treatment for Stage II colon cancer, the decision to treat remains controversial, and therapy needs to be tailored individually after patient-physician discussion of the benefits and risks of treatment.

Newer agents are being investigated for treatment of rectal and colon cancers. Preliminary results using capecitabine appear promising. Several current randomized trials are examining alternative agents, specifically irinotecan and oxaliplatin in conjunction with radiotherapy, for use in the neoadjuvant setting. Another trial compares capecitabine with infusional 5-FU in addition to preoperative radiotherapy. Several phase I and II trials have been performed using irinotecan-based therapy for locally advanced rectal cancer. The studies offer encouraging results and acceptable toxicity. Clinical studies using novel targeted therapies, specifically bevacizumab and cetuximab in combination with traditional cytotoxics, are underway, but none has yet been accepted as the standard of care.

Conclusion

Although this chapter has focused on adjuvant and neoadjuvant therapy for colon and rectal cancer, the importance of an adequate operative resection, for example TME, cannot be overemphasized. Our current regimen for adjuvant treatment of Stage III colon disease includes 5-FU/LV, capecitabine, or 5-FU/LV/oxaliplatin. For high-risk Stage II disease with poor prognostic features, our current practice is to consider these patients for adjuvant treatment with 5-FU/LV, capecitabine, or 5-FU/LV/ oxaliplatin. For patients with rectal cancer, our standard therapy is long-course preoperative chemoradiation for patients with Stage II and III disease, followed by postoperative adjuvant chemotherapy.

Selected Readings

Colorectal Cancer Collaborative Group (2001) Adjuvant radiotherapy for rectal cancer: a systematic overview of 8,507 patients from 22 randomised trials. Lancet 358:1291–1304

Andre T, Boni C, Mounedji-Boudiaf L, et al. (2004) Oxaliplatin, fluorouracil, and leucovorin as adjuvant treatment for colon cancer. N Engl J Med 350:2343–2351

Benson AB, 3rd, Schrag D, Somerfield MR, et al. (2004) American Society of Clinical Oncology recommendations on adjuvant chemotherapy for Stage II colon cancer. J Clin Oncol 22:3408–3419

Cassidy J, Scheithauer W, McKendrick J, et al. (2004) Capecitabine (X) vs bolus 5-FU/leucovorin (LV) as adjuvant therapy for colon cancer (the X-ACT study): positive efficacy results of a phase III trial. J Clin Oncol (Meeting Abstracts) 22:3509

Chau I, Norman AR, Cunningham D, et al. (2005) A randomized comparison between 6 months of bolus fluorouracil/leucovorin and 12 weeks of protracted venous infusion fluorouracil as adjuvant treatment in colorectal cancer. Ann Oncol 16:549–557

De Gramont A, Boni C, Navarro M, et al. (2005) Oxaliplatin/5FU/LV in the adjuvant treatment of Stage II and stage III colon cancer: Efficacy results with a median follow-up of 4 years. In: ASCO Annual Meeting Proceedings, p 3501

Folkesson J, Birgisson H, Pahlman L, Cedermark B, Glimelius B, Gunnarsson U (2005) Swedish Rectal Cancer Trial: long lasting benefits from radiotherapy on survival and local recurrence rate. J Clin Oncol 23:5644–5650

Gray RG, Barnwell J, Hills R, et al. (2004) QUASAR: a randomized study of adjuvant chemotherapy (CT) vs. observation including 3238 colorectal cancer patients. In: ASCO Annual Meeting,p 3501

Haller DG, Catalano PJ, Macdonald JS, et al. (2005) Phase III study of fluorouracil, leucovorin, and levamisole in high-risk Stage II and III colon cancer: final report of Intergroup 0089. J Clin Oncol 23: 8671–8678

Heald RJ, Husband EM, Ryall RD (1982) The mesorectum in rectal cancer surgery – the clue to pelvic recurrence? Br J Surg 69:613–616

Kapiteijn E, Marijnen CA, NagtegaalI D, et al. (2001) Preoperative radiotherapy combined with total mesorectal excision for resectable rectal cancer. N Engl J Med 345:638–646

Lembersky BC, Wieand HS, Petrelli NJ, et al. (2006) Oral uracil and yegafur plus leucovorin compared with intra-venous fluorouracil and leucovorin in Stage II and III carcinoma of the colon: results from National Surgical Adjuvant Breast and Bowel Project Protocol C-06. J Clin Oncol 24:2059–2064

LeVoyer TE, Sigurdson ER, Hanlon AL, et al. (2003) Colon cancer survival is associated with increasing number of lymph nodes analyzed: a secondary survey of intergroup trial INT-0089. J Clin Oncol 21:2912–2919

Mehta VK, Cho C, Ford JM, et al. (2003) Phase II trial of preoperative 3D conformal radiotherapy, protracted venous infusion 5-fluorouracil, and weekly CPT-11, followed by surgery for ultrasound-staged T3 rectal cancer. Int J Radiat Oncol Biol Phys 55:132–137

Minsky BD, Cohen AM, Kemeny N, et al. (1992) Enhancement of radiation-induced downstaging of rectal cancer by fluorouracil and high-dose leucovorin chemotherapy. J Clin Oncol 10:79–84

Minsky B, O'Reilly E, Wong WD, et al. (1999) Daily low-dose irinotecan (CPT-11) plus pelvic irradiation as preoperative treatment of locally advanced rectal cancer (meeting abstract). Proc Am Soc Clin Oncol

Moertel CG, Fleming TR, Macdonald JS, et al. (1995) Fluorouracil plus levamisole as effective adjuvant therapy after resection of Stage III colon carcinoma: a final report. Ann Intern Med 122:321–326

Moertel CG, Fleming TR, Macdonald JS, et al. (1990) Levamisole and fluorouracil for adjuvant therapy of resected colon carcinoma. N Engl J Med 322:352–358

NCCN (2006) Practice guidelines in oncology. Colon cancer 11:1010–1017

NIH consensus conference (1990) Adjuvant therapy for patients with colon and rectal cancer. JAMA 264:1444–1450

Poplin EA, Benedetti JK, Estes NC, et al. (2005) Phase III Southwest Oncology Group 9415/Intergroup 0153 randomized trial of fluorouracil, leucovorin, and levamisole versus fluorouracil continuous infusion and levamisole for adjuvant treatment of Stage III and high-risk Stage II colon cancer. J Clin Oncol 23:1819–1825

Quasar Collaborative Group (2007) Adjuvant chemotherapy versus observation in patients with colorectal cancer: a randomised study. Lancet 370:2020–2029

Sauer R, Becker H, Hohenberger W, et al. (2004) Preoperative versus postoperative chemoradiotherapy for rectal cancer. N Engl J Med 351:1731–1740

Saltz LB,ND, HollisD, et al. (2004) Irinotecan plus fluorouracil/leucovorin (IFL) versus fluorouracil/leucovorin alone (FL) in Stage III colon cancer (intergroup trial CALGB C89803). In: ASCO Annual Meeting Proceedings

Scheithauer W, McKendrick J, Begbie S, et al. (2003) Oral capecitabine as an alternative to i.v. 5-fluorouracil-based adjuvant therapy for colon

cancer: safety results of a randomized, phase III trial. Ann Oncol 14:1735–1743
Schrag D (2005) Improving rectal cancer outcomes with chemotherapy. Semin Colon Rectal Surg 16:162–169
Van Cutsem E, Labianca R, Hossfeld D, et al. (2005) Randomized phase III trial comparing infused irinotecan/ 5-fluorouracil(5-FU)/folinicacid (IF) versus 5-FU/FA(F) in Stage III colon cancer patients (pts). (PETACC3). J Clin Oncol (Meeting Abstracts) 23:LBA8
Wolmark N, Wieand HS, Kuebler JP, et al. (2005) A phase III trial comparing FULV to FULV + oxaliplatin in Stage II or III carcinoma of the colon: results of NSABP Protocol C-07. In: ASCO Annual Meeting Proceedings, p 3500
Willett CG, Badizadegan K, Ancukiewicz M, Shellito PC (1999) Prognostic factors in stage T3N0 rectal cancer: do all patients require postoperative pelvic irradiation and chemotherapy? Dis Colon Rectum 42:167–173

Part III
Gastrointestinal Bleeding

23 Lower Gastrointestinal Bleeding

Theresa W. Ruddy and Theodore J. Saclarides

Pearls and Pitfalls

- Lower gastrointestinal (GI) hemorrhage accounts for 1% of acute hospital admissions each year.
- The cause of lower GI hemorrhage varies by age group.
- Most lower GI bleeds (overall average 80–85%) will stop without any therapeutic intervention.
- Severe bleeding is that which continues for 24 h after hospital admission or that which recurs 24h after resolution.
- Methods of diagnosis in attempt to localize the site include endoscopy (upper, lower), RBC-tagged scintigraphy, capsule endoscopy, and angiography (if bleeding is severe).
- For severe hemorrhage, angiography offers the possibility of not only diagnosis but also therapy (vasopressin infusion or embolic therapy).
- Blind segmental resection for non-localized GI hemorrhage should be avoided because of unacceptably high rates of rebleeding.
- Total abdominal colectomy should be avoided until all attempts at localization of bleeding have failed because of the procedure's high mortality rate and the potential impact on GI function.
- Rebleeding may occur in a substantial percentage of patients.

K.I. Bland et al. (eds.), *Colorectal Surgery*,
DOI 10.1007/978-1-84996-444-9_23,

- Occasionally, patients with recurrent bleeding or transfusion-dependent occult bleeding of presumed small bowel source may require exploration with intraoperative enteroscopy.

Lower gastrointestinal (GI) bleeding originates from sources located distal to the Ligament of Treitz. Eighty-five percent of lower GI bleeds resolve without therapeutic intervention. For the majority of patients, there is time for resuscitation and localization of the source. Lower GI bleeding maybe occult or massive. It is essential therefore to have an orderly evaluation of lower GI bleeding which is tailored both to the individual patient and to the rate of bleeding.

Epidemiology

Lower GI bleeding can occur at any age, but most commonly it is found in the older adult population, with an average age range of 63–77 years of age. It has an annual incidence of 0.03% in the adult population and is more common in those with comorbid conditions. The reported mortality rate is 2–4%; however, it is rarely a direct cause of death. The mortality associated with lower GI bleeding is often due to other conditions for which elderly patients are hospitalized.

The most common causes of lower GI bleeding overall are angiodysplasia, diverticulosis, colonic neoplasms, and ischemic colitis. In adults less than 60years of age, inflammatory bowel disease must also be considered. In the very young, the common causes of lower gastrointestinal bleeding are anal fissures, Meckel's diverticulum, inflammatory bowel disease, and polyps.

Etiology

Most sites of lower GI hemorrhage originate in the colon or rectum. A small but substantial percentage (3–5%) come from the jejunum or ileum. Small intestinal hemorrhage is usually due to arteriovenous malformations, accounting for 70–80%. Other causes of small bowel bleeding include jejunal diverticula, Meckel's diverticula, neoplasia, Crohn's disease, and aorto-enteric fistula after the placement of a previous aortic graft.

A common cause of massive lower GI bleeding, i.e. bleeds requiring four or more units of blood in 24 h, is mucosal erosion of a colonic diverticulum adjacent to perforating vessels. Diverticulosis has a prevalence of 37–45% in the older population. Most people with diverticulosis are asymptomatic, but 3–5% will develop massive bleeding. This bleeding resolves without intervention 80% of the time. Ninety-nine percent of patients with these bleeds require four or fewer units of blood before they stabilize. Rebleeding occurs in 25–30% of patients after the first episode. If bleeding ceases spontaneously a second time, the recurrence rate is as high as 50%.

Angiodysplasia is also a common cause of lower GI hemorrhage. These lesions are acquired abnormalities involving vascular ectasis most commonly seen in the elderly and more often in patients with cardiac disease. Hemorrhage from angiodysplasia resolves without intervention 90% of the time but also has a recurrence rate of 25%. The most common location for angiodysplasia is in the ascending colon, but most affected patients have more than one site of angiodysplasia in their GI tract.

GI hemorrhage may also be the first presentation of inflammatory bowel disease, though it is quite rare. Bloody diarrhea accompanies ulcerative colitis more frequently than Crohn's disease, however, Crohn's is more likely to cause acute hemorrhage, because the lesions are deeper and transmural. With Crohn's disease, the sites of bleeding can also be in the small bowel. The patient with ulcerative colitis who hemorrhages usually has pancolitis. The recurrence rate of bleeding for inflammatory bowel disease is high, and operative resection is often necessary. Segmental resection is performed for Crohn's disease, while total proctocolectomy is preferred for ulcerative colitis.

Massive bleeding from colorectal neoplasms is rare, accounting for only 10–15% of lower GI bleeds in the elderly. In contrast, occult bleeding or spotty hematochezia is much more common. Patients may be anemic and can present with symptoms referable to their anemia such as fatigue, shortness of breath, and angina. Another cause of lower GI bleeding is anorectal disease, specifically anal fissures and hemorrhoids. This type of bleed is usually intermittent and associated with bowel movements, but it is rare, though possible, to have a large volume of bleeding with anorectal disease. Proctoscopy has an important role in ruling in or out an anorectal source of bleeding and should be part of the evaluation of every patient with a lower GI hemorrhage.

A common finding in patients with ischemic colitis is that of bloody diarrhea; however, this disorder usually does not lead to blood loss requiring transfusion. The presentation of ischemic colitis is different from the other entities described thus far. It is usually accompanied by left-sided abdominal pain and an increased white blood cell count. Ischemic colitis is due to small vessel disease, and therefore a causative lesion is difficult to identify during angiography. The rectum is usually spared because of its dual blood supply, specifically the mesenteric and internal iliac tributaries.

Polypectomy performed during colonoscopy can cause hemorrhage. The bleeding is usually self-limited and rarely requires intervention. When bleeding does not stop on its own, it may be amenable to endoscopic cauterization, repeated snaring, injection with epinephrine, or angiographic control. Only in rare situations would a patient require operative intervention for persistent post-polypectomy bleeding.

Non-steroidal anti-inflammatory drugs (NSAIDs) are associated with diverticular bleeding, as well as other lower GI causes of bleeding. NSAIDs can exacerbate inflammatory bowel disease, can cause a colitis resembling inflammatory bowel disease, and can cause irritation and ulceration of the bowel, especially the terminal ileum and cecum. There are other rare causes of lower GI bleeding, including Dieulafoy lesions and anorectal varices. Dieulafoy ulcers in the stomach much more commonly cause upper GI bleeding; however, these ulcers have been found in the colon and rectum and can cause massive hemorrhage. Anorectal varices are the result of portal hypertension, and although massive bleeding is rare, it is often severe when it does occur, requiring aggressive resuscitation and therapeutic intervention. Need for emergent colectomy has a 90% mortality with this condition related to the underlying liver disease. Strong consideration and therapy should be directed at portal vein decompression.

Other causes of lower GI bleeding include infectious colitis, with causative agents including *Salmonella*, *E. coli*, *Campylobacter*, and *Yersinia*. In the immunocompromised patient, one must also consider cytomegalovirus and *Mycobacterium avium* complex. Radiation can cause proctitis, leading to bleeding from 9 months to 4 years after treatment. Treatment should include argon beam coagulation, formalin instillation, and rarely proctectomy. Stercoral ulcers from constipation can also cause hematochezia, usually from the rectosigmoid area.

Evaluation

The history should focus on duration of bleeding, volume, and character of blood, specifically whether it is bright red, dark clotted blood, or frank melena. The presence or absence of abdominal or anal pain should be obtained. Previous similar episodes and known contributing conditions, including peptic ulcer disease, gastritis, and liver disease are important in determining the cause of the bleed. Other contributing factors can be a history of pelvic radiation or a history of constipation. Obtaining a history of previous GI tract surgery, previous operation for abdominal aortic aneurysms, and recent GI endoscopy is important. Medications, specifically anticoagulants such as clopidogrel, aspirin, and warfarin, can contribute to lower GI hemorrhage. NSAIDs, well known for causing upper GI bleeds, also have a strong association with lower GI bleeds.

The physical examination should begin by obtaining vital signs, taking note of parameters that may reflect hemodynamic stability, particularly hypotension, postural changes, syncope, and tachycardia. Associated findings include pallor and fatigue from blood loss. The abdomen should be evaluated for tenderness and distension. A digital rectal exam is necessary, along with rigid proctoscopy.

A complete blood count should be obtained at the onset of the evaluation. Other initial laboratory tests should include coagulation profile, electrolytes, and blood sample sent for type and crossmatch. Arterial blood gases can be helpful especially in determining the extent of the resuscitation that will be needed.

Hematochezia results from an upper GI bleed about 10–15% of the time. Therefore, the evaluation should begin by excluding an upper GI source. Nasogastric (NG) lavage is usually sufficient for this purpose. The lavage is considered negative for an upper gastrointestinal cause if bile and not blood is aspirated. Using NG lavage as a screening tool, the reported rate of missing an upper GI bleed is 16%. Therefore, esophagogastroduodenoscopy (EGD) can be substituted for NG lavage in the initial evaluation. EGD can, unlike NG lavage, provide both diagnostic and therapeutic intervention for upper GI hemorrhage.

Four diagnostic approaches can be used to evaluate the lower GI tract for bleeding, including colonoscopy, radionuclide scintography(tagged red blood cell scan), angiography, and wireless capsule endoscopy. Colonoscopy has a diagnostic accuracy of about 80%. It is most helpful when bleeding is not massive or has slowed, especially when the bleed is from angiodysplasia. Large amounts of persistent blood in the colon may make it difficult for the endoscopist to detect any mucosal pathology. Although blood is a cathartic and causes evacuation of the bowels, bowel cleansing will be helpful prior to endoscopy. Polyethylene glycol lavage by mouth or by nasogastric tube will cleanse the colon effectively. Conversely, complete bowel cleansing can hinder localization of the bleeding site if all bleeding has stopped and all signs of bleeding are washed away. Some endoscopists prefer to administer enemas prior to colonoscopic evaluation to allow for an immediate examination. Seeing blood on the left side of the colon and not on the right side may help isolate the location of the bleed, however, surgical decisions regarding the extent of resection should not be based on this observation alone. If angiodysplasia is the cause of the bleed, the site can be very difficult to find in unprepped bowel.

The diagnostic yield of colonoscopy within the first 24 h of admission for presumed lower GI hemorrhage is high. Jensen et al. reported on patients with known diverticulosis who underwent colonoscopy within 12 h of hospitalization for a GI bleed. The etiology of the bleed was found 71% of the time. Furthermore, some of the bleeds from diverticulosis were controlled successfully using colonoscopic modalities.

Radionuclide scintigraphy is performed preferentially as a technetium-labeled red blood cell scan. Although scintigraphy can also be performed with technetium-99 sulfur colloid, the free colloid is cleared rapidly by the reticuloendothelial system within 2–3 min of injection, and if there is no active bleeding at the time of injection, the diagnostic yield is low. The benefit of the technetium-labeled red blood cell scan is the that the test labels red blood cells for 12–24 h, and, thus, repeat scanning is possible. The technetium-labeled red blood cell scan can detect bleeding as slow as 0.1 ml/min and will show a bleeding source as quickly as 5 min after injection. If the patient is not bleeding at the time of the initial scan, the patient can undergo rescanning up to 24 h after the initial injection to determine the source of bleeding. This test can be very helpful if lower GI bleeding is intermittent.

Many surgeons are reluctant to advise operative intervention based solely on a tagged red blood cell scan because of the test's low sensitivity and difficulty localizing the source for both upper and lower GI bleeds. In one study by Olds et al., the scan detected only 39% of bleeds, and the site of the bleeding correlated with other diagnostic tests only 48% of the time and was not consistent with the documented site 10% of the time. The sensitivity of the study did increase, however, with increasing number of blood transfusions required. Therefore, technetium-labeled red blood cell scanning is usually not used as a guide for operative resection, but rather to determine other necessary studies or therapies. Its advantages are that it is minimally invasive, easy to do, and has a greater sensitivity for slow bleeding than angiography.

Selective mesenteric angiography requires the bleeding to occur at a rate at least 0.5–1 ml/min for it to be diagnostic. Angiography is invasive and carries a greater risk than nuclear medicine scanning; however, it is much more specific and allows an opportunity not for just diagnosis, but also for therapeutic intervention. Vasodilators, heparin, or thrombolytics can be used to increase its sensitivity. These agents may augment the extravasation of contrast, making the bleeding area more obvious. With these maneuvers, however, comes a higher risk of bleeding complications.

Angiography is most useful in lower GI bleeds secondary to diverticulosis, because the bleeding associated with diverticulosis is arterial and is more continuous and massive than other forms of bleeding. Angiodysplasia appears angiographically as clusters of tortuous vessels on the antimesenteric border of the bowel and usually has a prominent early draining vein. Identifying angiodysplasia does not guarantee it to be the source of bleeding. Angiodysplasia-induced hemorrhage is diagnosed reliably by the presence of contrast extravasation on angiography; however, extravasation is seen infrequently. Without this finding, the angiogram remains non-diagnostic in determining the source of hemorrhage. It is recommended by some that these lesions be treated when discovered during angiography for bleeding, even when they are not actively bleeding.

If the large bowel and upper GI tract have been investigated and no source of bleeding has been found, the small bowel needs to be evaluated. In the past, push endoscopy, visualizing the first 60 cm of jejunum, and enteroclysis were the only options available for small bowel evaluation; however, these tests provided a relatively low yield of information. Today, the use of wireless capsule endoscopy has revolutionized the diagnosis of small bowel pathology. This capsule represents an image-capturing system within an 11 x 30 mm capsule that is swallowed and travels through the GI tract, taking video image along the way. Over 50,000 images are captured by the capsule. A faster transit time, augmented by erythromycin and slowed by fleets phosphosoda, leads to a more complete small bowel study. Capsule endoscopy is capable of finding many lesions in patients who have had negative upper and lower endoscopic examinations. One drawback of capsule endoscopy is image read time. It can take 75 min to read one "scope." Small lesions are more likely to be missed, because they are found on single frame images. Other drawbacks include inability to obtain tissue samples or to reliably determine the site of bleeding in the small bowel and retention of the capsule at strictures (1% occurrence).

Treatment

Resuscitation is the key to the initial treatment of lower GI hemorrhage. Stabilizing a patient with GI hemorrhage requires continuous monitoring of heart rate and blood pressure (see Fig 23.1). A Foley catheter is helpful in tracking urine output, while large bore IVs are essential for adequate

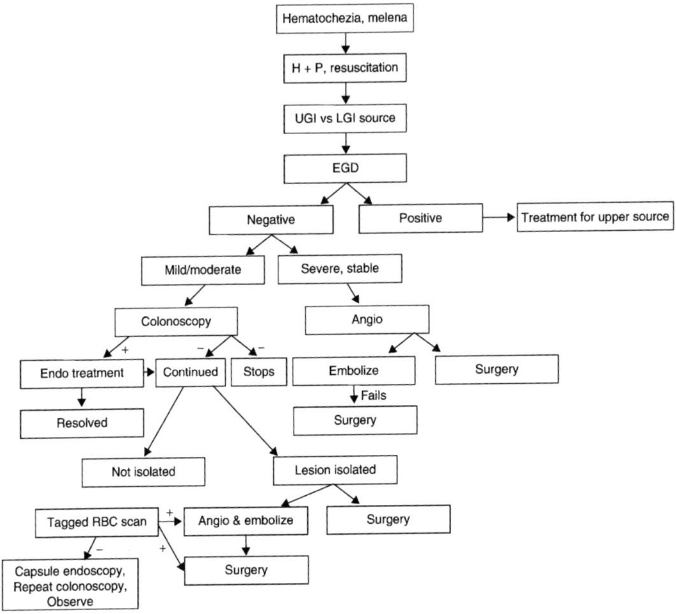

FIGURE 23.1. Approach to management of lower GI bleeding.

resuscitation. Resuscitation should begin with IV fluids. If hemodynamic compromise continues, patients should be cross-matched for blood. When the hemorrhage is massive enough that there isn't time for matched blood, uncross-matched blood should be used. Volume resuscitation should not be substituted by vasopressors. Platelets should be administered when the platelet count or quality is compromised. Fresh frozen plasma is necessary to reverse any coagulopathy noted on the initial assessment.

Lower GI bleeding can present with a wide variation of severity. Some patients need intensive care unit monitoring, especially the elderly or those with continuous and persistent bleeding. Also, patients with orthostatic hypotension should be monitored in a critical care unit. Once a patient has required more than 2 units of blood or has had a drop of 6% in hematocrit, he or she should be considered for ICU monitoring.

Multiple modalities are available to treat lower GI hemorrhage, but data comparing effectiveness of these modalities are sparse. Colonoscopy can provide not only valuable diagnostic information, but also therapy. Coagulation modalities used in endoscopy include heater probe, bipolar cautery, and Nd:YAG laser. These interventional techniques are most useful in bleeds caused by angiodysplasia and diverticulosis. Complications such as perforation associated with coagulation interventions are rare. Rebleeding can occur up to 50% of the time, but a second therapeutic intervention can treat the rebleed.

Angiography, as discussed above, can also be therapeutic. Selective infusion of vasopressin into the vessel supplying the site of bleeding can cause vasoconstriction to the area, controlling the bleeding. This technique is used most commonly for colonic bleeding from angiodysplasia or diverticula. The infusion is continued for 30 min, after which the angiogram is repeated to check for continued bleeding. If bleeding is controlled, the infusion is continued for 6–12 h and then weaned off over 12–24 h. At that time the catheter is removed. The initial success rate of vasopressin infusion is 80–90%; however, the permanent success rate is only 50% because rebleeding occurs in 30–50% of patients. After failed vasopressin therapy, operative colonic resection does not have an increased rate of mortality.

Selective transcatheter arterial embolization can also be used during angiography as a therapeutic intervention. Some materials used for vessel embolization include polyvinyl alcohol foam, dextran microspheres, microcoils, and/or gel foam. Although used originally for colonic bleeds, embolization can also be used selectively for small intestinal lesions. The most morbid complication associated with embolization is intestinal necrosis. Although the reported incidence approaches 20% in some early series, it has decreased with superselective embolization. Recent literature suggests that superselective transcatheter arterial embolization should be the first line of therapy for lower GI hemorrhage rather than reserved solely for those who are poor surgical risk.

Operative intervention may prove necessary for some patients with massive GI hemorrhage and persistent hemodynamic instability or recurrent hemorrhage after other therapeutic interventions. Bleeds that require 4–6 units of blood transfusion in 24 h or 10 units overall often require operative intervention. These parameters are met in 10–25% of patients with lower GI hemorrhage. Other than aortoenteric fistulas, most episodes of massive lower GI bleeding are colonic in origin.

Once operative intervention is required, the decision of which operation to perform must be made. This decision can be difficult because about 10% of lower GI bleeds are not localized prior to operation. Historically, left colon resection was performed, because the most likely source of bleeding was thought to be left-sided diverticula. This approach had a high morbidity (primarily rebleeding) and mortality and was then replaced by total abdominal colectomy. Rebleeding with this operation is very low, reported at less than 1%. In contrast, segmental resection should be performed when localization studies have identified successfully the site of bleeding. If operative intervention is necessary and localization studies have failed to identify the site preoperatively, consideration can be given to intraoperative colonoscopy in an attempt to localize the site of bleeding. This procedure is usually done immediately after an "on the table" colonic lavage. A balloon, Foley-type catheter is placed into the cecum and 3–6 l of balanced electrolyte solution is infused rapidly; a large rectal tube allows exit of the fluid from the rectum. Using hand assist, the colonoscopy is then performed immediately. This approach, although needed only rarely, may allow segmental resection, avoiding need for total colectomy and its postoperative morbidity. In contrast, if the site of bleeding remains unidentified and the patient has massive hemorrhage, then total colectomy with ileorectostomy is indicated.

Mortality after total abdominal colectomy has been reported as high as 27–57%, in contrast to the mortality after segmental resection of 10–15%. Rebleeding rates after segmental resection are less with a positive angiogram (12%). Mortality from total abdominal colectomy is less when performed earlier in the hospitalization after fewer blood transfusions.

Patients with recurrent episodic bleeding or persistent occult GI bleeding in whom the site cannot be identified may also be candidates for operative exploration. These patients usually have a small bowel source, because preoperative upper and lower endoscopy should be able to exclude gastroduodenal and colonic sources. Indications include transfusion-dependent bleeding or cardiac disease threatened by recurrent anemia. Operation in this small subset of GI bleeders (~1%) begins with a thorough intraoperative exploration, including the liver, biliary tree, and pancreas. If no palpable or visual abnormality is identified, then intraoperative enteroscopy can be performed. Intraoperative enteroscopy is best performed using a colonoscope with manual assistance by the surgeon. The coloscope can be introduced per orally, transanally, or via an enterotomy; the latter approach is much easier to manipulate and avoids stretching and trauma to either the gastro duodenum or colon. The success of intraoperative enteroscopy in finding the source of bleeding is only about 50%. If the small bowel is filled with blood, an "on the table" small bowel lavage will allow a much better endoscopic mucosal visualization. A balloon Foley-type catheter is inserted in the proximal jejunum, and exit of the lavage solution can be accomplished either by a transanal large bore rectal tube or by inserting a large bore chest tube into the distal ileum and directing the effluent into a receptacle beside the patient.

Conclusion

Lower GI bleeding can present both a diagnostic and therapeutic challenge. Fortunately, the bleeding usually stops spontaneously; each patient must be attended to with the assumption that the bleed will continue, however, because there are no proven parameters useful to make this determination. If bleeding is slow or has stopped, colonoscopy is the best initial diagnostic modality. Technetium tagged RBC scans detect bleeding occurring in very small amounts and can be helpful by virtue of their ability to allow repetitive imaging. Angiography requires a faster rate of bleeding for it to detect the source, and can be therapeutic by permitting selective infusion of Vasopressin and embolization. Capsule endoscopy can assess portions of small bowel not accessible to conventional upper and lower endoscopy. Operative intervention may be needed if the patient is hemodynamically unstable, if more than 6 units are required in a 24 h period, or if the bleeding quickly starts again after it seemingly had stopped. Segmental resections are preferable but only if localization studies have localized the source. Otherwise, a total abdominal colectomy is necessary. Rarely, patients with recurrent bleeding or persistent occult bleeding of a presumed small bowel source may require operative exploration with intraoperative enteroscopy.

Selected Readings

Bounds BC, Friedman LS (2003) Lower gastrointestinal bleeding. Gastroenterology Clin N Am 32:1107–1125

Davis BR, Harris H, Vitale GC (2005) The evolution of endoscopy: wireless capsule cameras for the diagnosis of occult gastrointestinal bleeding and inflammatory bowel disease. Surg Innov 12:129–133

Green BT, Rockey DC (2005) Lower gastrointestinal bleed-ing-management. Gastroenterol Clin N Am 34:665–678

Hoedema RE, Luchtefeld MA (2005) The management of lower gastrointestinal hemorrhage. Dis Colon Rectum 48:2010–2024

Jensen DM, Machicado GA, et al. (2000) Urgent colonoscopy for the diagnosis and treatment of severe diverticular hemorrhage. New Engl J Med 342:78–82

Kendrick ML, Buttar NS, Anderson MA, et al. (2001) Contribution of intraoperative enteroscopy in the management of obscure gastrointestinal bleeding. J Gastrointest Surg 5:162–167

Olds GD, Cooper GS, et al. (2005) The yield of bleeding scans in acute lower gastrointestinal hemorrhage. J Clin Gastroenterol 39:273–277

Strate LL (2005) Lower GI bleeding: epidemiology and diagnosis. Gastroenterol Clin N Am 34:643–664

Vernava AM, Moore BA, et al. (1997) Lower gastrointestinal bleeding. Dis Colon Rectum 40:846–858

24 Obscure Overt Gastrointestinal Bleeding

Genevieve B. Melton-Meaux, Mark D. Duncan, and Thomas H. Magnuson

Pearls and Pitfalls

- Approximately 5% of patients with gastrointestinal bleeding have obscure overt bleeding where no obvious source is found after initial upper and lower endoscopy.
- About 25% of patients with obscure overt bleeding will have successful localization with repeat extended esophagogastroduodenoscopy and colonoscopy.
- Angioectasias or arteriovenous malformations are the most common causes of obscure bleeding.
- Both small bowel enteroscopy (two-way enteroscopy or double balloon enteroscopy) and capsule endoscopy are new and promising second-line diagnostic techniques for obscure bleeding.
- While not therapeutic, capsule endoscopy offers a safe and minimally invasive modality to identify (but not localize) lesions throughout the small bowel.
- During intraoperative enteroscopy, the small bowel should be viewed during insertion rather than withdrawal to avoid misinterpreting iatrogenic mucosal injury.
- Only 40% of patients who undergo laparotomy and intraoperative enteroscopy are cured of obscure GI bleeding.

Gastrointestinal (GI) bleeding results in over 300,000 inpatient hospital admissions annually in the United States. While the great majority of patients will have GI bleeding which localizes

K.I. Bland et al. (eds.), *Colorectal Surgery*,
DOI 10.1007/978-1-84996-444-9_24,

with routine diagnostic work-up, approximately 5% of patients will have obscure GI bleeding, defined as GI bleeding that persists or recurs without a diagnosed etiology after initial routine work-up including upper and lower endoscopic examination. Obscure bleeding is further categorized as either obscure occult or obscure overt bleeding. The focus of this chapter is obscure overt bleeding, which is clinically obvious bleeding that persists or recurs in the face of negative endoscopic examinations. Obscure occult bleeding, in contrast, is the finding of persistently positive fecal occult blood testing without frank blood loss.

As a group, patients with obscure GI bleeding represent a diagnostic and treatment challenge to surgeons, especially because bleeding can be intermittent, variable in amount, and often occurring within the GI tract at sites not accessible by routine localization techniques. For these reasons, patients undergo extensive and repetitive testing frequently. Optimal care entails the use of a multidisciplinary team of gastroenterologists, radiologists, and surgeons and involves invasive and noninvasive approaches to identify the source of bleeding. Although not always available, recent advances in enteroscopy techniques and capsule endoscopy have expanded the armamentarium in the clinical

Clinical Presentation

Evaluation of a patient with obscure GI bleeding should first include a thorough history and physical examination. Although a patient's history may not always be helpful, important considerations include family history (inflammatory bowel disease, hereditary telangiectasias, known coagulopathies, or malignancies), patient age, obstructive symptoms, weight loss, previous surgery (including previous bowel anastomosis or aortic/other vascular surgery), and medications such as anti-coagulants or the use of nonsteroidal anti-inflammatory drugs (associated with ulcer formation). In addition to elderly patients, patients with renal disease, connective tissue disease, and von Willebrand's disease are at higher risk for vascular lesions.

Because approximately 50% of patients with obscure bleeding fail to localize despite a complete diagnostic work-up, it is difficult to know the exact incidence of different etiologies of obscure GI bleeding. In patients with an identified source, most have bleeding secondary to angioectasia (also known as angiodysplasia) or arteriovenous malformation (AVM), followed by neoplasms of the small bowel (Table 24.1). The incidence of angiodysplasia or AVM as a cause of obscure GI bleeding increases with age. In contrast, patients less than 40 years old are more likely to have Meckel's diverticulum, small bowel neoplasms, Dieulafoy's lesion, polyps from a hereditary polyposis syndrome, or Crohn's disease.

Table 24.1. Etiology of obscure overt gastrointestinal bleeding.

Common
Arteriovenous malformation
Angioectasias
True arteriovenous malformation
Neoplasms
Gastrointestinal stromal tumors
Adenocarcinoma
Lymphoma
Carcinoid
Small bowel ulcers or erosions (NSAID-related)
Uncommon
Lipoma
Jejunoileal diverticulosis
Dieulafoy's lesions
Cameron's erosion (in a large hiatal hernia)
Rare
Nevus lesion
Kaposi's sarcoma
Polyposis syndrome

(continued)

TABLE 24.1. (continued)

Meckel's diverticulum
Tuberculosis
Wirsungorrhagia (hemosuccus pancreaticus)
Hemobilia
Foreign body
Varices
Crohn's disease
Celiac sprue
Vasculitis
Aortoenteric fistula
Gastric antral vascular ectasia ("watermelon stomach")

As with other GI bleeding, initial evaluation includes localization of bleeding to above or below the ligament of Trietz, which may be determined partially from patient history or from gastric lavage. The great majority of patients with obscure GI bleeding present with bleeding per rectum (melena or hematochezia); hematemesis is rarely the presenting sign. The initial diagnostic endoscopic study should be directed above or below according to clinical suspicion. If it is still unclear whether the bleeding source is above or below the ligament of Treitz, both colonoscopy and esophagogastroduodenoscopy (EGD) should be completed on initial evaluation.

Those patients with ongoing active bleeding and negative initial endoscopic studies should next be evaluated with tagged red cell scan and/or possibly angiography (Fig. 24.1). In general, tagged red cell scans can demonstrate bleeding with rates in excess of 0.1 ml/min. Angiography provides a possible therapeutic modality and is more precise in localization than nuclear medicine bleeding scans, but localization with angiography generally requires a bleeding rate of 0.5–1.0 ml/min. Although not frequently employed, the use of provocative

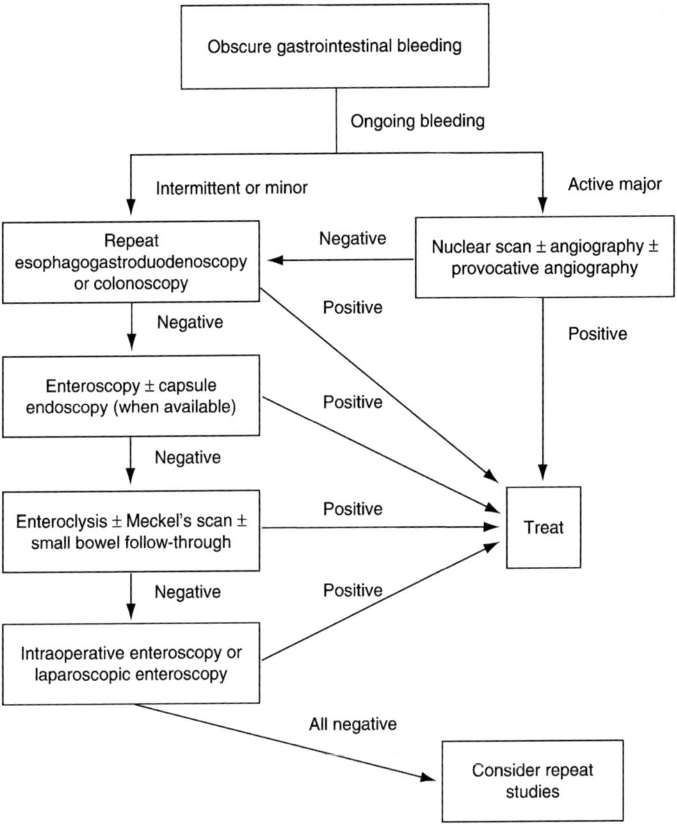

FIGURE 24.1. Algorithm for the management of obscure gastrointestinal bleeding.

angiography with the use of anticoagulants or vasodilators may improve the diagnostic yield at angiography.

Diagnosis

Several anatomic features of the small bowel, including its length (average 6.7 m), free intraperitoneal location, and active contractility make adequate endoscopic visualization of small bowel difficult. Although enteroclysis is superior to an upper GI contrast study with small bowel follow through for the GI bleeding localization, contrast studies are generally less than optimal for visualization of multiple overlying small bowel loops. The recent introduction and more common use of both two-way, double balloon enteroscopy and capsule endoscopy have improved our diagnostic ability with small bowel bleeding.

As delineated in Fig. 24.1, patients with active ongoing bleeding and negative nuclear medicine scanning and angiography should undergo repeat endoscopy. Similarly, those having intermittent or minor bleeding with initial negative endoscopic studies generally warrant repeat endoscopy. Other diagnostic tests include second line modalities such as enteroscopy, capsule endoscopy, enteroclysis, upper gastrointestinal study with small bowel follow-through, and possibly a Meckel's scan (Table 24.2). While some have used colostomies or enterostomies for the purposes of localizing GI bleeding, this is seldom necessary and generally not therapeutic.

Missed Lesions

A substantial proportion of gastroduodenal and colonic lesions are not appreciated on initial upper and lower endoscopy. Multiple reports with enteroscopy have demonstrated that approximately 25% of patients with initial negative endoscopic studies will have a "missed lesion" as a source of bleeding on later studies. For this reason, patients with minor or intermittent bleeding should generally undergo repeat endoscopy directed at the most likely bleeding source. Repeat endoscopy should also be performed in those patients with active bleeding who do not localize on nuclear bleeding scan or angiography. In particular, upper endoscopy can commonly miss Cameron's erosions in a hiatal hernia, gastric varices, Dieulafoy's lesion (afocal arterial bleed within a small mucosal defect typically in the proximal stomach), angiodysplasia, esophagitis, and gastric antral vascular ectasia ("watermelon stomach"). In the colon, the most common missed

TABLE 24.2. Diagnostic options in the evaluation of obscure overt gastrointestinal bleeding.

Test	Therapy
Repeat EGD	Y
Repeat colonoscopy	Y
Tagged red blood cell scan	N
Angiography	Y
Helical CT angiography	N
Provocative angiography	Y
Small bowel follow-through	N
Enteroclysis	N
Meckel's scan	N
Sonde enteroscopy	N
Push enteroscopy	Y
Double balloon enteroscopy	Y
Capsule endoscopy	N
Intraoperative enteroscopy	Y
Laparoscopic enteroscopy	Y

lesions are angiodysplasia and neoplasms. Bleeding from lesions associated with angiodysplasia and diverticular disease tends to be intermittent and recurrent, making both even more potentially difficult to detect.

Enteroscopy

Advances in small bowel enteroscopy have improved the management of obscure GI bleeding. Unfortunately, these techniques are not available in many hospitals. Sonde enteroscopy has largely fallen out of favor and has become mostly of historical interest. This modality is performed by introducing a long, thin enteroscope transnasally and allowing the enteroscope to advance using peristalsis. While it is often successful in reaching distal ileum, Sonde enteroscopy is limited in that it does not allow therapy, has long procedure times, and can cause patient discomfort.

Push enteroscopy (or so-called extended EGD) has been the standard and most common approach for examining the small bowel directly. This endoscopic procedure offers therapeutic intervention similar to standard endoscopy (biopsy, electrocautery, injection, and polypectomy) and can intubate to approximately 50–150 cm beyond the pylorus (approximately mid-jejunum). This technique is generally unsuccessful at detecting distal small bowel lesions. The yield of push enteroscopy is about 40%. Interestingly, many lesions detected by push enteroscopy are found within reach of standard EGD ("missed lesions" from endoscopy). Zaman et al. examined the outcomes of push enteroscopy in 95 patients with GI bleeding and demonstrated sources of bleeding in 35 (37%) of patients, of which 25 had lesions within reach of EGD. In a series of 545 patients who underwent push enteroscopy followed by Sonde enteroscopy, the yield was 41% compared to 65% respectively, with over 25% having lesions within reach of standard endoscopy. Complications of push enteroscopy are rare but include gastrointestinal mucosal tears, pancreatitis (from duodenal compression), pharyngeal tear, and abdominal pain. Although many vascular lesions may be treated with enteroscopy, only about 30% of patients who undergo treatment of a lesion at the time of enteroscopy have no further bleeding at follow-up.

In 2001, Yamamoto described and popularized the technique of double balloon enteroscopy, which utilizes two adjustable balloons that give the enteroscope traction along the lumen of the small bowel and allow the enteroscope to advance further and more effectively within the small bowel. As double balloon enteroscopy from above alone will typically allow advancement into mid-ileum and not the entire small bowel, two-way enteroscopy to access the remaining small bowel from below has also become increasingly used. The combination of two-way and double balloon enteroscopy has an excellent yield for accessing the small bowel in its entirety.

In a series of 123 patients undergoing double balloon endoscopy, visualization of the entire small bowel was achieved in 86% of patients.

Capsule Endoscopy

The introduction of capsule endoscopy in 2000 has added a significant expansion to the diagnostic options for obscure GI bleeding. Although capsule endoscopy has the inherent disadvantage of being a purely diagnostic test with no ability to biopsy or render therapeutic intervention or segmentally localize a lesion within the small intestine, capsule endoscopy is minimally invasive and very well tolerated by patients. Currently, the only wireless endoscopic device approved by the Food and Drug Administration is the GIVEN Diagnostic Imaging System (Given Imaging, Norcross, GA). The capsule is swallowed and travels by peristalsis through the GI system. Capsule endoscopy is contraindicated in patients with established GI obstruction or ileus; relative contraindications include GI motility disorders, history of GI fistulas or strictures, pregnancy, known small bowel diverticula, Zenker's diverticulum, active swallowing disorders, and presence of a defibrillator or pacemaker. The major source of morbidity associated with capsule endoscopy has been retention and aspiration of the GI capsule, together referred to as capsule entrapment. Entrapment occurs in 0.75–5% of patients. Most capsule entrapment occurs in the small intestine, often at the bleeding site. Other sites include impaction at the cricopharyngeus and retention in diverticula.

A recent study from the Netherlands comparing double balloon enteroscopy with capsule endoscopy in 35 patients for detection of lesions in obscure GI bleeding demonstrated detection rates of 60% and 80% respectively for the two modalities ($p < 0.01$). While 74% of patients treated during double balloon enteroscopy did not bleed further during initial hospitalization, only 51% of those patients remained stable without recurrent bleeding on follow-up. Because capsule endoscopy has very high diagnostic rates characteristically but no therapeutic abilities, some have suggested that capsule endoscopy should become an initial screening modality, with enteroscopy or operative interventions acting as focused diagnostic or therapeutic modalities after an initial capsule endoscopy.

Intraoperative Enteroscopy

In the past, one technique for localization of the site of bleeding has been colostomies or multiple enterotomies with the use of rigid proctoscopic luminal examination. Other techniques involved external occlusion of intestinal segments looking for bleeding into the isolated segment. neither of these approaches have proven very effective, therefore intraoperative enteroscopy has become the most reliable procedure for total visualization of the small intestine and should be considered if second line investigations have not yielded a bleeding source. Because intraoperative enteroscopy is inherently invasive, it is important to use a patient-centered approach, considering the potential risks and benefits of operative intervention compared with conservative management of intermittent transfusion. In those patients with ongoing transfusion requirements and no diagnosed bleeding site, operative intervention appears to be warranted. The surgical approach used traditionally involves an open laparotomy with enteroscopy.

As an initial step, intraoperative enteroscopy is performed typically by inserting a colonoscope orally and guiding it manually through the small bowel. As the enteroscope is passed intraluminally, the small bowel is pleated over the instrument; this maneuver must be done with care, as it may cause injury to the small bowel mucosa. Primary viewing of the intestinal lumen should be done during insertion rather than withdrawal in order to properly interpret these lesions as iatrogenic versus a potentially primary cause of the obscure bleeding. As an alternative method to peroral intraoperative enteroscopy or if peroral intraoperative enteroscopy does not gain access to the lesion, the enteroscope may be introduced via one or multiple enterotomies. While this technique minimizes potential injury to the small bowel and its mesentery, it increases the potential for operative intra-abdominal contamination. Transanal passage proximally has gone out of favor. Potential morbidities associated with intraoperative enteroscopy include serosal tears and mesenteric vascular tears, which may require resection. Published morbidity rates vary between 2–42%, but mortality is rare.

If a single specific lesion is identified with intraoperative enteroscopy, the involved bowel segment should be resected. In some patients, multiple AVMs may be diffuse or not confined to just a single segment. The recommended treatment in patients with unresectable diffuse disease involves cauterization or laser ablation of visible angiodysplasia without resection. This approach can be somewhat problematic, as diffuse disease usually results in recurrent bleeding. Several groups have reported on the use of intraoperative enteroscopy for obscure GI bleeding. Overall, about 70% of patients had a site-specific source of bleeding identified and treated; however, the therapeutic efficacy was only about 40% for prevention of recurrent bleeding.

More recently, laparoscopically assisted approaches have been used for both peroral enteroscopy and transabdominal (laparoscopy) enteroscopy in place of the traditional open approach. A laparoscopic approach should be considered only when the surgeon has considerable laparoscopic experience. The efficacy of open versus laparoscopic techniques has not been compared directly nor has the rate of associated morbidity with intraoperative laparoscopic enteroscopy been established.

Management

The management of overt obscure GI bleeding is dictated by both the primary disorder and the manner in which it is detected. While vascular lesions can often be cauterized or obliterated with laser therapy at the time of endoscopy, most patients continue to bleed after endoscopic treatment with only a third having no further bleeding. With respect to angiography, the use of therapeutic interventions such as embolization must be balanced with the possible complication of bowel infarction. Similarly, local infusion of vasopressin has been used with angiography but is associated with systemic effects (cardiac ischemia) and often only transient efficacy in the setting of acute bleeding.

Targeted operative therapy remains the mainstay of treatment for most identified focal lesions associated with obscure GI bleeding. Most of the lesions are amenable to resection via either an open or laparoscopic approach. The treatment for patients with multifocal or systemic disease, however, is less clear. Recurrent bleeding may be observed in patients who have undergone segmental bowel resection for focal angiodysplasia, because the disease is often multicentric.

Medical therapy is appropriate for patients with multiple vascular lesions, persistent bleeding after endoscopic or operative treatment, or when there is no identifiable bleeding source despite thorough evaluation. Several investigators have examined the use of combined hormonal therapy with norethindrone and mestranol but have demonstrated conflicting results. Barkin and Ross reported a series of 38 patients (25 with known AVMs and 18 with unidentified causes) treated with combined hormonal therapy and reported no patients with rebleeding at a mean follow-up of 2½ years. Recently, however, the use of hormonal therapy has been called into question. In a multicenter, randomized clinical trial of hormonal therapy with 72 patients randomized to combined estrogen-progesterone treatment or placebo, no significant difference between treatment or placebo groups with respect to rebleeding rates, number of bleeding episodes, or transfusion requirements was evident.

In summary, patients with obscure overt GI bleeding represent a unique and challenging group of patients from both a diagnostic and treatment perspective. These patients should undergo a regimented and thorough diagnostic work-up for GI bleeding using a multidisciplinary approach. Although there is no single uniform approach for obscure GI bleeding to apply to all patients, a careful workup involving repeat endoscopy, enteroscopy (push, two-way, and/or double balloon), capsule endoscopy, other potential imaging studies, and possible intraoperative enteroscopy may be warranted. The choice of interventions must be balanced with local expertise and the overall clinical picture of the patient. Once bleeding is localized, management is best tailored to the clinical setting, with either endoscopic therapy or operative therapy. The role of new technologies in the diagnosis and treatment of obscure bleeding, as well as current modalities such as capsule endoscopy and double balloon enteroscopy, remains to be delineated with future clinical investigations.

Selected Readings

American Gastroenterological Association (2000) American Gastroenterological Association medical position statement: evaluation and management of occult and obscure gastrointestinal bleeding. Gastroenterology 118:197–201

Barkin JS, Ross BS (1998) Medical therapy for chronic gastrointestinal bleeding of obscure origin. Am J Gastroenterol 93:1250–1254

Berner JS, Mauer K, Lewis BS (1994) Push and sonde enteroscopy for the diagnosis of obscure gastrointestinal bleeding. Am J Gastroenterol 89:2139–2142

Hadithi M, Heine GD, Jacobs MA, et al. (2006) A prospective study comparing video capsule endoscopy with double-balloon enteroscopy in patients with obscure gastrointestinal bleeding. Am J Gastroenterol 101:52–57

Kendrick ML, Buttar NS, Anderson MA, et al. (2001) Contribution of intraoperative enteroscopy in the management of obscure gastrointestinal bleeding. J Gastrointest Surg 5:162–167

Yamamoto H, Kita H, Sunada K, et al. (2004) Clinical out-comes of double-balloon endoscopy for the diagnosis and treatment of small-intestinal diseases. Clin Gastroenterol Hepatol 2:1010–1016

Zaman A, Sheppard B, Katon RM (1999) Total peroral intraoperative enteroscopy for obscure GI bleeding using a dedicated push enteroscope: diagnostic yield and patient outcome. Gastrointest Endosc 50:506–510

Part IV
Minimally Invasive Procedures

25
Laparoscopic Colectomy

David W. Larson and Heidi Nelson

Pearls and Pitfalls

- Laparoscopic colectomy is available for a wide variety of clinical indications in colorectal surgery.
- Technical challenges abound, but with experience and practice, this technique can be mastered.
- Multiple laparoscopic techniques (laparoscopic-assisted, hand-assisted, totally laparoscopic) can be utilized.
- Laparoscopic colectomy offers substantive improvement in post-operative recovery.
- The importance of training, experience, and credentialing is imperative.
- Conversion to an open procedure should be entertained whenever the surgeon is not fully confident of the findings or technical aspects.
- The financial considerations of laparoscopic surgery involve more costs for the operation itself (time, instrumentation) but marked financial savings in shorter hospital stay and earlier return to functional physical activity.
- Level 1 evidence is available for a laparoscopic approach to colon cancer for lack of an increased occurrence of port site recurrences or local and systemic recurrence and survival.
- The future? Questions remain about what to do about rectal cancer.

K.I. Bland et al. (eds.), *Colorectal Surgery*,
DOI 10.1007/978-1-84996-444-9_25,

Introduction

The technique of laparoscopic colectomy has been colored by its history. Over 15 years have passed since the first publication by Jacobs exposed the world to this novel technique. Although this approach has taken hold and expanded exponentially, many of its earliest controversies remain. Despite these controversies, laparoscopic colectomy has proven safe and feasible for nearly all operatively addressed diagnoses within the abdomen and pelvis. The use of laparoscopy has helped to alter the tenor of operative therapy to one committed to more minimally invasive approaches. With improving technology and operative experience, nearly all operations once performed in an open fashion can now be completed technically with these minimally invasive approaches. There remain, however, many important issues which the surgeon must weigh to implement these modern techniques in an appropriate fashion.

The use of laparoscopic surgery for colonic and rectal disease requires thought and consideration. Technically, the operation is much more demanding. Although the actual goals and principles of the operation have changed little from the open approach, the integration of imaging, instrumentation, and operative experience have added a dimension of complexity to the operation that many surgeons find unfamiliar. If one can overcome these obstacles, the results for the patient, as attested to by multiple publications, suggest very real improvements in postoperative outcomes. Although these improvements are well-documented, considerable caution and controversy persist regarding the role of such techniques in malignant disease. Issues such as credentialing, incidence and implications of conversion, cost, and outcomes remain the topics of the day. Through this chapter, we hope to present the general principles, techniques, considerations, and outcomes regarding the use of laparoscopic colectomy in the treatment of colorectal disease.

Diagnosis

The use of laparoscopic techniques has been included in literally every type of surgical diagnosis and indication for colorectal surgery. Multiple reports have been published of its use in the setting of inflammatory bowel disease (IBD), diverticulitis, rectal prolapse, and benign neoplastic disease, and, of course, especially in the setting of colorectal cancer. There is no question that malignant disease has received the most press and remains the most controversial topic. In the next few paragraphs, we center our discussion on the issues of laparoscopic surgery and cancer by reviewing the importance of the preoperative evaluation, technical approaches, and the pearls and pitfalls of the operation itself.

The controversy regarding cancer heightened the importance of the preoperative evaluation and staging. These issues become extremely important as the risk of unsuspected M1 disease at the time of operation was found by the Clinical Outcomes of Surgical Therapy (COST), Conventional vs. Laparoscopic Assisted Surgery in Colorectal Cancer (CLASICC), and Colon Cancer Laparoscopic or Open Resection Study Group (COLOR) trials to be 1–4%. The concerns voiced by many surgeons have centered on the lack of tactile sense available to the surgeon with the laparoscopic approach. Therefore, it has been our practice to aid the surgeon's senses by pre-operatively marking via colonoscopy the surrounding colonic wall of any tumor of interest with an ink tattoo. Likewise, standard radiologic staging of chest x-ray and staging CT of the abdomen and pelvis ensure adequate assessment of the patient preoperatively. Currently, only direct invasion of surrounding structures (T4 stage), which necessitates resection of adjacent invaded organs not amenable to a laparoscopic approach is a contraindication. A relative contraindication includes a bulky tumor exceeding 8–10 cm in size which makes the use of a laparoscopic approach less appealing given the large incision required to remove the tumor, thereby negating any benefits of the laparoscopic approach.

Treatment: Technique of Operations

The dissection and resection of any large intra-abdominal organ involving any quadrant of the abdomen and pelvis require the operator to overcome certain technical challenges. Because the colon and rectum have a large, extensive blood supply, development of special instruments to achieve intracorporeal division of blood vessels has been necessary (Fig. 25.1). The ability to move and mobilize the shear mass of this large organ in the abdomen requires an advanced level of expertise. The operative objectives

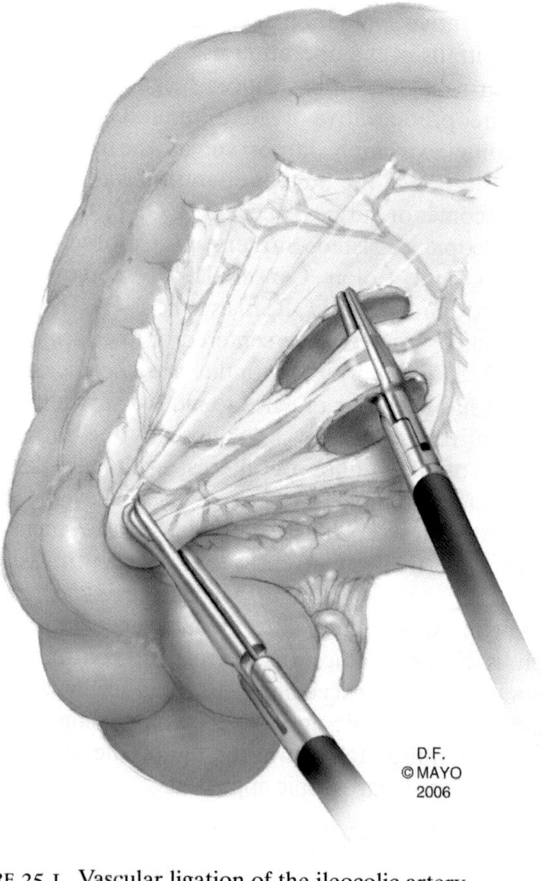

FIGURE 25.1. Vascular ligation of the ileocolic artery.

have been defined clearly by the results of the COST study. If one is unable to fulfill these requirements, then conversion is in the patient's best interest. Based on studies like COST, we know that the length of bowel resection, points of vascular ligation, lymph node harvest, and resection margins are critical to oncologic outcomes. The data from these trials have demonstrated that laparoscopic resection, completed by well-trained surgeons, can be achieved without compromising these factors.

The type of laparoscopic approach used to achieve these objectives has added a wrinkle into the fabric of this debate. The traditional methods of totally laparoscopic or laparoscopic-assisted procedures now also include hand-assisted surgery (HALS). HALS uses an abdominal wall port, large enough to admit the operator's hand, which provides an airtight seal allowing maintenance of a pneumoperitoneum. The traditional difficulty with retraction, lack of tactile discrimination, and the learning curve are improved markedly with this technique. To date, the results of multiple studies reveal that the postoperative, patient-related outcomes of laparoscopic surgery are not compromised based on this new technique. No studies, however, have been published of any significance which shed light on the oncologic outcome of HALS versus more traditional laparoscopic techniques.

The operative techniques of colonic resection and dissections go beyond this chapter but have been well-detailed previously. Regardless of the operation, certain technical points deserve mention. Positioning the patient can be of utmost importance. In general, laparoscopic colonic operations require a great degree of positioning extremes which maintain the patient in a safe and secure position.

Given these multiple changes of position, we use various methods to secure positioning, such as arm tucking, ankle straps, Allen stirrups, and a chest strap. The height of the patient's knees and thighs must also be considered because they relate to the abdomen. To position instruments properly through trocars in the abdomen and to prevent them from being obstructed by the patient's lower extremities, the knees and thighs must be level with the abdomen.

Laparoscopic exploration of the abdomen represents the first part of any operation to search for metastatic disease.

Beyond simple inspection, innovations such as intraoperative ultrasonography can be used to enhance visualization of structures such as the liver and pelvis. The second important function of exploration is its ability to allow the surgeon to determine promptly whether adhesions, altered anatomy, or characteristics of the neoplasm will require a conversion.

As in an open operation, identification of the ureters is a crucial component of colectomy, whether in the setting of a right (Fig. 25.2), left, sigmoid (Fig. 25.3), or rectal dissection.

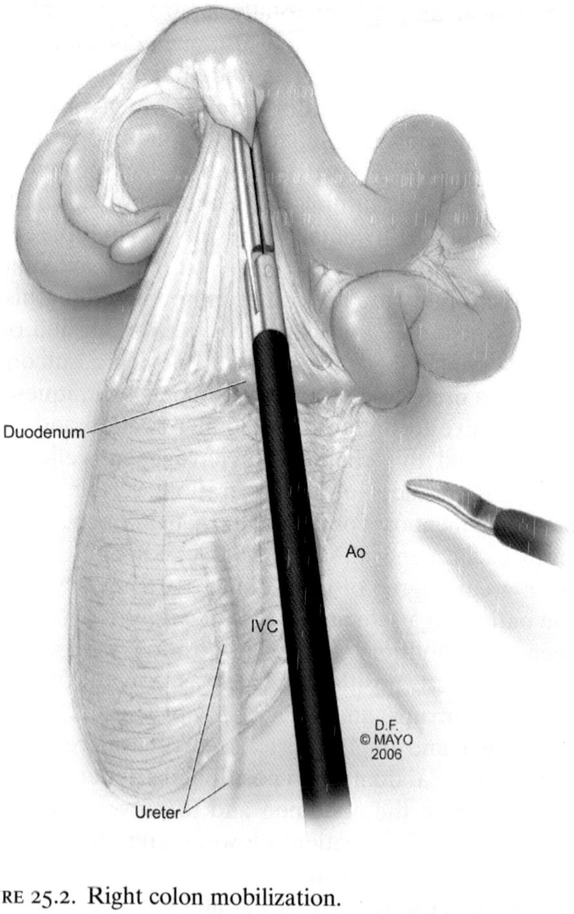

FIGURE 25.2. Right colon mobilization.

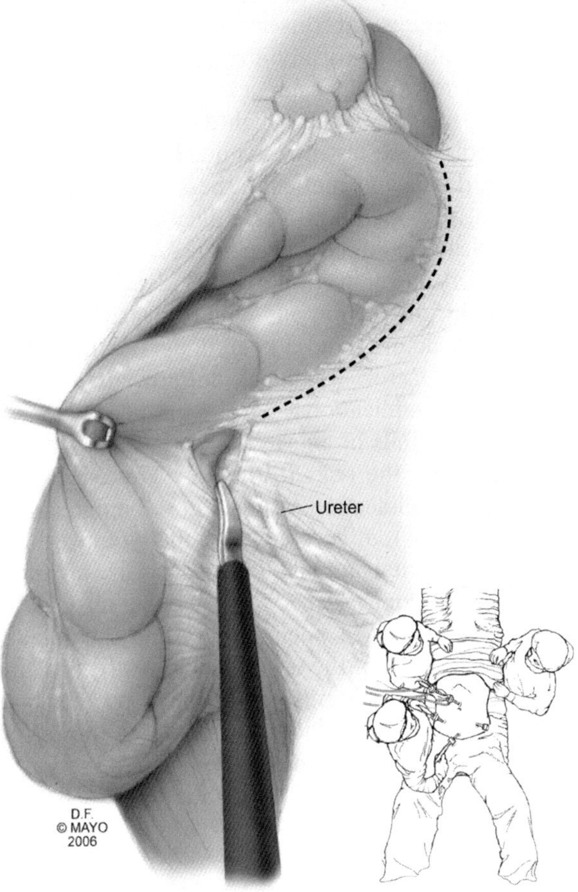

FIGURE 25.3. Left colon mobilization.

The simplest method of identifying the ureter is to follow its course at the level of the pelvic brim. In obese patients, it may prove necessary to score the peritoneum to identify the ureter. In difficult cases or those involved with inflammation or phlegmon, lighted ureteral stents may improve markedly the ability to identify these structures.

Over the past 5 years, advances in vessel sealing and laparoscopic devices for dissection have helped surgeons improve their abilities to mobilize and ligate large vessels. With this new technology came a host of possible complications related to the use of these high-energy devices. Although important tools, these instruments must be handled with the attention to detail and meticulousness that ensures a safe, complication-free operation. Vessel ligation in the setting of cancer is critical to allow for proper dissection and resection of the mesentery and appropriate lymphadenectomy. Standard surgical practice of traction and counter-traction, separation of important structures, and a keen understanding of spatial distance are key factors which prevent unwanted thermal or energy-related complications.

Beyond the pitfalls of energy devises, vessel ligation, and ureteral injury are the risks to the pelvic autonomic nerves during the pelvic dissection. As we know, benign conditions (IBD, diverticulitis) affect typically the young; therefore, preservation of sexual and bladder function are an important issue. As laparoscopic surgery has moved into malignant disease, the principles of open surgery and the standard of mesorectal dissection of the upper and lower rectum must be upheld (Fig. 25.4). Care must be taken to protect both the hypogastric nerves to reduce the incidence of retrograde ejaculation, and the anterolateral neural innervation to the rectum to prevent impotence during the rectal dissection.

Outcomes

Post operative recovery. The laparoscopic approach to colon and rectal disease offers several advantages demonstrated clearly in randomized trials comparing open and laparoscopic resection. Decreased post-operative pain and use of opiates and non-opiate analgesia have been well-documented. Decreases in infection rate also offer a benefit of this minimally invasive approach. It is, however, the issue of postoperative ileus and duration of stay in which laparoscopic surgery appears to have its greatest advantage.

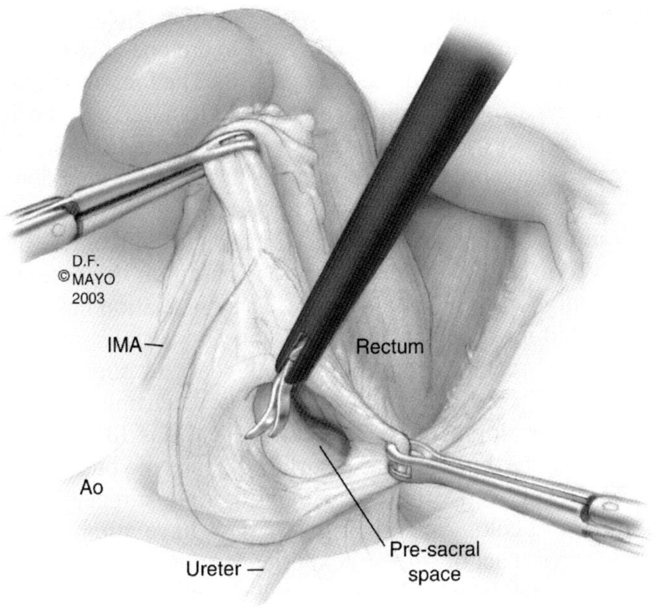

FIGURE 25.4. Rectal mobilization.

Using a variety of definitions for the return of bowel function, multiple studies have demonstrated a decrease in post-operative ileus with a laparoscopic approach. Most recently, the use of "fast track" protocols has contributed to the benefits of a minimal access approach on duration of hospital stay. These protocols have shortened stay not only for laparoscopic cases, but also for open colorectal procedures as well. It appears, however, that laparoscopic cases achieve a faster recovery versus their open counterpart. In addition, certain patients with co-morbid conditions, including cardiopulmonary disease, may benefit from this approach by reduced pain and narcotic use, leading to better preservation of pulmonary function. Because of this improved recovery time, patients are able to return to their social activities more rapidly. The short-term advantages of laparoscopic surgery have also been particularly important in the elderly who, in general, are less tolerant of the effects of major surgery. Several studies indicate significant decreases in morbidity, duration of hospital stay, return to pre-operative activity levels, and cost of care for elderly patients. The long-term benefits of a laparoscopic approach also lead to a decreased incidence of post-operative small bowel obstruction and a decreased incidence of wound complications such as incisional hernias compared with open operations.

Training and credentialing. Oncologic outcomes are improved in many surgical operations based on the parameters of surgeon or hospital volume. This association has been highlighted most convincingly in colon and rectal surgery in the area of rectal cancer. Historically, data to support this principle in colon cancer, however, have been minimal, but with the development of surgical innovations like laparoscopic surgery, this issue has resurfaced. Since the publication of the COST study, the use of laparoscopic surgery in the treatment of colon cancer has grown. Few have attempted to define the impact of surgeon experience, volume, or the need for credentialing in colon cancer. Not surprisingly, studies such as the COLOR and CLASICC trials have reported that hospital volume and surgeon experience appear to be important factors in predicting outcomes. Greater hospital volume in the COLOR trial appear to improve short term outcomes, and surgeon experience as defined by conversion rates improved postoperative morbidity and mortality in the CLASICC trial.

The level of experience required to perform laparoscopic colorectal cancer surgery is being defined currently. The American Society of Colon and Rectal Surgeons has recommended that surgeons perform 20 laparoscopic resections for benign diseases before undertaking procedures for cancer. A number of the trials, including the U.S. COST trial and the U.K. CLASICC trial have used this level of experience to define eligibility of a surgeon to enter these trials. In the COST trial, surgeons were required to provide proof of at least 20 laparoscopic colon procedures along with an unedited video. Such forms of credentialing may be needed in the future to assure adequate quality.

Risks of conversion. Conversion from a laparoscopic to an open procedure is a necessity in certain cases and occurs at a rate of 6–29% in published series. We know from randomized, controlled studies such as the CLASICC trial that conversion may be associated with increased morbidity and mortality. Reasons for conversion may include unexpected disease, extensive adhesions, or inability to identify confidently the vital structures, especially the ureters. A decision to convert is best made if these problems are encountered early in a procedure, so that prolonged attempts to achieve a laparoscopic resection, with the increased risk of complications are not made. This approach will minimize the rates of morbidity and mortality.

Cost. The expansion of laparoscopic surgery has been influenced by the costs of this approach. The need for new equipment different from that used for open surgery results initially in higher operative costs. Longer operative times have also added to the expense. The perception has been that this is an expensive technique with a subsequent argument that clinically significant benefit should be proven for laparoscopic surgery to balance the increased expense. Cost analyses are now widely available and suggest that overall costs of laparoscopic colorectal surgery are equivalent to, if not cheaper than, open surgery. Such analyses have shown clearly the cost reductions created by laparoscopic colorectal surgery because of decreased post-operative analgesic requirements, shorter hospital stays, and more rapid return to normal activities. Converted cases are more expensive due to costs of instrumentation and longer operative and post-operative periods. Thus, it is important to select patients carefully to decrease the need for conversion to an open procedure.

Outcomes in cancer. This topic has received prime importance. The concern initially regarding laparoscopic cancer surgery was the incidence of port site recurrence. Reports of port site recurrence were strikingly high in the early days of laparoscopic colectomy with incidence as high as 21%. Subsequent larger series, including the COST trial, have reported more realistic incidence of 0–1.2%, an incidence entirely comparable to open surgery. The issue of recurrence and survival in colon cancer have been most convincingly addressed by the COST trial, which included 66 surgeons in 48 institutions who had all performed more than 20 laparoscopically assisted colorectal operations prior to the study. After median follow-up was 4.4 years, recurrence and survival rates (overall and disease-free) were equivalent for both groups. This study provided major evidence to confirm the safety of laparoscopic-assisted surgery for colon cancer. Other randomized controlled trials, including the COLOR and CLASICC trials, have yet to report long-term survival data.

The role of laparoscopy in rectal resection is the newest field of debate. This debate centers around its technical demands and the lack of literature devoted to this operation. What is certain is that the same oncologic principles utilized in open rectal resection must be upheld when utilizing this technique in the setting of rectal cancer. Multiple feasibility studies have been published regarding rectal cancer and laparoscopic surgery. This limited academic work provides us with widely variable, short-term outcomes. Issues such as anastomotic leakage have varied between 0% and 21% indicating a spectrum of results which may or may not be as good as open surgery. Local recurrence rate, which is critical to long-term outcome, has varied from as low as 2% to unacceptably high rates. Concern has also been raised about possible increases in the rate of pelvic nerve injury leading to bladder and sexual dysfunction. A single, large, randomized controlled trial by Guillou et al. has published short-term outcomes regarding some of these issues in rectal cancer showing a decrease in sexual and erectile function in men after laparoscopic rectal cancer surgery and more positive circumferential margins after laparoscopic vs. open low anterior resections. Publication of other long-term, randomized, controlled data, along with completion of our own US trial, will define the place of this approach to rectal cancer.

Selected Readings

The Clinical Outcomes of Surgical Therapy (COST) Study Group (2004) A comparison of laparoscopically assisted and open colectomy for colon cancer. N Engl J Med 350:2050–2059

Braga M, Vignali A, Gianotti L, et al. (2002) Laparoscopic versus open colorectal surgery: a randomized trial on short-term outcome. Ann Surg 236:759–766

Guillou PJ, Quirke P, Thorpe H, et al. (2005) Short-term endpoints of conventional versus laparoscopic-assisted surgery in patients with colorectal cancer (MRC CLASICC trial): multicentre, randomised controlled trial. Lancet 365:1718–1726

Kuhry E, Bonjer HJ, Haglind E, et al. (2005) Impact of hospital case volume on short-term outcome after laparoscopic operation for colonic cancer. Surg Endosc 19:687–692

Lacy AM, Garcia-Valdecasas JC, Delgado S, et al. (2002) Laparoscopy-assisted colectomy versus open colectomy for treatment of non-metastatic colon cancer: a randomised trial. Lancet 359:2224–2229

Larson DW, Nelson H (2004) Laparoscopic colectomy for cancer. J Gastro-intest Surg 8:636–642

Veldkamp R, Kuhry E, Hop WC, et al. (2005) Laparoscopic surgery versus open surgery for colon cancer: short-term outcomes of a randomised trial. Lancet Oncol 6:477–484 (COLOR study)

Young-Fadok TM, Hall Long K, McConnell EJ, et al. (2001) Advantages of laparoscopic resection for ileocolic Crohn's disease. Improved outcomes and reduced costs. Surg Endosc 15:450–454

Index